*To Sarah
with love*

K S Hashmi

The medical and health procedures contained in this book are based on first-hand experience and recommendations of medical publications. The author and publishers, however, disclaim any responsibility for any adverse effects or consequences resulting from the misapplication or injudicious use of any of the material contained herein.

To

Nancy,

My wife

For Any Parent Ever Awakened by an Ailing Child

Here is
THE COMPLETE MEDICAL GUIDE OF COMMON CHILDHOOD AILMENTS
- How to diagnose
- When to call the doctor
- When—and how—to treat at home

How to Be Your Child's Doctor (Sometimes)

By A. S. Hashim, M.D.

"A. S. Hashim has one of the most entertaining ways of speaking to and writing for patients that I have ever seen."

—Glenn Austin, M.D.
editor of THE PARENTS' MEDICAL MANUAL
and THE PARENTS' GUIDE TO CHILD RAISING

© Copyright by the Author, 1984

© 1984 by A.S. Hashim, M.D. All rights reserved. Printed in the United States of America. No part of this publication may be reproduced, stored in a retrieval system, or transmitted, in any form or by any means, electronic, mechanical, photocopying, recording, or otherwise, without the prior written permission of the author.

ISBN #0-9611132-0-0

First Edition, 1984

Printed by the International Graphics Printing Service
4411 - 41st Street
Brentwood, MD 20722
(301) 779-7774

INTRODUCTION

Have you ever wondered what to do when your child wakes up at night with a croupy cough, an earache, or a spell of vomiting? Have you ever been puzzled by the colicky baby or the child with an unusual rash?

Have you ever worried whether to call the doctor at 2:00 am or wait until later in the morning, or whether or not your own treatment would be sufficient and adequate?

Such situations and many more face all parents (and every adult patient). This book is written to clarify the common diseases and to help you decide whether to call the doctor or treat at home with simple medications.

The material is concisely stated, and with only a few exceptions, two pages per disease was felt adequate for quick reference. Emphasis is put on prevention and preventive measures; I try to avoid unnecessary detail and unusual scary medical terms.

The material has proved to be a blessing to my own patients and it has cut down the number of my incoming phone calls by eighty percent. I am delighted and proud to see how well informed and less anxiety prone my patients have become.

I think this material will become a similar boon to all hurried parents who do not want any medical mumbo jumbo. I hope this book is a constant source of reassurance throughout your youngster's childhood.

A.S. Hashim, M.D.

CONTENTS

CHAPTER ONE
THE FIRST FEW WEEKS OF LIFE

Before the Baby Is Born 3
The Baby Is with You Home 3
Spitting Up 4
Colicky Pains 4
Bowel Movements 5
Constipation 6
Care of the Skin 6
The Belly Button 7
Bottoms 8
The Bleeding Vagina 9
Baby's Eyes 9
The Jumping Jack 9
Blemishes and Spots 10
Breasts 10
Sleep 10
Visitors 11
Relatives and Their Advice 11
Taking the Baby Out 11

CHAPTER TWO
FEEDING YOUR BABY

Breast-Feeding 15
Bottle-Feeding 18
Water 22
Orange Juice 22
Vitamins 23
Homogenized Milk 23
Solid Foods 24
Cereal 24
Fruits 26
Vegetables 27
Meats 27
Table Food 28
Eggs 29

CHAPTER THREE
WHAT IS EXPECTED

At the Age of One Month 35
At the Age of Two Months 38
At the Age of Three Months 40
At the Age of Four Months 42
At the Age of Five Months 44
At the Age of Six Months 46
At the Age of Eight Months 48
At the Age of Ten Months 50
At the Age of Twelve Months 52
At the Age of Fifteen Months 54
At the Age of Eighteen Months 56
At the Age of Twenty-One Months 58

At the Age of Two Years 60
Development of the Adolescent Male 63
Development of the Adolescent Female .. 65
Menstruation 67
Checkups 69
School Phobia 71

CHAPTER FOUR
CONDITIONS PECULIAR TO
BABIES AND YOUNG CHILDREN

Milk Allergy 75
Baby's Stuffy Runny Nose 77
Baby's Earache 78
Baby's Cough and Chest Trouble 79
Projectile Vomiting 80
The Cracked Anus (Fissure in Ano) 81
Sternomastoid Mass 82
Pin-Hole Meatus in the Male 83
Labial Adhesions in the Female 84
Spitting Up 85
Thumb-Sucking or Pacifier 86
Cradle Cap 88
Tooth Eruption and Teething 91
Care of the Teeth 93
The Watery Eye 95
Tongue-Tie 97
Thrush 98
Constipation in Babies 100
Diaper Rash 101
Jaundice 103
A Clean-Up Job 106
To Circumcise or Not 107
The Sore Bottom 109
Umbilical Hernia 111
Bruises 112
Accidents in the Very Young 114
ABC's of Child Safety 117
Accidental Poisoning 118
Contusions 121
Cuts and Lacerations 122

CHAPTER FIVE
FEVER AND INFECTIOUS DISEASES

Fever and Infections 127
To Bring a High Temperature Down 132
Febrile Convulsions 134
Viruses, Bacteria, and Fungi 136
Viral Infections 138
Flu 141
Why the Culture 143
The Strep Germ 145
The Staph Germ 148
Pneumococcus 149

Pneumococcus 149
Antibiotics, Use and Abuse 151
Roseola 153
Scarlatina 155
Chickenpox 157
Measles 160
Rubella 162
Mumps 164
Rheumatic Fever 166
Infectious Mono 168
Fifth Disease 170
Rocky Mountain Spotted Fever 172

CHAPTER SIX
THE EYES

The Eyes 179
Eye Checkups 181
Eye Drops and Ointments 183
The Eyes Are Crossed 186
Styes and Chalazions 188
Conjunctivitis (Pink Eye) 190
Black Eye 192
The Swollen Eyelid 194
Subconjunctival Hemorrhage 196
Eye Accidents 198

CHAPTER SEVEN
THE EARS

The Ears 205
Hearing 207
Earache 209
The Inflamed Middle Ear 211
The Gluey Ear 213
Discharge From the Ear 215
Diseases of the Outer Ear (Auricle) ... 218
Swimmer's Ear (Otitis Externa) 220
Ear Drops 222
Foreign Body in the Ear 224
Ear Wax 227

CHAPTER EIGHT
THE MOUTH AND THE THROAT

Mouth-Breathing 231
Geographic Tongue 233
Stomatitis (Trench-Mouth) 234
Aphtha (Canker Sore) 237
The Permanent Teeth 239
Tooth Abscess and Gum Boil 240
Accidents to the Mouth 241
The Throat 244
Lozenges, Gargles, and Mouth Sprays ... 246
Sore Throat 248

Herpangina 250
Acute Tonsillitis 252
T & A (Removal of Tonsils and Adenoids) 254
Hand, Foot, and Mouth Disease 256

CHAPTER NINE
THE NECK

The Neck 261
Wry Neck (Torticollis) 263
A Lump Under the Jaw 265

CHAPTER TEN
THE NOSE

The Nose 271
Colds 273
The Stuffed-Up Nose 276
Nasal Allergy (Allergic Rhinitis) 278
Postnasal Drip 281
Nose Bleeds 282
Fracture of the Nose & Deviated Septum. 284

CHAPTER ELEVEN
THE RESPIRATORY TRACT

The Respiratory Tract 289
Humidifiers and Vaporizers 290
Electronic Air Filters 292
Allergies of the Respiratory Tract 294
Allergy Shots 297
Cough 299
Cough Medicines 303
Upper Respiratory Infection 307
Laryngitis 309
Congenital Laryngeal Stridor 311
Croup 313
Tracheobronchitis 315
Asthmatic Bronchitis 317
Foreign Body in the Lung 320
TB (Tuberculosis) and Its Tests 322
Pneumonia 324
Pleurisy 326

CHAPTER TWELVE
THE DIGESTIVE TRACT

What Is the Digestive Tract 331
Appetite 332
Vitamins 337
The "Balanced Diet" 339
They Are Cute and They Are Chubby 342
Cholesterol and Our Diet 347
Food Allergy 349
Stomachache 352

What Is a Normal Stool 354
Acute Constipation in Children 356
Chronic Constipation 357
Vomiting 360
Gastroenteritis 362
Diarrhea 364
Dehydration 366
The Bloody Stool 368
Inguinal Hernia 370
Appendicitis 372
Round Worms 374
Pin Worms 376
Infectious Hepatitis 378
Diabetes 380

CHAPTER THIRTEEN
CHEST, HEART, AND BLOOD

The Chest 385
Tidbits About The Breasts 387
Chest Pains 389
Heart Rate 390
Heart Murmur 392
High Blood Pressure 394
The Blood 396
Low Blood (Iron-Dificiency Anemia) 398
Purpura 401
Anaphylactoid Purpura 403
Sickle Cell Disease 405

CHAPTER FOURTEEN
GENITO-URINARY SYSTEM

The Urinary Tract 409
Urine 411
Urinalysis, Urine Culture, IVP, etc. .. 413
The Bloody Urine 415
Urinary Tract Infection 416
Glomerulonephritis 418
Bedwettig 420
Meatal Stenosis 423
Hydrocele 425
Undescended Testicle 426
Vulvovaginitis 429

CHAPTER FIFTEEN
THE SKIN

The Skin 435
Dry Skin 436
Atopic Dermatitis (Eczema) 438
But It Is Only a Rash 440
Impetigo 441
Boils 443
Cellulitis and Abscesses 445

Lymphangitis (Blood Poisoning) 44
Ringworm 44
Hives 45
Pityriasis Rosea 45
Poison Ivy 45
Paronychia (Infection Around the Nail). 45
Hematoma of the Nail 45
Strawberry Hemangioma 46
Athlete's Foot 46
Bee Sting 46
Bites (Dogs, Cats, and Humans) 46
Urticaria Papulosa (Pets and the Itch). 46
Acne 47
Warts 47
Sunburn 47
Scalds and Burns 47
The Bald Spot 47
Lice 47

CHAPTER SIXTEEN
THE HEAD

The Head 48
Headache 48
Migraine Headache 48
Fainting Spells 49
Epileptic Fits 49
Nervous Tics 49
Hyperkinetic Child (Attention Deficit). 49
Concussion 49
Down's Syndrome 50
Meningitis 50

CHAPTER SEVENTEEN
ORTHOPEDICS

Bones and Growth of the Child 50
Growing Pains, Fact or Fiction 51
Sprains of the Joints 51
Fractures 51
The Swollen Joint 51
Flat Feet and Knock-Knee 51
Pigeon Toe 52
Osgood Schlatter Disease 52
Toxic Synovitis of the Hip Joint 52
Radial Subluxation 52
Scoliosis or the Curved Back 528
Kyphosis or the Round-Back 530
Lordosis or the Sway-Back 530
Congenital Dislocation of the Hip 532

CHAPTER ONE

EARLY BABYHOOD

THE FIRST FEW WEEKS OF LIFE.

before the baby is born
the baby is with you, home
spitting up
colicky pains
bowel movements
constipation
care of the skin
the belly button
bottoms
the bleeding vagina
baby's eyes
the jumping jack
blemishes and spots
breasts
sleep
visitors
relatives
taking the baby out

BEFORE THE BABY IS BORN

As a first pregnancy progresses toward the time for delivery, the future parents should select a pediatrician or a family practitioner. Get in touch with the doctor; visit the office if possible.

Ask about the doctor's routine; how he or she will handle the baby both in the hospital and at home. Talk about breast or bottle feeding, whichever you prefer. Ask about coverage with other doctors, at night, weekends, or vacations. Ask about his usual charges and about all other expenses you should expect.

When the excitement of expectation is over after the long-awaited birth, the doctor will check the baby in the hospital and then talk to the mother about baby care during the first few weeks of life. Some doctors will provide written material in this regard.

Remember, both of you will be nervous and unsure of yourselves. Having a baby is a pleasure, but also a big responsibility. If you need advice, please ask the doctor. Advice from friends may often be sound, but an occasional bad suggestion, however well-intentioned, can be dangerous.

THE BABY IS WITH YOU, HOME

Mother, father and baby leave the hospital. Both parents feel a sudden sense of responsibility. Many questions will come to your mind as you encounter some of the peculiar problems that a good many babies go through.

With feedings, there is the possibility that baby may spit up, have gas pains, and even develop colic. Not only that, but you may also notice irregular (sometimes very frequent) bowel movements, diarrhea or constipation. The baby will also need frequent diaper changes, skin care, baths and warmth.

Let us deal with some of these problems, one by one.

Spitting-up

As sweet as your baby is, let's face it: a baby is a baby and is likely to spit up and become sour-smelling. Spitting up is a very common thing and most babies will go through it sooner or later.

You feel you've paid so much attention: your baby has been fed, burped, and carefully laid down, when you suddenly notice some of the milk has been spit up all over his or her shirt. In most cases the spittting up is in small amounts, usually following a feeding, and it may come with a burp or a hiccup.

After their feedings, it is advisable to leave such babies propped up, i.e. in an infant seat. If the baby is left for about an hour in the infant seat, even if sleeping, the amount of spitting up will be much less. However, although this has worked with many babies, other stubborn cases necessitate changing of the formula to a different preparation, or to what the doctor recommends.

Please differentiate between spitting up and vomiting. With vomiting almost everything comes out. Vomiting can be serious in some babies, and can even indicate the need for surgery. Therefore, when in doubt, let your doctor know (see page 85).

Colicky Pains

These are very common, especially in babies who are hard to burp, and in those who have been underfed or overfed by their parents. Proper technique in offering the bottle is also quite important to avoid gas pains. Some babies may even have intolerance to the formula and may need a change to a hypoallergenic milk.

Occasionally all the above factors seem to be satisfied, yet the unhappy baby will keep on crying, sometimes for hours. Most babies have their crying sessions in the late afternoon or through the evening, just at the inopportune time when Mom and Dad are tired, and hungry! It will feel like insult added to injury when baby seems uninterested in your attempts at holding, patting, talking, burping and loving.

Such colicky pains usually start at around the third week of life, and often go on until he or she is three months old.

Most parents cannot stand these shenanigans and many become understandably uptight; the little one is driving them crazy. When baby is taken to the doctor, the doctor will determine whether or not he or she is being properly fed, given enough, is allergic to milk, and will pay special attention to the anus, since a tight anal ring may give rise to such problems too. When all seem okay, it may be determined that the baby is colicky. A medicine like Bentyl, Donnatal or something similar is prescribed in the proper dose, and quite often the baby will get some, if not a good deal, of relief.

If the parents are calm and handle their baby with love and understanding, the baby will reciprocate. The chance for colicky pains will be less. As stated before, most so-called gas pains are related to faulty feeding techniques, a tight anal ring, or milk intolerance or allergy. Before you become frightened that your baby has gas pains, however, don't forget that babies cry if they are uncomfortable too; any kind of discomfort. Some of them are particularly sensitive to ordinary discomforts. A crying baby may be quite hungry, need to be changed, or have some special important reason such as an ear infection. You will soon discover the difference between a discomfort cry and a pain cry and you will learn to respond accordingly.

Bowel Movement

The bowel movement of the baby will undergo transitional changes in the first few days of life. Babies who are breast-fed are more likely to have loose and frequent stools, just a few a day. Some of them may even have as many as seven or eight a day. In such babies, often the stools are soft, occasionally watery, and may be seedy; usually they are yellow in color, but it is not unusual to have a greenish-yellowish tinge.

A baby on formula will tend to have a soft or firm stool, and the smell is different from that of a breast-fed baby. Movements are not as frequent as in breast-fed babies either. Occasionally the stools become fairly hard.

Bottle-fed babies usually have one or two bowel movements a day, sometimes even three. Much of the consistency and frequency of the bowel movements depend on what the baby is eating and how much.

Constipation

In a breast-fed baby there should be no trouble with constipation; if there is, you'd better see the doctor.

Also constipation is not that common with the bottle-feeding. The consistency of the stools is important; if they are hard and the baby grunts and becomes red in the face before a hard bowel movement, you'd better call your doctor for advice. You may want to use glycerine suppository (nonprescription), or try putting the end of the thermometer in the anus.

Some such cases can be traced to a tight anus (what doctors call a tight rectum). In this case the doctor will show the mother how to dilate the area, once a day over a period of two weeks, and the trouble with constipation and gas pains will usually be over in a few days.

Some cases of constipation can cause a crack or a fissure in the anus, leading to a line of blood in the stools or the discharge of blood after the stool had passed. The baby will be in misery, crying like mad because of the pain. Many such cases can be prevented if you treat the constipation early enough (see page 100).

Care of the skin

When you take the baby home, the umbilical cord will still be attached. It is better not to bathe the baby in the usual manner until the umbilical cord falls off. Give a sponge bath to begin with. Continue that until the umbilical cord has separated and fallen off, usually around the age of ten days, give or take two days.

When the cord falls off, you can bathe your baby in the bathinette, making sure water and soap don't go into the nose or eyes. Many babies love their baths, even from the beginning, yet others sound their alarm and use their lungs to the fullest as long as they are being bathed.

Make sure the water is gently warm. Use mild soap such as Ivory or Johnson's baby soap. Dry the infant up well afterwards and try to prevent any unnecessary shivering.

It is better not to use baby oil at all, on the bottom, the

head, face or anywhere else. Baby oil is likely to block the pores of the sweat glands and cause some trouble. Instead, use powder. Apply it gently to your baby and don't make a cloud, because the powder particles can be inhaled into the lungs. Don't overpowder, because it will cake at the creases and may cause some skin trouble in those areas.

Caldesene powder is a favorite, but you can use any of the baby powders on the market. By the way, cornstarch powder, despite its popularity, should be avoided since it may promote the growth of bacteria. It is a digestable matter which the bacteria may use for food.

Some skin rashes are common in the first few weeks of life. One of them is pyoderma rash which consists of pussy blisters, i.e. blebs that are tiny, the size of a pinhead containing yellowish fluid. Pyoderma may show up in the diaper area and the lower part of the abdomen. It is caused by staph infection. If this type of rash occurs, take your baby to the doctor.

For description and treatment of cradle cap and seborrheic dermatitis see pages 88 & 90.

The belly button

The dangling shriveled umbilical cord may be an ugly sight, but you'd better leave it the way it is. It will usually separate and fall off before the baby reaches the second week of life.

When it falls off, the area left (the umbilicus) will look yellow and moist. You may want to dab it with some alcohol. Take a Q-tip, dip it in rubbing alcohol (not drinking alcohol, as one of my patients did), pull apart the skin around the belly button and touch the area with the alcohol-saturated Q-tip. You may do that three times a day for four to five days.

In some cases, a pea-sized bump, wet and glistening, gray in color may show up at the umbilicus (umbilical granuloma). The skin at the fold may be red and oozy and may at times even bleed a little since it is so fragile. If these circumstances arise, take your baby to the doctor, even if the baby doesn't seem to be in any pain. The area may have to be cauterized chemically with silver nitrate. This is a simple procedure that is completely painless.

If the umbilicus oozes liquid that is foul-smelling or smells of urine, the baby may need an immediate investigation and probably surgery.

If the belly button protrudes like a dome (though causing no pain) and becomes worse on crying, this indicates the presence of an umbilical hernia (see page 111).

Bottoms

Naturally the baby's bottom will demand a good deal of attention. Changing diapers, washing diapers, and buying disposable diapers command not an insignificant degree of time and care.

Babies will most likely cry or holler after they have wet or moved their bowels. Their bottoms will definitely suffer if diapers haven't been changed often enough.

When you clean your baby's bottom, don't smear the bowel movement all over the skin. Many parents do this unknowingly; it will lead to infection of the skin. If at all possible wash the bottom with a clean wet piece of cotton. You may even use Balneol or a similar nonprescription lotion. A clean bottom is less likely to develop diaper rash, especially if the baby is changed often enough.

When wiping the bottoms of baby girls, many parents unwittingly bring the bowel movement into the female genitalia. You can often see a resultant yellow stain at the sides of the genitalia, which can lead to infection and trouble. To avoid this, wipe her from the front to the back, and remove any bowel movement from the labia of the female organs with a Q-tip or a piece of wet cotton.

Also, obvious as it sounds, be sure to wash your hands afterwards. We have seen many parents neglect this. The result is an unhealthy and unaesthetic layer of bacteria left on the hands by the stool.

Powder or baby lotion is more than adequate for the bottom. Make sure to put on only a thin layer of powder, and do not put so much that it cakes at the creases. Caked powder at the creases will irritate the skin.

If a pink bottom develops, use A&D, Desitin or a similar ointment. These tend to protect the sensitive skin of the baby from the effect of wet soggy diapers. However, don't use baby powder in conjunction with A&D or other ointments, because together they are likely to make an unusually gritty concoction. Use either the powder by itself, or the ointment by itself, and keep to it. Don't use boric acid powder, boric acid ointment, or boric acid solution for the bottom; they can lead to toxic absorption.

For more details about diaper rash see page 101.

The bleeding vagina

Baby girls may have a small amount of vaginal discharge, usually thin and clear. This should be no cause for alarm; such discharge usually stops when the baby is a few weeks old. In occasional cases, however, this discharge will look bloody. This is usually related to the fact that the baby is experiencing a withdrawal of the mother's female hormone that had been received during pregnancy. The discharge can be ignored, and it will go away.

Baby's Eyes

In the hospital, the newborn's eyes may be swollen and slightly red. This swelling goes away after a few days. Occasionally some yellowish white material appears at the corner of the eyes; it is harmless and should be removed with a Q-tip.

The eyes should not water. However, if one or both eyes seem to water continually, there may be an obstructed tear duct (see page 95).

The white of the eye may have a red spot (usually one), as if there has been some bleeding underneath. This is no cause for alarm and is likely to go away after a few weeks (see page 198).

The color of the eye will gradually change, and by the time the baby is eight weeks old (give or take two), the eyes will have attained their permanent color. Your baby will see you only as a hazy figure until the age of three or four weeks; his or her eyesight will gradually sharpen until the age of three months. Afterwards eyesight should be quite good.

The Jumping Jack

Babies get startled when there is a sudden noise or jarring

movement. They will jump, their arms extending then going in an embrace, and may cry afterwards. This is called the "startle reflex," and it is a normal process that should be present from birth and up to a few months of age.

Blemishes and Spots

A good many babies have red spots of varied size at the forehead and the base of the nose, often extending down to the eyelids. If you look at the hair line, at the back of the neck, you may find a similar spot. This is common and temporary, and usually gradually disappears around the time of the baby's first birthday. There is no need for treatment; please learn to ignore it.

Among some dark-skinned babies, i.e. those of Mediterranean ancestors and some Blacks there may be another skin condition. Near the bottom of the spine there may be a slate-colored spot, of variable size and no particular shape. In some babies it is about one or two inches in diameter, but in others it may be quite big. This is called the "Mongolian spot," and it is perfectly normal. It usually goes away by itself much later in life.

Breasts

Many babies, boy or girl, will have a swollen breast, at times almost as big as a walnut. It doesn't hurt, and on rare occasions even some thin liquid may come out of it. It is best to leave this alone, since it will gradually shrink to normal size and shape before your baby is about two months old. Massaging or squeezing it may cause it to be infected.

Sleep

Babies who are fed well and changed properly will sleep soundly. They should be covered well but not smothered, and left alone without much noise.

Most babies sleep eighteen hours a day and even more, but some live-wires are not geared for that much sleep. Either way, let mother nature decide by allowing as much sleep as he or she wants.

Visitors

Your baby is the center of attention attracting oodles of friends, relatives, and acquaintances with gifts and frequent visits. But please be careful of those who have colds, flu, upper respiratory infection and other communicable diseases. Those who come to see the baby, but have infections with sneezing, coughing, spitting, etc., are doing a disservice to you and the baby. Mention to them gently that a baby is more likely than an adult to catch infection, that you appreciate their gifts, and that the baby will appreciate seeing them in the near future when they are healthy.

Relatives and their advice

Parents-in-law, friends, and neighbors are all loaded with unasked-for advice. Be patient, considerate, and agreeable; their advice is loving and heartfelt. Although most of their advice is harmless, it may also be at best useless; follow, instead, the advice of your doctor or the applicable advice of this book. Occasional well-meaning unprofessional advice, when taken, can lead to a lot of damage to your baby.

When shall I take my baby out?

When the baby is four to six weeks old, weather permitting. If it is nice outside, not raining or snowing or too cold, your baby can be bundled up well and taken for a stroll. Many babies enjoy the outside when they are three months old and after, but should not be taken out excessively or unnecessarily before then.

Exposed to direct sunlight, babies can easily sunburn, even in wintertime (see page 474).

Covering his or her face to protect it from the wind may be of some help, but avoid smothering. Too many clothes are as bad as too few. Become a good judge of appropriate dress for the weather.

Taking your baby out from home to a warmed car during wintertime, then from the car to another warm place, can be done at any time, at any age. That is because you are not really exposing him or her to the outside atmospheric condition.

CHAPTER TWO

FEEDING YOUR BABY

breast-feeding
bottle-feeding
water
orange juice
vitamins
solid foods
cereal
fruits
vegetables
meats
table food
eggs

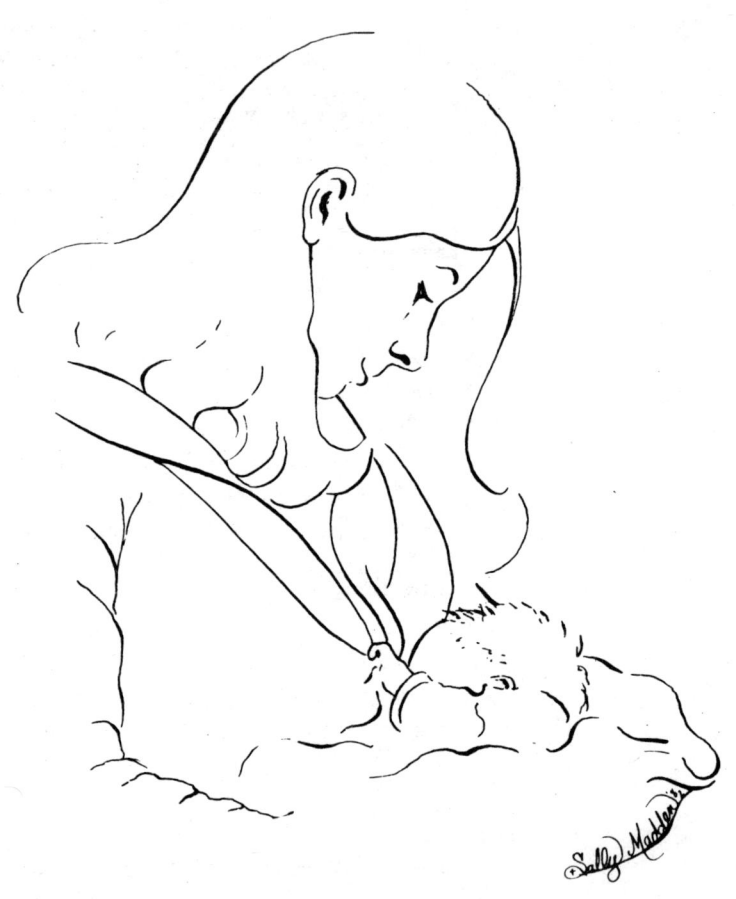

BREAST-FEEDING

Breast-feeding is the natural way, highly recommended, and the best for the baby. Billions of mothers do it and have done it through the ages; you are urged to join them. Consider your circumstances and your wishes carefully, and if it seems feasible, go ahead with it. You will have a good sense of accomplishment and gratification. The breasts offer a free and ready supply of milk, sterilized and warmed, well supplied with all forms of nourishment, ready for your hungry baby. Unlike bottle-feeding, breast-feeding has a spirit in it; it is not mechanical. It has a touch of charm, a measure of love, and a means for a strong bond with your little baby.

How often shall I nurse?

Don't go by the clock. Offer the breast when the baby is hungry; this will be about every three hours, to begin with. Later on the baby may demand it less often. Let him or her take one breast for ten to fifteen minutes. When the baby stops nursing, he or she is ready to be burped. After burping, offer the other breast and repeat the procedure. If the baby sucks at the nipple for longer than ten to fifteen minutes, he or she may be playing, and not taking more milk.

About three to four hours after this feeding, the baby will be ready for the next feeding. Offer the last breast you used during the last feeding, to be followed by the other breast. Be sure to treat both breasts equally. Some mothers prefer to have one breast completely emptied in a full feeding; with the next feeding they will offer the other breast. This is an acceptable alternative.

How about vitamins and iron?

Breast milk has an ample supply of biologically effective vitamins and iron. But if circumstances require vitamins and iron to be used in a breast-fed baby, your doctor will advise you.

Many doctors use vitamins with fluoride (prescription) for all breast-fed babies until the baby is old enough to drink a sufficient amount of water. If the water the baby is drinking is fluoridated, the vitamins with fluoride should be discontinued. If your town doesn't have fluoride in the water, keep giving vitamins with fluoride, or fluoride alone, until the child is ten years old.

Can I use the bottle in addition to breast feedings?

Yes you can, depending on your circumstances. Breast milk is usually sufficient in most cases, if not in all. Occasionally, however, a fast-growing baby with a ravenous appetite will be demanding the breast all the time. In such a baby the weight gain compared to that of the height may not be good enough. It may be necessary to use a supplemental feeding with a bottle.

The bottle can also be given when the mother goes out to work or leaves the house for other reasons, and one or two breast feedings are missed during her absence.

How can we give supplemental feedings?

If the baby seems to need more than what the breasts can offer, you may want to use a formula such as Enfamil, Similac, or SMA.

Offer one of these formulas after the baby is done with the breast. If after the breast-feeding the baby takes one or two ounces of formula, that is O.K., but if he or she takes three to five ounces it will mean the breast milk is seriously lacking in quantity. Supplemental formulas may then be given routinely; many a hungry baby will be happy with this arrangement. Giving the feedings on demand will help stimulate the breasts for good production, as well as satisfy the baby better. Most breast-fed babies will not need solid foods until about six months of age, though some doctors may start them earlier.

How long shall I continue with the breast-feeding?

To be meaningful, it is best to breast-feed until the baby is at least six months old, preferably until twelve months of age. We have seen babies who were on the breast up to the age of five years, and others for a mere five to six weeks! Either way is extreme if not excessive and unnecessary.

From a physiological and nutritive point of view, breast milk is ideal especially during the period when the baby needs it most, i.e. the first year of life, more so during the early few months.

Upon dicontinuing the breast-feeding, go to a formula if the baby

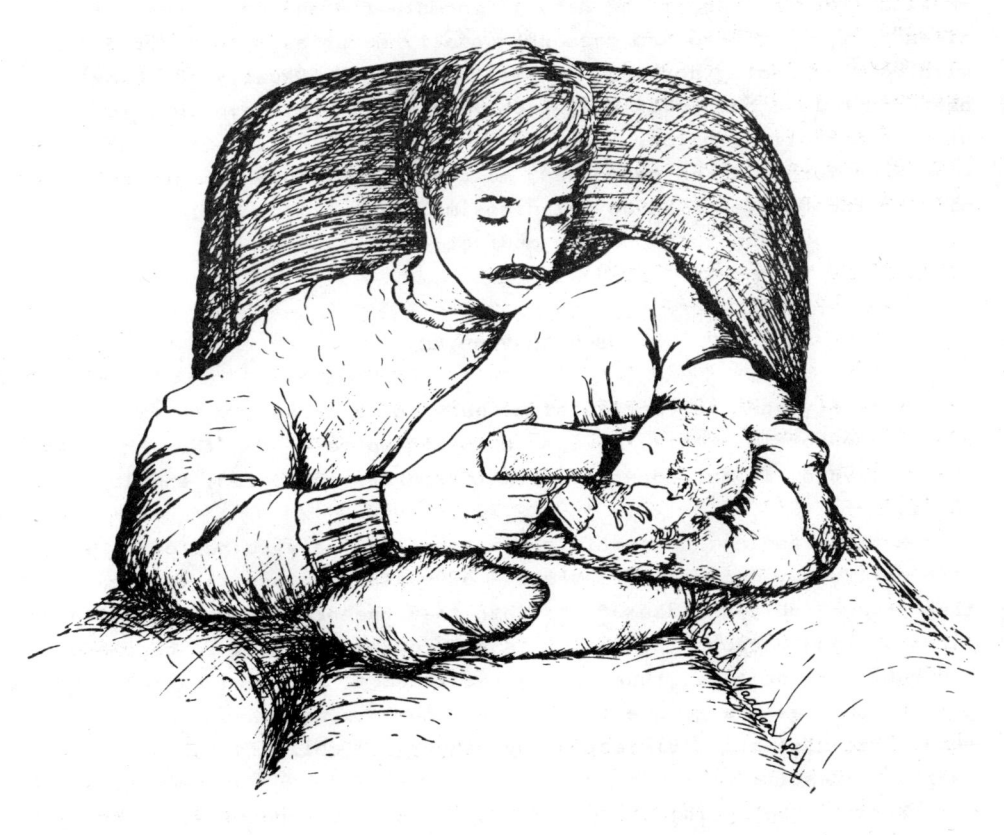

is less than one year old. Don't jump to homogenized milk right away; you may use it later on. Continue to use the formula until the baby is about one year old, then switch to homogenized milk.

Can the breast-feeding affect the baby in some unforeseen ways?

Yes, they can. The baby's stool will be soft if not liquid, will smell different than if the baby is formula-fed and occur several times a day. Spitting up does not usually occur as much as it does with bottle-feeding nor does it smell the same. Usually the baby needs much less burping. Very rarely will the baby develop milk allergy or colicky pains.

When mother takes medicines, most such medicines go through the milk to the baby, but in an infinitesimal proportion. Talk to your doctor if you need to be on any medications.

BOTTLE-FEEDING

A fairly good percentage of mothers in this country continue to prefer the bottle. This, of course, is in spite of the fact that breast-feeding is far superior both for mother and child, and is the ideal.

Bottle-feeding, however, is practical and easy to perform. It is also desired by many mothers because of social factors (i.e. because they have a job), because of the fear that the breasts will lose their firmness, and because the mother is afraid that she has to be close to the baby all the time, thus losing her freedom. As long as the mother prefers and desires to use the bottle, there is no reason why she shouldn't; ultimate satisfaction by mother and child is the most desirable result.

From the beginning of this century until now, bottle-feeding has undergone gradual and steady improvement, and it has reached by now a very good level of sophistication. The advantages of breast-feedings over bottle-feedings have been narrowed somewhat.

What is on the market?

Basically, there are two kinds of "bottles," the Playtex and the regular, and there are numerous variations within each.

The Playtex bottle consists of a rigid plastic "bottle" without a bottom, some thin plastic bags, a nipple that is shaped very much like the nipple of the breast (yet not of the same elasticity), and a cover for the nipple.

Using the Playtex bottle is preferable, because there will be less likelihood for the baby to swallow an extra amount of air, thus avoiding a possibility for gas pains.

However, some babies don't go for the Playtex nipples no matter how hard you try. Whatever the reasons, you may find it necessary to go to the older method-the familiar bottle with the long nipple.

Most nipples for such bottles have holes at the base. When you tighten the plastic ring that holds the nipple to the bottle, don't tighten it too much; just make it snug. When done this way, the holes will continue to be open, and they will allow bubbles of air to go through the milk as the baby sucks at the bottle.

If you tighten the plastic ring excessively, it will close the holes at the base of the nipple. As a result, no air bubbles will go through the milk during sucking. Therefore, the baby will have to:

1. suck very hard at the nipple and in the process get tired easily;
2. interrupt the sucking to let the air enter the bottle through the holes at the tip of the nipple;
3. swallow air, thus becoming liable to develop some gas pains.

None of the above problems show up with the Playtex bottle.

Are there other kinds of bottles?

Yes, they come in kit forms, and you will have to take your time to read the directions carefully and follow what they suggest.

What kind of milk shall I use?

There are many kinds of milk in the market. The preference of most pediatricians is the prepared formula. There are of course a good many prepared formulas, and each company claims that its own is the best.

The most well known formulas are Similac, SMA, and Enfamil. These formulas also come in different variations (plain or with added iron).

Prepared formulas come in liquid form and in powder form. The liquid form is the preferred one and is also the most popular. The powder form comes in a can or in a packet, is less expensive, and is useful when space is a problem.

Liquid formulas also are sold either as concentrated or fully prepared. The latter is usually sold in large cans, and you don't have to add water to it or sterilize it.

By the time the baby is twelve months old, you may give straight homogenized milk (a few doctors start homogenized milk at an earlier age).

How about formulas with extra iron?

An example is Similac with iron. They are good for prematures and twins because such babies need the extra iron. They are also good when there is doubt that the baby's nutrition will be adequate enough. Many pediatricians use them routinely. Follow your doctor's suggestions, since he or she knows you and your baby best.

How should I offer the bottle?

Hold the baby lovingly, prop him or her up a bit, and be gentle, comfortable, and calm. Offer the bottle at an angle, let the nipple touch the infant's searching lips, and let him or her gobble up the milk. Avoid giving the bottle while the baby is flat on his or her back; this may lead to an ear infection.

Please don't allow distractions and/or too much noise, and don't be in a hurry. The strong bond between you and your baby is working well by now, so make use of this chance.

Your baby may be very hungry and may finish off the feeding in as short as a ten- to fifteen-minute period! Most babies however, take as long as twenty to twenty-five minutes before they finish. Beyond twenty-five minutes is time lost; the infant will only be playing with the nipple.

How much milk shall I give the baby?

The amount varies according to the need of your baby, and there is no set limit. Let his or her stomach be the judge. Increase the amount of milk in the bottle if the baby completely finishes off the bottles of a few previous feedings. That is to say, if a three-week-old baby takes four ounces of milk to the last drop, and does so for several feedings, then the parent is to increase the amount to five ounces in each bottle for the next day's formula.

By and large, babies take four ounces a feeding until three to four weeks, five or six ounces a feeding until seven to eight weeks old, then six to eight ounces a feeding from two months and up. Don't offer more than eight ounces at a feeding.

In one whole day, a two months old baby or older is satisfied with twenty-six to thirty ounces of milk. To go beyond thirty ounces a day is overfeeding.

Some babies who are on solid food refuse to take more than sixteen ounces of milk a day, and the parents can become understandably concerned. But such babies do well with this amount. Actually, this amount will give the baby enough calcium and protein, so don't worry.

How often should I offer the bottle?

The golden rule is to let the stomach of the baby decide. The average baby will demand a bottle every three to four hours, but a small one who is two to three weeks old may demand it more often.

Don't follow a strict time schedule; remember, your baby is not a machine.

If the baby demands the bottle too often, e.g. every two hours, it means that he or she is thirsty, or ready for more milk or more solid food.

How long will they demand night feedings?

Usually the smaller the baby at birth the longer it will take before he or she sleeps through the night. An average baby will sleep through the night by the age of five to six weeks, give or take two weeks. (Sleeping through the night means that after a full meal in the evening, the baby will sleep until around 6 am.)

How shall I know when the baby needs to be burped?

The best way is to let them tell you: let them keep sucking the breast or bottle until they slow down and stop. In so doing they will have taken enough milk and air to distend the stomach. Take the breast or the bottle away (they will gladly let you), then prop them up or let them be on your shoulder; with a few taps on the back they will burp -one or two, loud and musical. By then they will be ready for more breast milk or formula, but not as vigorously as before. When they finish, another burp can be expected. It usually takes less than two to three minutes to do the job of burping.

Please don't mechanically interrupt their feeding every so often for the sake of burping. Don't yank the breast or the bottle out of the mouth of a still vigorously sucking baby, and then try to burp the little one. This doesn't work well at all, because the baby is not ready for it yet; he or she will get tired in the meantime and some problems of feeding irregularities will start buiding up.

One burping session in the middle of the feeding and one at the end is all that most babies need.

The formula is not agreeing with my baby; can I change?

By far the majority of babies will do well on whatever formula you choose for them. Changing formula from one to another should vigorously be discouraged. Generally, babies who are unhappy or uncomfortable are either too hungry, overfed, or affected by some other specific trouble. (See section on milk allergy and changes of formula, page 75).

How about water for the baby?

You can offer water to the baby; if he or she takes it, fine; if not, there is no reason for alarm. Babies on the breast are less likely to want or need water.

However, babies in non-air-conditioned houses during summertime (or overheated during wintertime), will be more likely to need a four ounce bottle of water. Make sure the water has been sterilized for five minutes, and it is O.K. to add one teaspoon of sugar to it.

How about orange juice?

You may offer the baby orange juice once a day. Start at the age of six months or beyond (some doctors advise earlier). Dilute the juice with equal amounts of water. Look for signs of trouble when you first offer it, since orange juice is allergenic in some babies. Stomachache, gas, diarrhea, or rash may indicate an allergy.

By the way, you don't have to insist on orange juice everyday.

Since we offer vitamins every day (which contain vitamin C), orange juice has lost much of its prestigious position.

Tell us more about vitamins:

Vitamins with or without iron, come in different forms and varieties. It is often advised that all babies be given the multiple vitamins, once a day, for the first two years of life. The multiple vitamins contain vitamins A, D, B complex, and C. Poly-Vi-Sol, Abdec, and Vi-Daylin, are but a few names. Tri-Vi-Sol and Vi-Daylin ADC lack the vitamin B component. If you use the drops, give one ml, once a day.

You may say, "But the prepared formulas already have vitamins in them." You are right, and you may want to ignore the additional vitamins until the baby is changed to homogenized milk or you may want to use half the above dose. Either way is O.K. If you give the baby vitamins while he or she is on prepared formula, the excess of certain vitamins will be excreted in the urine.

When shall I shift to homogenized milk?

You can do that at the age of twelve months or anytime after, though a few doctors prefer to do it earlier.

It is good to be cautious though, and try for a day or two to alternate the feedings between the formula and the homogenized milk. This will make the transition easy, and help detect any signs of trouble the new milk may give.

When shall I stop the sterilization?

You can discontinue sterilization by the time the baby is five months old if you have city water. For those who use well water, it is better to sterilize the water or the constituted formula up to the age of one year, because some well waters are likely to get contaminated.

Naturally you don't have to be concerned about any of this if you use "ready-to-feed" formula in a Playtex bottle.

SOLID FOODS

<u>I am anxious to start the baby on solid foods, when shall I start?</u>

If your baby is thriving well, and acts contented, continue with the breast or formula alone. If the baby's growth is satisfactory, and if everyone is satisfied, then wait until there is a definite need for the solid foods (usually around the age of six months).

Many babies will act hungry at an early age, and somehow milk by itself will not seem to satisfy them that well. They cry in demand, they go wild after the bottle, and they guzzle it down as if there is no tomorrow. Many even demand to be fed as often as every two hours if not more often.

If such is the case with your baby, it is good to start him or her on baby cereal. The earliest that this should be started is at the age of a few months.

<u>Why the baby cereal first?</u>

Baby cereal has three points to its credit:

1. It offers calories and nourishment to the baby;
2. It has added iron which helps prevent anemia;
3. It has bulk, and this makes the stomach full and the bowel movements more substantive.

Rice cereal or barley cereal are best at the start. They are to be followed by oatmeal and mixed cereal. Rice cereal tends to bind the stools, oatmeal tends to loosen them. If the stools get too hard, stick to oatmeal cereal. If the stools tend to be too loose, offer rice cereal.

<u>How can I prepare the cereal?</u>

If you buy boxed, powdered cereal, put the cereal in a bowl, add milk or formula slowly, and stir the mixture. Keep doing that until the cereal is of the consistency of applesauce; then the cereal is ready to feed. Don't make the cereal too runny or too thick; either way the baby will not like it.

Cereal may come already mixed with fruits. This is more

expensive and it has fixed proportions of the cereal and the fruits, making it harder for you to alter the ratio.

If you offer the cereal and the baby doesn't seem to like it, you may forget about it for a week or so, then try it again. Or you may add some fruits to it, thus flavoring it. It is rare that a baby will refuse to take cereal; the majority like it, especially with fruits mixed in.

How shall I offer it to the baby?

Prop him or her up in your lap, and support the head nicely. Use a small spoon for the cereal. A hungry baby will open his or her mouth readily like a baby bird. Fill the spoon with the cereal, put it at the back of the tongue, and the baby will down it with a beautiful gulp.

If you put the cereal at the tip of the tongue, more likely than not the baby will put the tongue out, and the cereal will slobber down the chin. Don't be discouraged by this; if it happens, scoop it up and put it back, at the back part of the tongue. Mealtime can be messy, but messes can be fun too.

How often and how much cereal shall I give?

To begin with offer about one tablespoon twice a day. Gradually increase the amount, and about two or three weeks after, you may offer two to three tablespoons twice a day. Eventually you will be offering a bowl (three to four tablespoons) of cereal for each feeding.

Some parents do strange things: some dump the cereal in the bottle and mix it with the milk. Some go so far as to cut the nipple of the bottle at its center, so that the milk, thickened with cereal, will be easy to take.

Please avoid these extreme practices. There is nothing sacrosanct about a baby taking the cereal like clockwork; if the baby doesn't want to take it in the usual manner, don't insist.

Cereal is easy to digest and filling. It is not as nourishing as meat, but the baby will not need meats that early in life. It is rare to see intolerance or allergy to cereal, so it is relatively safe to use.

Should fruits be offered next?

Fruits have a pleasant taste, and a good balance of minerals and vitamins; some are even rich in calories, such as bananas.

Because they are easy on the stomach, and add bulk to the contents of the intestine, no wonder fruits come as a good choice after the cereal.

How should I feed them to the baby?

Mixed with cereal fruits offer flavor and substance.

Bananas can be used in conjunction with the cereal. Bananas are easily tolerated by all except about one percent of babies. Besides the other qualities fruits have, bananas are rich in calories and will thus offer a feeling of fullness to the baby. To begin with, add about a 1/4 of a jar of baby bananas or 1/4 of a mashed fresh banana to each feeding of cereal. As the baby grows and the demands for food become increased, you may increase the amount to about 1/2 a jar with each cereal feeding, i.e. three times a day when the baby is about four to five months old or older.

Applesauce and pears can of course be used for variety. They are good, the baby's lipsmacking may even be heard from a distance. They are least likely to cause trouble with the bowels, and they are quite safe to give.

Are there fruits that may give trouble?

There are four fruits which should be watched, since they may give rise to gas pains, stomachache, and loose bowel movements in some babies. These fruits are: prunes, apricots, plums, and peaches.

When you want to start them, start one at a time. If after three or four days there seems to be no trouble, you may start the next fruit in line.

Also remember, if your baby has constipation, feeding prunes and/or other fruits may help the bowels. As a matter of fact, prunes, prune juice, or prune/apple juice are often given to treat constipation in a small baby.

How long shall I wait before I use vegetables and meats?

Cereal and fruit may be used until the baby reaches the age of six months, give or take two weeks.

By then, the baby's system will be ready for the extra protein provided by meats. Vegetables are similar to fruits in their content of vitamins and minerals, although some vegetables do contain amino acids, which are a component of the protein.

When the vegetables and meats are started, they can be given together, and they will constitute the midday or evening meal. This way, the baby will have cereal and fruit in the morning, vegetables and meats at noon, and cereal and fruit before bedtime.

Are there any vegetables we ought to be careful about?

Yes; carrots and legumes. Carrots contain a substance called carotene, which becomes converted into vitamin A. An excess amount of carotene will cause a noticeable yellowing of the skin, sometimes all over, but especially at the tip of the nose and ears. This condition looks like yellow jaundice without its effects on the white of the eye. It is called carotenemia.

If you stop giving carrots, the yellow color of the skin will slowly disappear over a period of a few months.

Legumes are greens such as green beans, peas, etc.; they are quite valuable and nourishing to the baby because they contain an abundance of proteins which are important for growth. However, in some babies they produce gas pains and stomach upset, and may even cause diarrhea. Therefore, introduce them cautiously, one at a time, and watch for signs of intolerance.

How much of the vegetables shall I give?

Usually half a jar a meal is enough, yet you may have to keep offering until the baby rejects it. Most, if not all babies have the sense to do that. Some will clamp their mouths shut, others will spit it out, and others will shake their heads as if to say, "cool it, I'm loaded."

You ought to keep in mind that some babies simply refuse vegetables no matter what kind they are, and others refuse fruits completely but are more receptive towards vegetables. This is not much of a problem, since you may interchange fruits for vegetables and vice versa at any time, and the resulting nourishment will be the same.

How about meats?

As mentioned before, meats are rich in proteins, and proteins are needed as building blocks for the baby. When the baby reaches the age of around six months, the need for the proteins will be larger, and the protein in the milk may not suffice. The proteins in the meats and in green vegetables will fill the bill. Meats and vegetables also have a good supply of iron, and the baby's body will welcome this addition.

By the age of six months, most babies will take the meats well and will not mind its sticky consistency or its unusual aroma. Occasionally a baby will prove sensitive to a particular kind of meat.

Start with lamb or chicken at first, and if it is well tolerated, continue with another kind of meat.

How much meat shall I give my baby?

Offer the meats in combination with the vegetables until the baby shows signs of being full enough or resists taking any more. Most babies are satisfied with half a jar of vegetables and half a jar of meats for a meal, but their needs vary depending on how hungry they are, how big they are, how old they are, and a host of other factors.

My baby is six months old; how about some table food?

For some babies it is time to introduce some table food. The medium that we depend upon is the mashed potato. Since the baby's digestive tract is mature enough to handle table food by this age, and since the only component missing is the presence of enough teeth to chew with, it would be good to start with table foods that are not chunky. Mashed potatoes will fit the bill nicely and it is the best item to start the baby on.

If the baby takes it well for a few days, you start adding whatever items of food you have on the table. Make sure that you also mash the foods until they are of the consistency of applesauce. Mix those foods with the mashed potatoes, then offer it to the baby and let him or her enjoy it.

As the baby grows, you may want to start offering some meats from the table. At the age of seven or eight months and beyond, many babies can easily take small chunks of meat, often mixed with mashed potatoes. Hamburgers that have been fragmented with a fork, hot dogs that have been cut into very small pieces, and chicken that has been chopped into small chunks, can all be eaten and enjoyed.

The same thing applies to vegetables you cook for the family. Just mash the vegetables with the back of a fork or spoon, mix the mashed vegetables with the mashed potatoes, and offer them to the baby.

My baby is eight months old; how much table food should he or she have?
Again it all depends on your baby and the gag reflex. If the baby seems to accept table food increasingly well, keep offering it in bigger and bigger proportions, taking care not to push.

Many babies will take one or two whole meals a day from the table around this age.

As your baby grows to the age of around ten months, he or she is more likely to accept, if not demand, two meals from the table.

How about eggs?
Eggs are nourishing, but they may ignite reactions in babies who happen to be allergic to them.

Start introducing eggs when the child is six to nine months old, not earlier. If there is a family history of allergy to it, it is better to wait until a few months later.

Start cautiously by mashing the yolk of a semi-hard-boiled egg with a fork, and offering it mixed with applesauce or simply by itself.

Look for signs of reaction, such as gas pains, stomach upset, vomiting, diarrhea, rash, etc. If these symptoms appear, the baby will be considered to be allergic to eggs and will have to avoid them.

If there is no allergy to the egg yolk, try a whole soft-boiled egg and also watch for the same signs of reaction. If reaction shows up, the baby will be considered to be allergic to the white of the egg and ought to avoid it.

If the baby is not sensitive to eggs (and most of them aren't) one or two eggs a week is reasonable.

A soft-boiled egg mixed with chips of bread, or even scrambled eggs with some bread, are enjoyed by many babies in the morning.

Please remember not to give too many eggs, i.e. every day, since they might lead to trouble with cholesterol deposit later in life (egg yolk is extremely high in cholesterol). Moderation pays off in most instances.

Can I give my baby ice cream if he or she is now on whole milk?

Sure, let the baby enjoy life and be sticky and messy. Ice cream and milkshakes are as nourishing as milk and well-liked by most babies.

The same applies to many goodies in life. You can offer soups or desserts and pies, etc., but simply make sure solid food is mashed or in the form of small crumbs.

Vegetables or foods that cannot be mashed easily (such as corn, nuts, bacon) should be avoided until the baby is beyond the age of eighteen months. Also avoid raw honey until the child is one year old (this will avoid infant botulism).

My baby gags on table food; what shall I do?

A few babies are born with a sensitive gag reflex, and this condition will persist with them for the rest of their lives (see page 54). Such babies cannot take table food easily. These babies can take the relatively chunky food approximately three to six months later than an average baby, i.e. at about nine to twelve months of age.

An average baby is fully on table food by the age of twelve to thirteen months if not earlier, but a baby with a sensitive gag reflex cannot be fully on table food until eighteen to twenty-four months of age. There are, however, a number of eager beavers who are on complete table food at the age of seven to eight months if not earlier. These are of course exceptions.

What shall I do in case may baby has a sensitive gag reflex?

In such cases, slowly add "junior food" (see page 48) to take the place of the baby food, starting at the age of six to nine months. Over a period of a few months you will have shifted completely from the baby food to the junior food. This is to be followed slowly (and as much as the baby's condition can bear) by a shift from junior food to table food. You have to experiment repeatedly as to when your baby will be able to swallow and accept table food without much gagging.

Junior food should not be used extensively or routinely for every baby, because it is not needed in general and is both an extra expense and an extra effort.

Can I fix junior food at home?

Fixing junior food at home is easy; all that you need is a blender. In the blender put whatever food you want to process, add some water or milk, turn the machine on, and in a few minutes the food is ready to be used by the baby or for storage in the refrigerator.

Buying junior food will of course save you the bother of extra work, but it means more expense.

When shall I stop offering the bottle?

By the age of one year you ought to cut down on the number of bottles the child takes. Most of the one-year-olds take two bottles a day; one when they wake up in the morning and one before they go to bed. Some will want a third bottle during midday. To cut down on the bottle, offer milk from a cup.

A few weeks later, the bottle in the morning will have to be stopped, and believe it or not the baby usually doesn't miss it!

By the time the toddler is fifteen to sixteen months old, the bottle at night will have to be stopped too. It takes three nights of fussing and restlessness before the child becomes used to this idea. But after that, the era of the bottle will be behind us.

When shall I stop mashing the baby's food?

As the baby grows up, and as the jaw teeth start coming in (i.e. ten months of age and beyond), there will be less need for mashing the food. At the child's first birthday, he or she is fairly able to take care of the food without your help, i.e. with his or her teeth. Those who are slow teethers, however, may still need your help, and you may have to prolong the process of mashing and chopping the food for a while. It is very rare for a toddler who is eighteen months of age to need any assistance from a parent in that regard.

How about nibbling on cookies, zweiback, crackers, etc.?

Many parents think it is good for the child to nibble on such food items and may even believe that it helps with the teething.

On the contrary, such a practice ought to be discouraged and if possible stopped. It is a messy thing at its best, and it interferes with the little one's appetite at the expense of a well-proportioned diet. It can also lead to a marked degree of tooth decay even at such an early age.

Sometimes I see pieces of fruits in the baby's stools:

This can happen easily if you offer fruits that have not been mashed. Some parents offer a piece of melon, peaches, etc. to a baby who has no more than the front teeth and maybe one jaw tooth. The baby will of course not be able to chew the fruits well, and may swallow it whole. This piece of roughage will have to pass through the intestines undigested. This will not harm the baby, though at times it may cause some stomachache and or gagging. It is better not to give fruits as such, and when given, to be in the consistency of applesauce.

CHAPTER THREE

WHAT IS EXPECTED

at the age of one month
at the age of two months
at the age of three months
at the age of four months
at the age of five months
at the age of six months
at the age of eight months
at the age of ten months
at the age of twelve months
at the age of fifteen months
at the age of eighteen months
at the age of twenty one months.
at the age of two years

physical development of the adolescent male
physical development of the adolescent female
menstruation
checkups
school phobia

WHAT IS EXPECTED
AT THE AGE OF ONE MONTH

Development:

One month olds are a little more lively now than at birth. At times they look at you with a gaze as if trying to see who you are, though you will not be in sharp focus. If you talk to them, they respond by what looks like a smile.

If their eyes are caught by something interesting to them, and that object is moving slowly, then their eyes will follow the moving object to some extent.

They may respond with a sudden jerk to any jarring movement or sudden noise; the response may be in the form of reaching as if to embrace. This tendency is present from birth, and it will continue for the first few months of life. It is called the "startle reflex," and is normal.

They may vocalize (coo) at times, and later on they will do this more often.

Lastly, if put on their stomachs, they may try to lift their heads up about forty-five degrees. They are trying to take a look around, and are showing some muscle control of the neck.

How about their eating?

The odds are that they are quite satisfied with milk, be it breast or formula. However, if they act hungry and demand feedings too often, they may have to be fed more formula with each feeding. This sometimes happens in babies who tend to grow fast, or who move a lot.

At checkup time, they will have gained about one or two pounds since leaving the hospital, and about one or one and one half inches in height.

Upon seeing the doctor:

The doctor will ask about the development of the baby, measure weight, height and head circumference, check about the feeding and sleep schedules, and take care of problems. The baby will be examined all over, and the rectum maybe checked too. A blood specimen from the heel for PKU and other tests will be taken.

The doctor may also discuss future checkups and shots and immunizations to be given. Your doctor may give you pamphlets or printed papers to aid you in the care of the baby.

Some tidbits:

The umbilical cord will tend to fall off by the time the baby is two weeks old, if not before then (see page 7).

When it comes to bathing, you may sponge bathe the baby at first, that is until the umbilical cord falls off. After it falls off, you start giving the baby a full bath. Use mild soaps, and bathe only briefly. Soaps like Johnson's, Dial, and Neutrogena are quite good.

Grunting at this age is quite common, as is hiccupping and sneezing. They can be annoying at times, but they will not be that obvious in a few more weeks.

Some bottle-fed babies are more likely than others to get colic. The colicky pains usually show up around the age of three weeks or so, and they will continue for a good many weeks (see page 4).

Babies' stools may be soft or seedy at this age, and they may have them once or twice a day. If they have them less often, and the consistency is soft, then parents needn't worry (see page 5).

Babies at this age may exhibit a rash on their cheecks and chin; this rash is mild, but may become more pronounced later on (see page 89).

Make sure to clean the diaper area well, especially after a bowel movement. Don't just wipe the material in such a way as to smear the whole bottom with it. You have better results if you "clean-wash" the area (see page 8).

Remember that dry bottoms are much healthier than constantly wet ones, and they are more resistant to diaper rash. Change the diapers when they become wet, and do it as soon as it is feasible for you (see page 8). Baby powders, especially Caldesene powder, are good to use; so are lotions.

Most babies will still wake up at night for feedings (if yours does not, then congratulations, you are lucky). This habit will stop around the age of six to seven weeks in most cases.

About DPTs

DPT stands for diphtheria, pertussis (whooping cough), and tetanus respectively. Upon receiving such shots, if your baby develops high temperature, loud crying spells, convulsions or any untoward symptoms, please be sure to notify your doctor. The doctor may elect to give a DT shot next time, i.e. one without whooping cough vaccine. A reaction, especially severe enough, should be a warning to give a DT next time, not DPT.

Please note that the American Academy of Pediatrics and the overwhelming majority of pediatricians, reaffirm the recommendation of giving the DPT, especially in view of the seriousness of whooping cough in unimmunized infants.

WHAT IS EXPECTED
AT THE AGE OF TWO MONTHS

Development

Two month olds are more active by now and more likely to smile by themselves. At times they may even laugh loudly, making you and those around quite happy. They may squeal too, sometimes often and sometimes loudly.

They follow a moving object all the way (180 degrees) with their eyes. They are becoming more aware of their surroundings and show signs of participation in the activity around them. They may discover their hands; they may hold them together or look at them.

If put on their stomachs, they can raise their heads a full 90 degrees to look around. And if put in someone's lap, they are able to hold their heads up rather than let their heads flop. In other words, they have better control of their neck muscles than ever before.

The average weight at this age is eleven and one half pounds, and the average height is twenty-two and one-half inches, but there are, of course, variations from baby to baby.

How about their eating?

Appetites vary; each baby has individual needs and demands. By this age, the baby will be needing more milk than before, and if he or she is on the bottle, you will see that a seven to eight ounce bottle becomes necessary. Do satisfy your baby's thirst, or else he or she will holler for satisfaction! Usually, an average of twenty-four to thirty ounces of milk over twenty-four hours is sufficient. You may offer four ounces of water, once a day.

Upon seeing the doctor:

Aside from checking the baby up and discussing any possible problems, the doctor may administer the baby's first DPT shot and oral polio vaccine,

"DPT" stands for diphtheria, pertussis (whooping cough), and tetanus. The baby is supposed to have a total of three DPT shots, one shot every two months, though a minority of doctors prefer to give them once every month. This is to build a good immunity level against these three troublesome diseases.

The polio immunization is to be given by mouth (Sabin vaccine), and it offers immunity against the three different varieties of the poliovirus.

Will there be any reactions?

Most babies who get the immunization will have no reaction. Occasionally however, a baby will become fussy and irritable and may have some fever. Usually this happens the day the shot is given. You may give the infant 0.3 ml of Tempra drops, or 0.4 ml of Tylenol drops every four hours if he or she is fussy enough or feverish to need it.

Occasionally, a baby's buttock will react to the shot, and it may become sore, or somewhat swollen. This can also happen locally in other areas where the shot maybe given (such as the arm or the thigh). To help relieve the soreness, you may apply heat for twenty minutes, three to four times a day for one to two days. Hot water bottles or a heating pad will do. Later on, you may discover a small lump, the size of a pea or slightly larger, just at the area where the shot was given. Don't worry, it will go away after a few months.

Some tidbits:

At the age of two months, a number of babies with tender skin may develop some rash on the cheeks, chin, or forehead. The rash may show up as a few spots, then become worse in a few day's time. This rash is pink in color, slightly rough, and may be glistening. Putting the babies on their stomachs may make them rub their cheeks against the bedsheet, irritating the area and making the rash worse. The same thing happens if they lay their cheeks against their parent's sweater or jacket, since wool and synthetic fiber can irritate also.

This problem is called seborrheic dermatitis (see page 90). The baby is very likely to outgrow it in a few months. By the way, food has nothing to do with the rash, so don't worry about milk or food allergy being the cause.

Babies with such a rash are also likely to develop cradle cap (see page 88). A mild cradle cap will wash away with mild shampoo such as Johnson's Baby shampoo. Don't apply baby oil on the head and face if this problem appears; it often makes it worse.

Diaper rash becomes more prevalent from this age on. If it is mild and if the area smells of ammonia, you may use A and D, Desitin, or Caldesene ointments among others. Also frequent changes of diapers, as soon as they get wet, will help a lot (see page 101).

Many babies at this age will attempt thumb-sucking (see page 86). This is a golden opportunity to discourage your baby from doing that, so don't miss it. Taking a pacifier is the lesser of two evils.

Some degree of spitting up, mainly in bottle-fed babies, is not unusual at this age, but it becomes more of a common thing from the age of three months and beyond (see pages 4 and 85).

WHAT IS EXPECTED
AT THE AGE OF THREE MONTHS

Development:

Three month olds can recognize people and respond to them; they can laugh and squeal and fill hearts with delight.

If you put your finger, or a rattle, in their hand, they will hold tightly to it. They are interested in seeing things at this age, and may gaze at any new object, even if it is as small as a raisin. By this age, they can see things quite clearly. The color of their eyes by now is almost permanent.

They have good control of their eyes and head and may even attempt to reach nearby things of interest to them. In adult laps, they are able to hold their heads steadily and even look around. If you put them on their stomachs they will be strong enough to push themselves up and look around. A good many babies roll over from back to stomach or stomach to back, although some prefer not to.

Many babies will also enjoy standing up if you hold them by their sides. This is perfectly all right and it will not hurt their legs at all, nor will it hurt any of their bones.

The average weight at this age is twelve and one half pounds, and the average height is twenty-three and one half inches, but keep in mind that variations from these figures do exist from baby to baby.

How about eating?

They are happy when their stomachs are full. They will continue to be on breast milk or formula, though a number of parents will want to try starting cereal and fruits. By the way, vegetables and meats are not needed by the baby's system until around the age of six months, therefore you do not have to rush. As a matter of fact most babies do not need to be started on solid food until they are five or six months old.

Some fast-growing babies will demand solid food. If such is the case, you start with a small amount and slowly increase it, until the baby takes as much as three or four tablespoons of cereal at a time, along with one half a jar of fruits. Not only will they take this helping, but they may take two or three ounces of milk after that (to "wash it down"). More than this amount of milk may cause spitting up.

Upon seeing the doctor:
After checkup and discussion, some doctors give the second DPT shot at this age. It is too early to give the second polio at this visit. Your doctor, like most others, may not give any immunizations this time, prefering to give the second DPT shot and the oral polio together at four months of age.

If there were any reactions to the DPT in the previous month, please mention them to the doctor. He may, instead, give the DT shot (DPT not including the whooping cough vaccine).

Some tidbits:
From now on, babies will slobber a good deal. They will want to bite on things, and will want to chew on their fists often. Slobbering is not a sign of teething; it so happens that at this age babies produce plenty of saliva they prefer not to swallow.

A good many babies tend to spit up by now too, mainly if they are on the bottle. At times the spitting up can even be excessive. This tends to become worse in the few weeks to come, then it will slow down gradually until it stops when they are seven to nine months old.

If they had been colicky, the colic will tend to disappear by this age. If they are on medicine for colic, it is time to stop this medicine by now.

By the way, many an older brother or sister is likely to become jealous of the baby. They might sneak in and hurt the infant somehow, so be on the alert. These siblings can also quickly transfer colds, infections and other diseases to the baby. The answer to this problem is to keep the baby away from any sick child or from an adult who has a cold, cough, sore throat, or any other disease.

WHAT IS EXPECTED
AT THE AGE OF FOUR MONTHS

Development

Four month olds are more agile than ever before, more active and playful. They may turn their heads towards the source of some noise or voice. They reach for things easily enough, though hesitatingly at times.

They like to put weight on their legs, and they seem to enjoy stiffening up and standing if you hold them by their sides. If they are on their backs, and you pull them by their hands to sit them up, you will see that they will make an effort to help you. In other words, their heads will not lag passively.

At this age, they will do more of their laughing, squealing, looking around, putting things in their mouths, and enjoying all this socializing.

The average weight at this age is fourteen pounds, and the average height is twenty-four and one half inches. This, as said before, varies a lot from baby to baby. You may be surprised to see that your baby is much bigger than the above figures both for height and weight. In this case, he or she is simply bigger than the average and that is okay.

However, if your baby happens to be too heavy for his or her height, there are simple ways to trim the baby down now before it becomes too late. This will be discussed later on.

What will the baby eat?

By now, a few parents want to shift their babies to homogenized milk or two percent skim milk against their doctor's advice. Such a shift is likely to result in an anemic baby. It may also lead to a degree of constipation in some and spitting up of a smelly, cheesy substance every once in a while. Rather than shifting to homogenized milk, it is better and wiser to continue with the breast or formula until the baby is twelve months old.

Some doctors put babies on juices by this age, recommending orange juice alone or in combination with other juices. Use the juices that come in cans, i.e. prepared special for the babies. (If you give the orange juice you drink, the baby may develop some stomachache.) Use a diluted juice at first, one half juice and one half water, and offer three to four ounces a day. After a few weeks, use straight juice without dilution. When starting an infant on juice, look for signs of reaction such as stomachache, loose bowel movements, gas, rash, and ulceration around the anus among others. These symptoms indicate allergy to the orange juice. Most doctors prefer to start orange juice when the baby is six months old and beyond.

Upon seeing the doctor:

At this age, besides checking and discussing the baby, the doctor will give the next DPT shot along with the oral polio.

If the doctor has followed the regimen of giving a DPT shot and oral polio every second month, the baby will have taken the second DPT and oral polio by now.

If the doctor has followed the regimen of giving a DPT shot once a month, all three DPTs will have been given by now, and two oral polios.

Tidbits about common problems:

If the stools become hard and not frequent enough, they can crack the anus, and give lots of problems (see page 81).

Remember to clean the area of the genitalia and around. If your baby is an uncircumcised boy, try to pull the foreskin back as much as you can to help stretch the opening of the prepuce (see page 107).

In girls, make sure to clean the smegma from near the clitoris and lips of the genitalia (see page 102).

If the area around the anus becomes sore and excoriated, use Balneol lotion or zinc oxide ointment (nonprescription) to soothe it and make it less sore. Desitin or A & D ointment may be used afterwards.

WHAT IS EXPECTED
AT THE AGE OF FIVE MONTHS

Development

Everything goes in one direction-their mouths! If they have something in hand and you want to take it away, they will cling to it. They may even be able to transfer something from one hand to the other. They may drive you crazy by scratching (using their hands as rakes) on anything and everything.

If they are interested in something nearby, they will fix their eyes on it for a while. They begin to reach for toys that are of interest but are out of reach. Upon hearing a voice they often turn their heads toward the source of the voice.

They may be able to stay in the sitting position for a second or so, on condition that you separate their legs. They also love to stand up holding on to your hands.

The average weight at this age is fifteen pounds, and the average height is twenty-five inches, bearing in mind some variations from baby to baby.

What will they eat?

Some babies may have been started on solid food, usually consisting of cereal and fruits. At this stage of their growth, they begin to need extra protein beside that of milk. That is why meats and vegetables become important from now on, especially after the age of six months. Start these now if you have not done so already.

A few parents will have tried feeding a taste of mashed potatoes or something similar, and the baby may respond enthusiastically to it. But don't go too far with table foods yet, wait until the age of six months or after.

By this age, you don't have to sterilize the bottles anymore-what a relief. If you drink well water, however, you will have to continue to boil the water until the infant is one year old.

Upon seeing the doctor:

Besides the usual checkup, the doctor will discuss any problems that cross your mind. If the baby proves to be too heavy for his or her height, this is a good time to do something about it. For such a baby, some doctors may suggest reduction of the amount of food intake. Other doctors have their own routines, but all aim towards reducing calorie intake.

The doctor will also do developmental exams, as before, but with more emphasis.

The doctor will explain about feeding instructions in the next six months; discussed will be table food, eggs, blended food and junior food. He or she may also give a special plastic bag to collect the baby's urine, along with an explanation on how to use it.

Tidbits about common problems:

An annoying problem may show up at this age. A number of babies will start waking up at night, thus interrupting the sleep of members of the family. The odds are that the mother or father will respond to the little one's demand by changing the diapers, offering a pacifier or a bottle, or simply lifting the baby up and love him or her. The baby will love all this attention and in the process, a habit may form, and the baby will keep waking up every night demanding some attention.

To stop this habit early, it is better to let the baby cry it out after awakening. Check on the baby only from a distance. It takes an average of three to four nights of this procedure before the habit stops, and the baby will begin to sleep through the night henceforth. The baby must be left crying up to about one hour's time. This treatment may sound cruel, but it is necessary. It is much better to go through it than to have the alternative.

At this age too, babies put anything and everything in their mouths, and will spit up often.

Your baby's gums may become ready for the onset of teething. They may swell slightly, their edge may become round, and the infant may love to chew on your finger. As a matter of fact, it may even hurt a bit, though the bite will be a toothless one (see page 91).

WHAT IS EXPECTED
AT THE AGE OF SIX MONTHS

Development:

By this age they may have a toothy smile which will delight parents to no end. With two teeth showing up, they become the subject of a good many pictures.

They are more active and more agile than ever before. They are noisy, and may say "dada" or "mama" without knowing who either is. They will also enjoy "peek-a-boo."

More than ever before they will reach for toys, hold tight to them, transfer them from hand to hand, and put them in their mouths, if the toys are too big, they will still open their mouths and try to put them in!

Some babies may show signs of being shy with strangers when they see them at first. This will become worse in the coming two to three months.

They are capable of sitting up without support for a short while, and this capacity will improve a great deal in a few weeks. They will also love to stand up holding onto something, but usually they are not able to pull themselves to a standing position as yet.

The average weight is sixteen pounds and the average height is slightly less than twenty-six inches, bearing in mind some variations from baby to baby.

What will they eat?

If you intend to discontinue breast-feeding at this age or after, put the baby on formula (see page 18). Don't start homogenized milk yet, wait until the baby is one year old.

It is time you introduce vegetables and meats at this age if you haven't done so already. Also, you may try introducing some table food; mashed potatoes is a favorite. Over a period of few weeks you may gradually introduce some vegetables from the table, mashing them with a fork or a spoon, along with the mashed potatoes. You may also offer meat cut into tiny pieces, perhaps mixed with the mashed potatoes.

If you offer any table food, make sure it is in the consistency of mashed potatoes, and either give it alone or mixed with the potatoes. Remember that though the baby's stomach is strong enough to digest the food, there are not enough teeth to do any of the grinding or mashing.

By the time babies are seven to eight months old, they usually take one whole meal from the table (either lunch or dinner).

If they gag on the table food, this means they have a sensitive gag reflex to rough food. In this case, don't insist on giving the table food, but keep trying periodically to introduce it. It will take longer for these babies to get used to it.

You may start cautiously feeding them eggs at this age, though some doctors prefer to do that later on. On rare occasions a baby proves to be allergic to them.

Introduce the egg yolk first, and look for signs of trouble such as gas pains, stomachache, vomiting, diarrhea, or rash. If you keep using the egg yolk for three days, and if it seems to agree with the baby, then he or she is not allergic to it. Buy the egg yolk from the grocery store, where it is sold in a jar as so many baby foods are, or use the yolk of a hard boiled egg (see page 29).

Upon seeing the doctor:

Besides the checkup and discussing any problems, the doctor will give the last of the DPT and the oral polio doses. If your doctor has decided on a monthly DPT shot but oral polio every second month, he or she will give the third polio this time.

Some doctors will do urinalysis now; others do it when the baby is eight months old. The urine will have been collected in a special plastic bag that you will have to put in place. Your doctor should have supplied you with it during your visit the month before.

The urine is checked for albumin, sugar, pus cells, red cells, and examined for many other aspects. This is a base study that will be compared to later tests, and it is important to do.

Tidbits about common problems

Many babies will have one or two teeth by now. The gums become round-edged, and may require some massaging or something firm to bite on, such as a teething ring (see page 91).

Some babies don't have their teeth until much later and that is perfectly normal. Many doctors have known of a good many late teethers, even up to the age of thirteen months!

Keep an eye on some yellowing of the skin, especially the tip of the nose and ears. This is an early stage of carotenemia, a condition caused by the child eating too many carrots, beets or certain other foods for the young system to handle (see page 27).

WHAT IS EXPECTED
AT THE AGE OF EIGHT MONTHS

Development

They are becoming more capable by now and they can help themselves to a sitting position. They may even pull themselves to a standing position and be proud of it. It is not unusual to see them taking a few steps by holding onto something like a coffee table.

They have good control with their hands too. They like to play pat-a-cake- and bang objects together. They will use a thumb-finger grasp to pick up tiny things.

Many prefer to scoot, others prefer to crawl, yet some prefer to do neither.

These newly acquired skills will make them aware of their abilities, give them a feeling of participation and accomplishment, and make them enjoy socializing a great deal.

The average weight at this age is eighteen pounds and the average height is twenty-seven inches, allowing for some variations from baby to baby.

What will they eat?

Some babies are ready in a few weeks for a total of two meals from the table, i.e. lunch and dinner. Some are already on such a schedule, yet others cannot because they have a sensitive gag reflex.

Those who gag on table food and cannot take it, may be put on blended food or junior food that you buy from the grocery store. Even so, you should persist in offering table food often enough so that the young one gets used to it.

Most babies, however, will take to the table food, and you will be encouraged to give more and more varieties. They can take just about anything, but you should avoid offering foods that are harsh to digest, such as corn. Corn, large chunks of fruit, and similar foods can be given in mashed forms, but not whole, the way people with teeth can eat them.

Upon seeing the doctor:
Besides checking up the infant and discussing the various aspects of his or her needs and development, the doctor will either do a urinalysis or a blood test. If a blood test is to be done, it is to see if the infant has normal blood, is anemic, or is a borderline anemic.

Blood tests are good to do. Small babies-prematures, twins, babies who have had many infections already, babies who prefer to drink milk all the time, or babies born to a big number of siblings-are more apt to develop anemia (see page 398). The treatment for such things is easy at this age.

Tidbits about common problems:
There will be less drooling by now, and very little spitting up if any at all.

It is better not to use walkers at all. Using a walker will give the baby a sense of mobility, but can also lead to accidents. If you decide to use it anyway, supervise the youngster, and don't let him or her be in it for more than a total of one hour a day. The reason is that bones at this stage are still easily malleable, and being in a walker will put a wide wedge between the young legs. This, in time, is likely to lead to bowing of the legs (a form of pigeon toe).

The baby may still wake up at night and interrupt your rest and sleep. If this has been going on for too long, you may feel as if you have had it by now. To break the habit, (see page 59).

You may buy booties but not the recommended shoes as of yet. More about this point on page 53.

Last but not least don't forget the vitamins!

WHAT IS EXPECTED
AT THE AGE OF TEN MONTHS

Development:

Ten month olds see the parents, and specifically call them mama or dada. They are noisy at times.

They have gone through a stage of being quite shy with unfamiliar people or strangers. This shows up initially when meeting strangers.

Not only do they enjoy pat-a-cake, but they also like to play ball if the ball is rolled slowly toward them or near them.

Some babies are capable of drinking from a cup by this age, but if not, they will soon do so if given the chance to practice.

They are more capable with their fingers and more exacting. They demonstrate neat pincher grasp with thumb and index finger and can easily pick up a raisin. They are also more balanced, and may be able to stand up for a second or two. It is true that babies vary a lot in the timing of these milestones of development, and your baby may be able to walk at the very early age of seven or eight months, or as late as fifteen to sixteen months, but most babies are just able to stand up for one to two seconds by this age.

The average weight at this age is twenty pounds and the average height is twenty-eight inches, give or take a little.

What will they eat?

Most babies by now will have been on table food, if not for two meals a day, then for three. If they have not been taking the kind of breakfast you take, it is time you introduce it to them.

The food will still have to be mashed, because a few front teeth won't be able to chew the food well enough yet. A number of babies will refuse taking a bottle by now, so don't fight it. Offer the formula or juice in a cup. Some babies may not want to take as much formula as you like them to. Remember that a minimum of sixteen ounces (one pint) of milk a day, including that in their cereal, is enough for them. One pint (not a quart) of milk a day has sufficient protein and calcium to fill their demand.

Upon seeing the doctor:
    Apart from checking the baby up and discussing any problems with you, the doctor will do the blood test (see page 398) or TB test (see page 322).

Tidbits about this age:
    As your child stands up more and more firmly, you will see that his or her feet look flat. This flatness is normal now. You don't have to buy shoes at this age unless your toddler is able to walk without help.
    If the baby clings to you excessively, and is quite petrified when being held by strangers, it may mean that he or she is too attached to you, and that you subconsciously encourage this. This extreme condition can lead to a good deal of trouble in later years. School phobias may even start here, as well as other antisocial habits. Try to break this habit now and nip it in its bud. You (and the child) will receive a sweet dividend later on (see page 71).
    To break this habit, you have to leave the baby with other people as long and often as you can. Don't pamper the child too much, and do leave him or her in the care of other people as you go about your errands. Try to lessen his or her tenacious dependency on you as much as possible.
    Many babies show signs of temper tantrums. If this happens, play it cool and act as if nothing is happening. In other words, simply ignore the child. The inability to get attention from you will help the baby wise up and decide that tantrums are not of value.
    Quite often babies prefer to feed themselves by this age. This is a phase too, and it may last for several months. They will insist on picking the food, then throwing it to the floor and looking at the mess beneath. Don't be alarmed about this, since most babies at this age go through it. Let them feed themselves, and you will be surprised to know that they will manage to eat quite enough to satisfy themselves.
    Parents must keep an eye on toddlers at this age since they are more mobile than ever before. This will mean that the chances for accidents will be higher. Their curiosity is fairly high and they may play havoc with the TV or hi-fi knobs; they may even put their fingers

in electric sockets. Watch them carefully and prevent accidents as much as you can (see page 114).

WHAT IS EXPECTED AT THE AGE OF ONE YEAR, HAPPY BIRTHDAY!

Development:

Only a year ago they seemed so tiny, so helpless and so precious. Now they have become tigers and are able to do so much.

Not only can they say "mama" or "dada" and mean it, but they may be able to say one or two other words too, such as "bye," "bird," etc. They are playful, they can go after a ball, and they can easily drink from a cup. In other words, they are less sloppy. If they want something, they will point to it to let you know, and will not cry for it. They can scribble with a pencil or a crayon to some extent. They are neat pinchers.

By now, they can stand up by themselves for a short while, though hesitatingly at times. They can stoop and pick up something from the floor then stand up again. If they are not too cautious, they may be walking well by now. They cannot run well yet, but they can walk slowly and steadily. They have indeed come a long way in only one year.

The average weight at this age is twenty-one and one half pounds and the average height is twenty-nine and one half inches, give or take some.

What will they eat?

They enjoy everything from the table. They don't show much in the way of likes or dislikes, but if they do their wishes should be respected, because they are responding to their bodies' natural demands.

At this age the child can be changed from formula or the breast (if still on the breast) to homogenized milk. If they do not want much milk, that is okay, since one pint of milk a day gives enough calcium and protein. If they take cheese, cottage cheese, buttermilk, or yogurt, these must also be figured in the total milk nourishment.

Upon seeing the doctor
    Other than the usual checkup, the doctor will do the TB tine test. It is a base study for future comparison's sake. It is to see if there has been exposure to the TB germ (see page 322).

Tidbits about this age
    Be careful about the fit and make of shoes. This is important from now up to the age of two years. You may buy your child either:

1. A firm, (not hard nor soft) soled shoe, but it should be high-top, or
2. A soft-soled shoe, but it should be low-top.

    The fit of the shoe is important. It ought to be: one small-finger-breadth wider than the foot, and one index-finger-breadth longer than the foot. By so doing, you will give enough space inside the shoe for the toes to grip and for the foot to grow. If you insist on this fit, you may need only one pair of shoes now, and another one five or six months later.
    Some good makes are Stride Rite, Buster Brown, and Edwards.
    After the age of two years, any make of shoe will do, as long as it fits well.
    It is time to stop use of the pacifier by this age. Simply get rid of it. Your child will miss it and will cry occasionally for it, but in a day or two it will be forgotten.
    Most infants by now will be off the breast feeding, and taking one or two bottles of milk a day. They will usually take the bottle when they wake up and before they go to bed. If yours seems to want the bottle more often, i.e. three to four bottles a day by this age, try to cut down on it; this will prepare the child later on, when you stop the bottle.
    The child is not ready to be toilet-trained yet. It is better to wait until the correct developmental stage (age eighteen months and after).
    Babies at this age are active -walking, exploring- and are proud of themselves. They are likely to lose their balance and fall, or cut themselves or put loose pills in their mouths. The age of accidents

has really begun (see page 114).

WHAT IS EXPECTED
AT THE AGE OF FIFTEEN MONTHS

Development:

By fifteen months they are very active, full of life and vitality, and you are after them constantly. If they walk, they run. If this fast mobility doesn't show by now, it will show up in a month or two from now. They are mastering walking quite well. They can walk backwards too, and are even able to go up steps.

They are able to say a few simple words, which sometimes only the parent can understand. If you ask them where a part of their body is, such as the nose, they may point to it. Some of them may follow one or two commands from you.

They can use their hands well also. They take delight in dumping things e.g. emptying a bottle! If you let them play with blocks, they will try to build a tower of cubes (one block on top of another). If you give them a pencil or crayon, they will scribble with it in a haphazard way.

They may also take delight in taking off their shoes, socks or some other clothing. They can use a spoon, though not in a well-coordinated manner. They may even try to imitate simple housework, such as sweeping or dusting.

The average weight at this age is twenty-three pounds and the average height is about thirty-one inches, give or take a little.

What will they eat?

The majority of infants at this age will have been taking food from the table for some time. A few ones, however, will still only cautiously take table food. These are the ones who have the sensitive gag reflex. They are the ones who could stand the junior food for only the past few months, but by now they have become somewhat able to consume the table food. Be patient if your child is one of them; gradually they are able to take more and more table food, and the process may not be complete until the age of twenty-one months or after!

If your child is still taking the bottle, you may discontinue the morning bottle by now. Offer only one bottle a day, before he or she goes to bed. They can take the milk through the cup, and will not miss the bottle at all.

Upon seeing the doctor:
Other than the usual checkup, the doctor will administer a shot called MMR. This shot will confer immunity against measles, mumps, and rubella (German measles). The immunity will last for life, and about ninety-five to ninety-eight percent of the children who receive it will develop this immunity.

Only ten to fifteen percent of children show a reaction to the MMR. If such reactions show up, they do so about a week after the shot has been given, and will be in the form of some rise in temperature, a runny nose, cough, shiny eyes and may be even some blotchy pink rash. This reaction may take a few days before going away. For the fever give the child an antipyretic such as one baby aspirin or .8 ml of Tylenol drops every four hours.

Some doctors prefer to give the MMR immunization in three separate shots, i.e. measles shot, then mumps shot, then rubella shot at various intervals in between them.

Some tidbits:
Having reached this age, fifteen month olds have become old enough to understand discipline. You cannot let them loose to do whatever they please, otherwise they will hurt themselves. The process of discipline and rule-setting is long and changeable. It all depends on a child's age, temperament, and points of weakness and strength, but every child needs some discipline.

By this age, they are like live wires. They tend to be into everything. They can fall, hit, bite, put their fingers in an electric socket, and do lots of things that you would never have dreamed of before. This intense activity and curiosity will go on and on, month in and month out. Although accidents can happen, most of them are mild and babies will learn through the pain of having them.

You cannot prevent all accidents, but you can prevent a good many. Study the house, and try to eliminate anything that is likely to cause accidents.

Cluttered houses, loose bottles of medicines or chemicals here and there, unattended hot objects (coffee, a pan of boiling water), wide-open staircases, etc., are all frank invitations for accidents. With careful thought you can easily correct many such would-be hazardous situations and prevent the chance for accidents (see page 114).

By this age, one bottle of milk a day, before bedtime, is enough. Stick to this amount.

Temper can fly and your child may take advantage of your tender heart. Remember to ignore all tantrums and the toddler will come out of it in time. This age is tiring but it's lots of fun!

WHAT IS EXPECTED
AT THE AGE OF EIGHTEEN MONTHS

Development:

Eighteen month olds are advancing fast. They can say a number of words, sometimes even combining two words together, such as "bye-bye" or "come here." They may follow two or three directions if they please. They can easily identify parts of their bodies such as the ear or bellybutton. They may even identify a picture of a cat or a dog.

They have good control of their balance by this age and are able to kick a ball and even throw a ball overhand. They can easily take a step or two backwards, and also be able to walk up steps.

They can build a tower of four cubes, one on top of the other and are also good at making messes and scribbling with crayons and pencils, so beware.

They can use the spoon more accurately, and they can help in the house by doing some simple tasks. They are also good at taking off more of their garments! some of them love nudity.

The average weight at this age is twenty-five pounds and the average height is thirty-two inches, give or take a little.

What will they eat?

Stop giving the bottle completely by now. They are too old for it. They will not miss it and it is quite likely they will stop wanting it themselves. Don't make a mistake of giving your child (before bedtime) a bottle of juice instead, it may affect his or her teeth and lead to a good deal of tooth decay. This is also true at any age.

Their mouths are toothy by now, they can take rough foods quite easily. They may eat less than what you expect, but they will be taking enough food for their requirements. Don't worry.

Upon seeing the doctor?

Other than checking the baby and discussing any concerns that you have, the doctor will give DPT booster shot. This shot will give a boost to the effect of the three DPT shots your child had before. If any reaction had developed when the child had the DPT series before, please tell the doctor about it before this booster shot is administered.

The doctor will also give an oral polio booster. The polio booster (Sabin) will boost the effect of the polio series that was given before.

Tidbits:

Most toddlers are developmentally ready to be toilet trained now, not before this age.

If you start the toilet training at this age, there is a reasonable chance for gradual success. Toddlers pass through the stage of awareness of the problem, to the stage of informing the parents, to the stage of successful accomplishment. This may take a variable period from only a few weeks to much longer.

If your baby tends to be chronically constipated, you may want to add roughage to his or her diet (see pages 356 and 357).

Chewable vitamins may be preferred at this age and may be bought without prescription (see page 337).

Parents may start brushing the child's teeth by now if they have not started this earlier. Use soft tooth brush of the appropriate size.

By this age the toddler will need another pair of shoes. Their feet will have started to show an arch. Going barefoot indoors and outdoors as long as practical is good for their feet. Walking on tiptoe will help their development by pulling at the arches of the feet. Therefore, it is good to encourage your child to tiptoe as much as is practical.

If the skin seems too dry, make baths less frequent. You may use Keri lotion after the bath to soften the skin (see page 436).

Keep vigilant about preventing accidents, and read any booklets you can find about that subject. Don't neglect your library for this information.

Toddlers may not need as much sleep at this age as they used to. They may give up a nap, or their naps may become shorter. They may go to bed later, but if you calculate the number of hours of sleep they get, it may amount to about twelve hours, plus or minus two hours. If your child starts waking up at night, do not respond. If your child wants to sleep with you, be firm and take the little one to his or her own bed. This firmness and perseverance in all but the rare case, can correct the problem early enough in the child's life.

WHAT IS EXPECTED
AT THE AGE OF TWENTY-ONE MONTHS

Development:

By now they are beside themselves, excited with new discoveries about what they can do. Quite often they can combine two different words, have a vocabulary of a respectable number of words, but say things that are not intelligible. They follow commands when they wish, usually two out of three times!

They may try to wash and dry their hands, though not as neatly as you like them to. They are able to take their shoes off (if they are not tied), and can play games with others, if they are in the mood.

They are not only good at kicking and throwing a ball, but they enjoy jumping in place too. If they have some blocks to play with, they may build a tower of four to six blocks, one on top of the other.

At this age their scope of activity is expanding, and so is their power to participate and their will to impress you. They like and cherish your admiration, and try their best to attract your attention at times.

The average weight at this age is twenty-six pounds and the average height is thirty-three inches, give or take a little.

How about their eating?

Just about every child at this age will be eating from the table. They may start to have some favorite foods. Try to respect their likes and dislikes to a certain extent, and try to influence their likes by what you offer.

Upon reaching this age, many of them will be less interested in eating. At first you will not notice it that much, but soon this will be obvious and may start to worry you a great deal (see page 332).

Upon seeing the doctor:

Other than checking the child and discussing any possible problems, the doctor will do the TB tine test and the blood test (hemoglobin and/or hematocrit).

The doctor will pay more attention to the child's feet and legs this time than before, and will probably discuss the child's appetite, caring for the teeth, accident prevention, and other subjects of importance at this age.

Tidbits:

If you haven't let your toddler go barefoot often enough, it is time you do. This will help the arches of the feet to a good extent. The child may go barefoot indoors, but may not like it outdoors, especially on the grass. Most of them get used to it after a while, however.

From now on, a good many children want to walk holding the parents' hand. At times the child may sag to the ground for some reason, and the parent will respond by pulling his or her hand reflexly, trying to prevent a fall. If you discover that the child doesn't use that hand afterwards, this often means radial subluxation (see page 526).

At this age, the child's biting, kicking, and hurting others can be fairly bothersome and embarrassing. Discipline is the answer, and you may have to do it in such a way as to hurt the child some. Let the child know you mean business. Repeat it as often as the child keeps the nasty habit. It won't be long before the child finds out that biting is not profitable, and will decide to stop the nasty habit.

A number of children will be scared at night. Some will want a regular bed. Others will want a night light in the room or the door to be slightly open. Many of them are simply scared being in a room that looks so big and formidable. Because of this, a small percentage of them will decide to go to the parent's bed and sleep there. This of course will disrupt privacy and the usual routine of the parents in their bedroom. To stop this before it becomes a bad habit, try to be firm but loving and take the child to his or her room. Don't be too lenient. The youngster will get the message and cooperate. In case yours is one of the diehards who absolutely refuses to go to his or her room, allow the privilege of being in your room for a few nights before taking the child back.

WHAT IS EXPECTED AT THE AGE OF TWO YEARS; HAPPY BIRTHDAY AGAIN!

Development:

By this age two year olds have come a long way in their development, and can do many things, skillfully and well. They are bouncing tigers and are happy with themselves. They can balance on one foot for a second or so. They like to jump in place (and may fall), and they may attempt to pedal a tricycle, even though they may not be able to.

They are more precise with their hands, and if given blocks to play with, they will build a tall tower of seven or eight blocks, one on top of the other. If they have a crayon or pencil in their hands, they can imitate a vertical line. They can wash and dry their hands well. They are better at playing with others, and they may separate from their parents easily but not for long.

Their vocabulary will have expanded by now (though there are extremes: some will say only a few words and some will be able to make sentences). Quite often they are able to use plurals too.

These great strides will give them a feeling of pride and sureness of self, and when this is accompanied by a feeling of curiosity, they will be on the go, exploring everything. It will be tiring just to look at them and think of the energy expended.

The average weight at this age is twenty-seven pounds and the average height is thirty-four inches, give or take a little.

What will they eat?

They can eat any foods, since they now have a mouthful of teeth. Surprisingly though, they prefer to eat very little. Their appetites will have dropped a good deal (there are exceptions of course), and their low food intake may worry you very much.

Some will go for cookies and candies and many parents will keep accomodating. This is unhealthy, not only for the teeth, but more so because the cookies and candies can block the appetite. Thus, the child will end up taking less of the nourishing food, and more of the "empty" calories. By allowing these foods, the parents are cheating their child without knowing it.

Instead, offer sweets only infrequently. This way, cookie-taking becomes neither a "privilege" nor a habit. This is true of all ages.

Upon seeing the doctor:

Besides the checkup, the doctor will discuss the appetite or any problems that cross your mind, and will do a urinalysis or a screening urine culture (see page 413). The odds are that this is the last of this series of checkups at such frequent intervals; many a doctor will see the child once a year from now on. The above frequency of checkups will also vary from doctor to doctor.

Some tidbits:

With only some exceptions, the central theme about this age is that the children don't like to eat much. The appetite drops to a low level, because the rate of growth has slowed down a good deal. This means that their needs for food and calories are such that they don't have to eat like you do, and they may not need three meals a day (see page 332)!

It is time to buy a soft toothbrush, and let them try to brush their teeth with one of the fluoride toothpastes. They may do it clumsily at first, may suck at the toothpaste, but be patient and do help out (see page 93).

You may have quite a time disciplining them. It is not easy, and it may hurt you to do so, but it is for their own good. Don't overdo it, but also don't be too permissive or they will take advantage of you.

You have allowed your child to sleep in your bed because he or she was too scared to be alone in another room, the beginning of a new bad habit might have started. Nip it in its bud; be firm about the child's sleeping in his or her own bedroom. You may read to the child before sleep, but be careful that there are as few distractions as possible, such as loud music, TV or other noises. Give some assurance, ask if he or she wants a door slightly open or some light in the room. The odds are that the child will oblige, and the habit will disappear ......so that a new one can show up!

PHYSICAL DEVELOPMENT OF THE ADOLESCENT MALE

The onset of puberty in boys is quite variable, which can make the "late bloomers" dismayed and disheartened. Some boys may start their adolescent physical changes as early as eleven years of age, while others will not begin to develop until they are fifteen.

Why the variability in age?

There are many factors at play, the most important of which is the genetic. Although poor nourishment, the presence of a chronic disease, or endocrine disease can all play a part, the timing of puberty and the ultimate growth is far more related to heredity and genetics than anything else. Therefore, knowing the age at which puberty began in parents, grandparents, and other members of the family will help a lot in guiding our thinking about the onset of puberty in the offspring, since the ultimate height of the boy is related to the height of the close members in the family.

What changes shall I expect?

The earliest change in the boy is that the testicles will gradually increase in size, and will be slightly sensitive to the touch. The scrotum will also change in texture and will be somewhat reddened. Along with that, or soon after, the penis will increase in length. After some time the penis will increase in width, until it assumes an adult's size.

As these changes take place, pubic hair will also develop. At first it will be thin and sparse, with an occasional dark curly hair, but gradually it will increase in amount and distribution. When the growth in height accelerates, the growth of the pubic hair will accelerate too, soon reaching adult quantity and distribution.

How about axillary (underarm hair) and facial hair?

Usually the axillary (underarm) hair begins to develop about eighteen to twenty-four months after the first sign of the pubic hair. Facial hair follows almost the same pattern. However, the timing of the appearance of the facial and axillary hair is fairly unpredictable, and it often follows the same pattern as that of the father, grandfather, and other males in the family.

How about the voice changes?

Usually the voice change shows up at the peak of the accelerated growth. Because the quality and caliber of the voice are so uncertain, this may be an uncomfortable period for the adolescent boy. After the growth spurt has reached its peak and is leveling off, the boy's voice will usually become stable, deeper, and similar to an adult's.

Along with these changes, usually acne will show up to a various extent. It may be bothersome to many boys if it is severe, and if so, it ought to be controlled by medications or treatments prescribed by a doctor.

How about breast tissue?

In a high percentage of adolescent males, there is some enlargement of one or both breasts. This shows up in the middle of adolescence, and it is usually a result of enlargement of the tissue underneath the nipple. The size can be from that of a hazel nut to that of a walnut, and it can be somewhat tender. Often this lasts for about nine to twelve months. The boy may be embarrassed or worried about it, but an explanation by the doctor will help allay the fears (see page 387).

How about changes in height?

For a late bloomer, the pubertal changes start perhaps at age fourteen-and-a-half to fifteen years. Because he looks so small and because he and his parents become so restlessly anxious about whether or not there is something wrong, a visit to the doctor may prove to be very important. Examination, X-ray for bone age, and some blood tests may be recommended to make sure everything is O.K.

During adolescence, the spurt of growth will accelerate a lot, making the boy outgrow his pants and clothes fairly often. Not only will he raid the refrigerator often, but he will sleep a lot. These two points are physiologic requirements which practically all teenagers experience. As this heightened growth reaches its zenith and beyond, the boy will start to experience wet dreams and have seminal discharges. It would be wise that the father sit down with his pre-teen boy to inform him about what is ahead without embarrassment. This is preferable to the inaccurate and often exaggerated information from his friends and peers.

Each boy has his own way of developing; therefore, if your boy develops somewhat differently from the above, don't worry or panic unless this deviation is very obvious. In that case consult with your doctor.

PHYSICAL DEVELOPMENT OF THE ADOLESCENT FEMALE

With the onset of puberty, a good many physical changes will become obvious, including the start of the monthly period. As is the case in boys, the physical changes come more or less in a specific order, until the girl changes to have the appearance of an adult female.

The onset and the sequence of these changes, however, are fairly variable from one girl to another.

How do the changes vary?

Although most girls start their puberty at or around the age of eleven years, a few may start a year or two earlier or later. The late bloomers will worry because they see themselves far behind their friends in the level of their development; they may not start their puberty until the age of fourteen to fourteen-and-a-half years.

What kind of changes shall we expect?

The development of the breasts is usually the first sign of puberty, in the form of visible elevation of the area of the nipple and tissues underneath. It may show up in one breast at first, to be followed by the other within a few months. Quite often, however, it seems to involve both breasts at the same time.

Over a period of many months, the breast tissue will slowly become more visible, round, and elevated, to finally assume the adult's shape and size.

The young girl may be embarrassed about this new development, in spite of the fact that she has full knowledge about it through her mother's talk, friends' confidentiality, reading, etc.

It is interesting to note that it takes an average of four years for the breasts to develop completely and to assume their adult size and shape.

Is breast development always the first visible sign of puberty?

In about one out of five girls, rather than budding of the breasts, the appearance of pubic hair will be the first sign of the onset of puberty.

However, even the majority of girls-whose first sign of puberty is budding of the breasts-experience some growth of fine pubic hair at the same time. The hair will accelerate in its growth, and in about five to six months it will become coarse and curly, and will expand in its distribution. The pubic hair won't assume the adult's quantity and distribution until almost three years later.

Axillary (underarm) hair is fairly variable in its onset. When it is seen, it will mean that puberty is proceeding normally.

How about growth in height?

As pubertal changes take place, there will be a steady acceleration in growth. The velocity of height growth will be at its peak within a year or so from the onset of puberty. The growth will then continue at a slower rate for two to three years, after which it will slow down even more until adult height is attained.

How about menses?

Menses usually starts about two years and three months from the time the breasts bud, give or take a few months. This varies from one girl to another. Menses usually shows up after the velocity in the rate of growth has been reached. Once the girl has started her period, the rate of her growth in height will not be as fast as it was before (see page 67).

Are there any other changes?

Yes, there are changes in the shape and proportions of the external and internal parts of the genitalia (mainly the latter).

Acne may be bothersome and worrisome to some girls, and if it goes beyond certain limits it ought to be controlled by medication.

Changes in the size of the hips are some of the earliest manifestations associated with puberty; they are not that noticeable by most people.

As mentioned in the section about boys, each child has a unique way of developing, so if your girl develops slightly differently from the way described above, don't panic unless this deviation is very obvious. In that case, have your doctor check.

MENSTRUATION

Menstruation is caused by delicate but precise interaction of the hormones of the pituitary gland (which lies under the brain) with those of the ovaries. This interaction is also affected by conditions of other body organs, including the brain and adrenal glands.

The deliberate variation in the levels of these different hormones will produce certain changes in the wall of the womb (uterus) leading to the monthly period, along with changes in the ovaries to lead to the release of an egg (ovum). However many of the monthly periods of the first year or two are irregular and they are often not associated with release of an ovum.

Why are early periods irregular?

This is a form of adjustment of the body to the new experience, and may happen not only during the first year of menstruation, but also to some extent during the second year.

The flow might be heavy and it may continue for several days, or it might be scanty and short-lasting. The girl may start her first period or two, to be followed by an interval of months before another period shows up.

However, after the first year of menstruation, if more than six months pass by without a period showing up, a visit to the doctor is advised. In such cases, the girl will be examined in an attempt to look for a cause, and a gynecologist might need to be consulted.

Can the early periods be regular too?

While the majority of girls have irregular periods during the first year of their menstruation, some experience good regularity.

This is true of the intervals in between, the duration of the menses and the amount of the flow.

When do girls start their periods?

This varies greatly. Most girls will have started menstruating between the ages of eleven and sixteen years. It is said that only one out of one hundred girls will start her period before the age of eleven years or after the age of sixteen years. The majority of girls will experience their first menses at the age of thirteen, plus or minus one year. It is important to know that if the mother started her monthly periods early or late, her daughter usually follows suit.

What if the girl hasn't started?

If the girl reaches the age of sixteen years and hasn't started her monthly period at all, she should consult the gynecologist. This is true whether or not the girl has developed the secondary sexual characteristics (budding of the breasts, pubic hair, etc.).

How about the discomfort and the abdominal cramps?

The presence and severity of such cramps are variable from one girl to another. Medications such as Motrin (prescription) are readily available and quite successful. During the first year or two of having the monthly periods, when the menstruation is often not associated with the release of an ovum (called anovulatory cycle), there are usually no concomitant pains. Later on, and especially after the second year of having monthly periods, the menstruation becomes associated with release of an ovum (ovulatory cycle), and the cramps or pains begin.

Shall I consult a doctor if her periods have become irregular?

The monthly period is a mirror of the good function of certain hormones and the organs involved. Once the menstruation becomes regular, it usually continues to do so unless there is something wrong.

Therefore, if in such cases the period is missed, there may be a chance for pregnancy or something else. If there is continuous or unusually heavy bleeding, too much irregularity, too much pain, etc., call the doctor. A visit to the gynecologist may become necessary.

Pelvic exam, tests, etc. may be needed.

CHECKUPS

The schools will send you forms for checkups, and camps and sports teams will also require them. Sometimes it is quite confusing as to how many checkups the poor child has to go through.

Are the checkups really necessary?

A checkup is a nice investment in health. It is true that you can forget about checkups for several years, but that is taking a gamble on your child's health.

During a checkup, the height, weight, physical appearance, and all the systems are examined, and any special problems are discussed. Many a case of a hernia, enlarged spleen, or fluid in the ear can be detected as well as trouble with the spine, legs, feet, eyes, etc. if these checkups are done. If problems are detected early, they can easily be treated, before any major consequences have time to develop.

How often does the child have to have a checkup?

Usually once a year, except in case of babies. There are some convenient ways to remember these checkups. Some parents time them to occur around the child's birthday. Others wait until the school sends a notice, or until the child is ready to go to camp (in such cases, it is better to have one checkup done both for camp and school). Other parents prefer having two or three children checked up at the same time. It is preferable, from a physician's point of view, to do the checkup during spring or summer, when there is less pressure on the child's time and less infection going around.

Are any special tests done with the checkup?

Most doctors will do the following tests along with the checkup:

1. Hemoglobin and/or hematocrit test to see if the child has anemia. Strangely enough, a pediatrician detects four or five cases a year through this routine (see page 398). The number is higher in underpriviledged areas.

2. Urinalysis, to examine for albumin, sugar, pH, specific gravity, pus cells, red blood cells, etc. When the urine shows pus cells, a complete urine culture has to be done to prove the presence of infection. A screening urine culture is done on females. On the average, about five cases of urinary tract infection a year are detected, many without any symptoms (see page 413).
3. TB tine test, to see if the child has converted from having no reaction to the TB test, to having a positive reaction (see page 322).

How about shots?

Of course if the child needs DPT booster, DT booster, Polio booster, measles, mumps, or rubella vaccine, he or she will be given accordingly.

How about smallpox vaccination?

This is not given anymore, since it is said that no countries in the world harbor smallpox anymore. Only if the family is traveling to countries where sanitation is quite poor do they elect to have the smallpox vaccination.

I have too many children and I hate to have so many checkups:

Families with a big number of children will find it expensive for all the children to have regular checkups every year. For these, however, you can divide the number of children into two groups each of which has a checkup during alternating years. Very large families (nine to ten children) may find it necessary to subdivide the children into three annually alternating groups.

The school wants a checkup, but the child had one sometime ago:

If the child was checked recently (within a few months), there will be no need for another checkup.

But if the child has not had his or her checkup for about a year, then another checkup will have to be done. You can never tell whether some recent problems have developed (such as a hernia) in the meantime, unless you do the checkup again.

SCHOOL PHOBIA

The child seems to be scared, and tries to find excuses for not going to school. He or she may succumb to gentle encouragement and go to school. But next morning the whole bothersome show will repeat itself.

This kind of scene may show in the first week or so of the school year, but more likely it comes few weeks afterwards. It may persist for as long as two months or even longer. Such school phobia can be quite severe at times, and may make you very concerned and perplexed.

How severe can it be?

Severe ones may start earlier than usual, take longer to go away, and have more menacing daily scenes. In such cases the child may act as if he or she is expecting trouble even before breakfast. The child is uneasy and may either prolong or delay eating breakfast. When the school bus arrives, the child will "freeze," so to speak, and will refuse, fight, cry, and use whatever means at hand to convince the parents to let him or her be at home rather than go to school. Some of them cling to mother tenaciously, others act nauseated, shake, sweat, or even vomit once or twice, leaving parents without any choice but to agree to the demands.

When it is Saturday or Sunday, and there is no school to go to, the rascal seems to be chipper and in tiptop condition!

When does school phobia usually show up?

Most school phobias are mild, they start almost imperceptibly in the first grade, become obvious in the second and third grades, and become almost imperceptible again in the fourth grade.

If the child has a more advanced case, he or she may start in the kindergarten if not even earlier, and may continue up to almost the fifth grade!

Why do some children have school phobia?

It usually shows up in children with an abnormally strong bond to the mother. Often such a bond starts in the first year or two of the child's life, when he or she clings to the mother too much and gets loving response. School means mother-child separation, and the consequent fear of the unknown. This fear will make the child mad at the world.

What do you do for it?

If we see a case where mother-child interdependence is potentially troublesome (no matter how early in the game), we usually try to explain to the mother about the future possibility of school phobia. Even if the child is as young as two to three years old, we may tell the mother to ease off and not overindulge or overprotect the child, but rather allow freedom, and exposure to other people as much and as long as possible, be it friends, relatives, or babysitters and encourage enrollment in nursery school. This preventive piece of work has led to good results.

Many times we see a child who is already seven or eight years old having a bad case of the phobia. For such a child, we suggest the parents be cruel, and firmly insist that he or she goes to school. They should also encourage the child to make friends in the school and even invite some of them to come home and play.

Such treatment usually succeeds in most, but it takes several weeks of morning scenes until the situation reaches normalcy.

In all cases of school phobia it is best to consult the doctor. In severe cases, however, the child may even need psychotherapy. Tranquilizers and other drugs are to be avoided; they are only very rarely needed in the treatment of phobias. It is difficult to be cruel and "force" a scared child to go to school. It is difficult to insist that a shaky child face a strange world. But unfortunately it is the best way to treat most school phobias, and most of them respond to it in the long run.

CHAPTER FOUR

DISEASES PECULIAR TO BABIES AND YOUNG CHILDREN

milk allergy
baby's stuffy runny nose
baby's earache
baby's cough and chest trouble
projectile vomiting
the cracked anus
sternomastoid mass
ammoniacal diaper rash
pin-hole meatus in the male
labial adhesions in the female
spitting up
thumbsucking or pacifier
cradle cap
tooth eruption and teething
care of the teeth
my baby's eye keeps watering
tongue-tie
thrush
constipation in babies
diaper rash
jaundice
a clean-up job
to circumcise or not
the sore bottom
umbilical hernia
bruises
accidents and their prevention in the very young
ABC's of child safety
accidental poisoning
contusions
cuts and lacerations

MILK ALLERGY

Although only a few weeks old, your baby may develop gas pains, a gurgling stomach, some passing of gas, and intermittent general discomfort. The story may repeat itself almost every day. The baby's bowel movements may be affected too, often appearing soft or even watery.

In more severe cases there may be diarrhea of various degrees, even with mucus or (rarely) blood. Spitting up and occasional vomiting can occur. The baby's pains cause frequent, intermittent discomfort and fretfulness.

<ins>Are these all the symptoms of milk allergy?</ins>

No, not necessarily. In addition to the above, milk allergy can often affect the respiratory tract. Some babies will come down with runny noses, will cough on and off, and will seem to have colds all the time. Visits to the doctor become frequent, and medicines become prescribed fairly often. Although wheezing is not that common with milk allergy, it may occur in more advanced cases.

<ins>How soon can milk allergy be discovered?</ins>

Milk allergy and its early symptoms may show up in the first few weeks of life in some cases, earlier in severe cases, and much later in mild cases. The symptoms are subtle; therefore only after a number of visits to the doctor does the suspicion of milk allergy arise, until finally a trial of a new kind of milk is made.

<ins>Does milk allergy show up in breast-fed babies?</ins>

Breast-feeding is one of the best ways to avoid having trouble with milk allergy. It is very rare that a baby has allergy to the breast milk. If breast-feeding is the means of nourishing, and if your baby still develops stomach or respiratory trouble, the chances are high that this trouble is caused by something other than allergy.

Milk allergy is mostly due to sensitivities to the protein of cow's milk, i.e. the milk designed by nature for nonhuman species. Fortunately most children are not allergic to cow's milk or the formulas, which are modifications of cow's milk. However, be aware of the symptoms, just in case.

If the baby is on the breast, what substitute milk may I use?

If you and the baby are happy with breast-feeding but you must be away from the baby for a while, you may use substitute feeding. If you desire, you may pump the breast milk in a sterile bottle and keep the bottle in the refrigerator, for later use. If this is too much trouble, you may offer, instead, a bottle of formula to substitute for one or two breast-feedings. Formulas like Similac, Enfamil, SMA and others may be used.

What shall I use if my baby is allergic to the milk?

Soybean formulas are fairly good, and may be used on a trial basis whenever milk allergy is suspected. In these formulas, the protein of cow's milk is substituted with soybean protein. The nourishment is good, and if the baby was allergic to the previous formulas, the symptoms will disappear when he or she is put on soybean formulas, usually within two to three weeks' time. Good examples of soybean formulas are: ProSobee, Isomil, Soyalac, and Nursoy. Though these are all soybean formulas, the quantity of their different components vary among them.

Goat's milk formulas and meat-base formulas are not as desirable, and should only be used in special circumstances. Your doctor will explain the situation should it arise.

How long shall I use the anti-allergenic formula?

If your baby is indeed allergic to cow's milk or regular formula, but proves to be doing well with anti-allergenic formula, keep using the latter for quite some time. Some babies may not "outgrow" their milk allergy for a long time, perhaps two years or more.

For a baby on anti-allergenic milk, it is wise to try regular formula for three to four days every two to three months to see if the baby has outgrown the milk allergy. While doing so, look to see if the allergy symptoms show up again. If so, go back to the anti-allergenic formula. You may repeat this procedure every two to three months, until a time comes when the regular formula does not bring out the symptoms of milk allergy anymore. By then, chances are he or she has outgrown the milk allergy. Remember though, some seem to be over their allergy to milk for years but show those symtoms again later in life.

Will some children be always allergic to milk?

A high percentage of children with milk allergy will "outgrow" their allergy by the age of twelve to twenty-four months. The more severe cases will have various degrees of sensitivity to dairy products, especially milk, and may take much longer to "outgrow" this tendency. On rare occasions, a child may continue to be allergic to milk for almost a whole lifetime. Understand that such persons will avoid taking milk or dairy products, and must not be pushed into it, otherwise some problems might arise.

BABY'S STUFFY RUNNY NOSE

The cold season may be upon you, and your baby hasn't gone beyond a few weeks of age. Anxious brothers, sisters and others who love to handle the baby may happen to have common cold.

Your baby is likely to pick up the cold and start having stuffiness in his or her nose, and some degree of trouble breathing. Of course, a stuffy nose can come from other conditions too, notably allergy to milk.

Babies don't learn to breathe through their mouths until they are a few months old. Therefore, a stuffy nose can cause some difficulty in breathing for quite some time in a baby's life.

Can I use nose drops to open the nostrils?

In a small baby, medicinal nose drops such as Neosynephrine should be avoided if at all possible. The reason is that upon using it, the baby may soon develop what is called the "rebound phenomenon", a troublesome condition that is more likely to show in a small baby. In such cases, the nose becomes more stuffy after the nose drops have been used for a short while, i.e. the nose drops cause the stuffiness.

Instead, use salt-water, or saline, nose drops. They will only wash away the mucus from the baby's nasal passages and will not affect the lining of those passages, as Neosynephrine or similar drops do.

The way to fix the saline drops is quite simple: Add 1/4 teaspoon of regular table salt to one cup of water. Mix and it will be ready to use. The usual dose is four to five drops in each nostril every three hours or so, as needed.

Don't use decongestants or antihistamines in very small babies before consulting with the doctor.

Baby's earache

The baby may scream bloody murder, hour upon hour, and may truly drive you bananas. A few months old baby will not say "my ear hurts," nor even pull at the ear, for that matter. There may not be any fever or other symptoms of significance.

Out of desperation, you take the baby to the doctor, suspecting something terrible taking place. The doctor will determine if the crying is due to an ear infection and will tell you so. In rare cases, however, the baby fusses only a little or not at all, yet ear infection will be discovered accidentally during a regular checkup!

Although there may be no symptoms other than constant crying, many babies may in addition have symptoms of colds, have a cough, perhaps feel slightly warm to the touch, and refuse to eat as much.

<u>Why are you telling us all this?</u>

For one thing, to make you alert to the fact that ear infections in babies are not rare. But more importantly, many mothers often think that the baby is crying mainly because of teething. They patiently tolerate the screaming and crying, and meanwhile lose precious time. If not treated in time, the infected middle ear will bulge with pus, and the pus may come under pressure and lead to a rupture of the eardrum. If this happens, there will be a constant pussy drainage from the ear canal, sometimes profuse. It is much better to treat ear infections early with antibiotics. A ruptured eardrum from infection of the middle ear will heal, but not that well, because a "thin" scar will develop at the spot of the rupture. A number of scars in the eardrum can have cumulative effect and can affect the hearing.

The moral to all this:
If the baby screams constantly, it is not because of teething, he or she may be having a severe earache. If the baby has a cold for a few days, is fussy, and starts to cry excessively, make sure to consult with the doctor.

BABY'S COUGHS AND CHEST TROUBLE

Your baby is a few weeks old, and has had a cold for only a few days. The cough hasn't seemed too bad, with only an occasional hack. You use the salt water nose drops, the humidifier (see page 290), and perhaps a decongestant (see page 305), yet the cough continues.

All of a sudden the baby is much worse. The cough is tighter and deeper, and breathing is difficult, with some huffing and puffing. The color of the baby's face becomes slightly gray, and he or she is not interested in the surrounding or in taking the breast or bottle. His or her temperature may either have gone up or remained normal. Chest and abdomen continue to heave with breathing which seems to you to be quite labored.

You know deep in your heart that by now there is more trouble than usual. Being an observant parent, you make an arrangement with your doctor right away. After checking your baby up, the doctor may discover a bronchiolitis or possibly pneumonia.

Babies' lungs and bronchial tubes are not as strong as ours, and complications of colds can lead to trouble. Trouble like bronchiolitis, pneumonitis, severe croup, pneumonias and other major respiratory conditions ought to be treated promptly and energetically.

Are you trying to scare me?
Not at all. There are troublesome conditions that can affect the baby's lungs, and that you should be on the alert. Make an appointment to take your baby to the doctor if:

1. the baby has a sudden, frequent hacky cough that goes on and on,
2. there is croupy breathing (see page 313),
3. there is difficulty taking a breath in and out, and the lower part

of the chest moves in and out with the breathing,
4. the color of the baby is gray or dusky.

Whether, in addition, fever is present or not doesn't make a bit of difference; the criteria above ought to be your guideline. As usual, with early management, many a complication can be prevented-your baby will suffer less and you will not go through as much.

BABY WITH A SPECIAL KIND OF VOMITING: PYLORIC STENOSIS
Projectile vomiting

Projectile vomiting is a condition that occurs when the vomited material shoots out one or even two feet from the baby, quite forcefully. It usually starts around the age of three weeks, and it will persist and even increase in frequency, to two or three times a day or more. Everything in the tummy seems to shoot out. There will be no fever and no other troubles, but the baby becomes hungry and demands the breast or the bottle more often. The baby's stools become drier and harder, yet there are no gas pains.

If there is no letup after a few days, you take the baby to the doctor, who diagnoses it as "pyloric stenosis."

What is that?

In pyloric stenosis, a lump develops at the lower end of the stomach. The lump becomes as big as or bigger than an olive. In many cases this lump can be felt, usually above the belly button and slightly to the right. Your doctor may stoop, looking intently at the belly of the baby, who is placed on his or her back in the nude with a bottle in mouth. Your doctor may show you how to spot some slow waves on the baby's belly, one coming after the other in a gentle manner, moving from the left side of the stomach to the right. Those waves show up at the lower margin of the chest on the left, then move towards the umbilicus.

What can I do about it?

Such cases belong to a surgeon. The small olive-sized lump has to be cut in half, because it has been partially blocking the flow of food from the baby's stomach to the intestine.

It is not a serious operation and most babies will be back home after a short hospital stay.

Suppose we don't operate?

The baby may starve to death. The more you wait the more the chance the baby's condition will deteriorate, and an emaciated baby will be more difficult to treat, because the baby will have to build up before the operation, and maintain a good condition in the days to follow.

So don't wait too long if there is projectile vomiting, even if it proves to be caused by conditions other than pyloric stenosis.

THE CASE OF THE CRACKED "ANUS"
Fissure in ano

Bowel movements cause a remarkable degree of pain and discomfort. The baby wants to "hold its bowel movement in," but of course will have to let go, along with a loud shrieking cry that will continue for a short while after.

You notice a bright red line of blood on the surface of the stool. It looks like fresh blood to you, not dark and digested. Sometimes the blood comes at the end of the bowel movement, or may dribble a drop or two after the movement has passed.

The doctor says this is "Fissure in ano"

What this means is that the baby has developed a crack in the anus (many people refer to the anus as the rectum). This crack or fissure is a result of a hard, wide, constipated stool that stretches the anus beyond its limits of stretchability. As a result, the anus gives in and develops a crack. The crack becomes stretched with each subsequent movement, causing all that crying. The blood comes from this crack, which acts like an opened wound whose tiny blood vessels have been "busted."

How are you going to treat it?

Fortunately, practically all such cases heal with simple treatment. The stool must be made loose, so softeners such as Milkinol (nonprescription), will usually suffice. This ought to be used consistently for a prolonged period of about two months.

To treat the fissure itself, a local anesthetic such as Nupercaine (nonprescription) is quite adequate, and should be applied to the fissure before the baby indicates a need for a movement. This is usually necessary for about two weeks.

It might help promote the process of healing to put the baby in hot sitz baths, two to three times a day for four to five days.

Will the fissure come back?

It all depends on whether your baby is going to have a hard wide stool that may crack the anus again. So, you should monitor bowel movements and try to keep them on the soft side.

By the way, many times a small skin tag will show up at the anus; it is called sentinel pile. You don't have to remove it or do anything about it.

STERNOMASTOID MASS, OR WRY NECK WITH A LUMP IN THE MIDDLE

Fortunately this is not too common a condition. A baby who is two to three weeks old and beyond may start developing a lump on the neck. The lump may gradually become as big as a walnut, and hard to the touch; what we call "rubbery firm consistency." It is not painful and it doesn't seem to bother the baby at all. Yet, the baby will gradually hold the head more and more toward the side of the lump, and will have more difficulty turning his head to the other side.

If it doesn't bother the baby why should I then bother about it?

If you ignore the condition, and the baby keeps holding the head towards one side, then a "wry neck" effect will develop. The face will gradually shape itself to the new position in such cases; thus, it will gradually become asymmetrical or lopsided. In some extreme cases the baby will not be able to move his or her head freely upon growing up, thus leading to psychological aftermaths.

How can I discover it?

Simple; put your palm below the upper part of the back, lift the back a little, and let the baby's head drop slightly. Look for those lumps at either side of the neck, i.e. in the muscle that extends from the center of the neck at the collarbone up to behind the ear. If there is a lump, it will stand out prominently. Feel it and make sure it is there. This condition has the fanciful name of sternomastoid mass.

Can anything be done about it?

When the diagnosis is confirmed, and if your baby is still a few weeks old, you stand a good chance to effect a complete recovery. Your doctor may tell you that you have to massage the lump three or four times a day, ten to fifteen minutes each time. He may also tell you to help turn the head of the baby to the other side, and even to let the child sleep on that side. The twisting of the neck is the troublesome complication here, so it is best to help prevent it.

It takes a few weeks before the lump "melts away" and disappears, but the wry, or twisted neck may linger and it may take much longer before it is gone.

The older the baby at the time treatment begins, the more difficult and even the more prolonged the treatment will be. In some "late" cases, even an extensive surgery in the neck, followed by orthopedic management, may become necessary.

THE TIP OF THE BABY'S PENIS AND AMMONIACAL DIAPER RASH

Be they circumcised or not, some baby boys can develop some problems. If a diaper rash develops, especially if it starts smelling of ammonia and even burns your eyes with the smell, then a tender spot like the tip of the penis is likely to be affected.

If the boy has not been circumcised, the tip of the foreskin may become red, slightly swollen, and even ulcerated to some degree. The baby will try to protect the sore area. If the baby is circumcised, the area where the urine comes from can become red, slightly swollen, and ulcerated somewhat, i.e. as if the area is being "chewed up."

Naturally with the ammoniacal diaper rash, the bottom may look "scalded," red, and sore. But this is not always necessarily so, and trouble with the tip of the penis may be the earliest sign of ammoniacal diaper rash (see page 101).

Another problem with baby's penis is pin-hole meatus

This is a fairly common condition, and all male babies ought to be checked for it. See if the hole that the urine comes from is tiny. If it is tiny, it may be so tiny that it may look like a pin hole. Most doctors look for such a thing as a matter of routine.

Such a condition can lead to obstruction to the flow of urine, and the urine will back up. In doing so, trouble with the bladder or kidneys may lie ahead; and a great deal of damage may result. If this pin-hole meatus is fixed, then you will have saved yourself all the possible troublesome consequences.

What can be done about it?

A small operation is needed to enlarge the hole to the normal size. A surgeon or urosurgeon is usually consulted, and the matter is usually handled in the office or the outpatient department of the hospital.

"LABIAL ADHESIONS"

The female baby of course cannot escape some possible minor problems with her genitals either. Labial adhesions are a common problem and should be watched for.

In some baby girls, the two sides of the female genitalia seem to become glued together; as a matter of fact, in some cases nothing can be seen except a tiny hole where the urine pours through.

Strangely enough, most mothers skip noticing such an obvious thing, and it is usually detected by the doctor during the usual checkup of the baby.

Can it cause any trouble?

Not that much, yet it is an abnormal situation, and these adhesions ought to be broken up. This is done by the doctor in his or her office. Sometimes a special ointment has to be used. The adhesions are nothing but a very thin membrane that glues the two sides of the female genitalia together.

What will you do?

Almost all such cases can be dealt with in the office. The mother will stand by and hold the baby's bent legs apart. With one quick jerk using an "ear-speculum", the adhesions are easily broken by the doctor. The baby will jump in a startle but will hardly cry, and a normal external female genitalia will appear.

A small "raw" area will be left at the labia and the parent is to use Vaseline on that area once or twice a day for about a week. Some doctors may prefer applying special female hormone ointment to the area.

Can this come back?

Yes it can, and the doctor will have to take a look at the area whenever checking the baby. Parents should look for it too.

Remember, this condition is less likely to show up if you put Vaseline on that area after the membrane is opened. In case this condition comes back, using the hormone ointment is more likely to do a good preventive job.

SPITTING UP

Spitting up is very common. Will be upsetting to you for sure, and the infant may start to smell of sour milk, yet the doctor seems to be calm and unconcerned. This is because it shows up often, and in most cases the infant proves to be perfectly normal. The spitting up varies in amount, and doesn't follow any special pattern. It usually increases in frequency and amount around the age of four to five months, when it reaches its zenith. After that, it decreases slowly and almost imperceptibly until the infant reaches the age of eight to nine months, when you will hardly notice it, and you will almost forget about it.

Why not be concerned about it?

Most babies keep on gaining in weight and height as other infants their age do and though they seem to mess up everything around them, the amount coming out is usually not that much.

Can I help?

Try the following suggestions:

1. It is worth experimenting by putting the baby in an infant seat after mealtime, even to sleep in. This may reduce the degree of spitting up.
2. After feeding a solid meal, don't give more than two ounces of milk to wash it down with.
3. Occasionally, some doctors use 1% or 2% skim milk in older babies. Though this is not recommended, you may give it a try for a few days, and if it works keep using the skim milk. If it does not work, go back to the previous formula.
4. Patience, please; it is a virtue.

THUMB-SUCKING OR A PACIFIER

They may look cute with thumb in mouth. They may suck at it vigorously, especially when tired. They may perpetually suck at it whenever bored, using the thumb as a means of comfort.

Many babies start this habit during the first few weeks of life, others at a later age; when they discover their thumb, they try to satisfy their sucking urge. But if this continues for some weeks, it will become a habit. The habit then continues until the child is about three to four years old or beyond.

The frequency and intensity of sucking the thumb varies from baby to baby. Vigorous thumb-suckers (babies or toddlers) are likely to develop some calluses on their thumbs. Fortunately the majority of children are not that vigorous thumb-suckers, and they are satisfied with doing it only occasionally, mainly upon going to bed. Such a mild degree of thumb-sucking can be tolerated since chances are high that they will forget about this habit when they are one to three years old if not younger.

Is vigorous thumb-sucking bad?

A baby or child who vigorously thumb-sucks can develop excoriation, infection, and/or calluses on the poor thumb. Many times the callus becomes fissured, thus making it painful to suck the thumb at night. The latter will then interfere with the sleep.

What is more bothersome is that the teeth will mold themselves to accommodate the thumb or fingers that are so often inside. The upper front teeth will protrude forward, and the lower front teeth in some children will go backward for the same reason. Children who use fingers other than the thumb may end up with a fairly advanced degree of teeth misalignment.

Vigorous thumb-suckers are overly stuck on this habit. Because of that, chances are that they may continue to suck their thumbs beyond the usual period when thumb-sucking is stopped by other children (two to three years). In such cases, the other structures in the mouth often become affected and malocclusion shows up. Although malocclusion of the teeth is not always a result of thumb-sucking, if it does occur it will require treatment by an orthodontist later on.

The vigorous thumb-suckers form a very small percentage of all thumb-suckers. They are more likely to continue to suck their thumb until they are in school, and some rare ones until adolescence!

How can we stop this habit?

A good many thumb-suckers will stop this habit by the age of twelve to eighteen months, by themselves. These usually are the mild cases. Hardier ones will continue the habit through the second and third year. By then it is better to try to stop the habit, though the child will resist your attempts.

"Thum" is a mildly bitter medicine that contains some spicy material. If it is used to stop thumb-sucking, put it on the thumb and fingers three to four times a day at first, then twice a day. Most children don't like the material, and when first applied they may cry every time they put their thumb in their mouth. They will have restless nights for the first three or four nights. You better make sure to use the stuff during daytime too, so that they will not suck their thumbs during daytime. A course of a few weeks of such use is needed.

What if it doesn't work?

A number of children will not respond to the above attempts. A few children may even like the taste of "Thum!" It is still best to be persistent. Sometimes using mittens at night will work, but the child has to be willing to cooperate. This may be more successful when the child is of school age.

If the child is a vigorous thumb-sucker, he or she will continue the habit until becoming too embarrassed in school to suck the thumb; suddenly there will be cooperation.

How about prevention?

Now you are talking. Most cases of thumb-sucking start very early during infancy. If babies have something in their mouths, they are satisfied.

If, as soon as they seem to discover a thumb, parents offer a pacifier instead, they will have completely prevented thumb-sucking. It is rare in our office to see a baby or small child who sucks his or her thumb.

Not all babies will accept and take to pacifiers, but the parents can persist. If babies do not take to one kind of pacifier, parents may try a different one, whether it's the regular or the "Nuk" type. The "Nuk" pacifier is preferred because its shape is such that it may aid in the development of bony structures around the mouth. However not all babies will accept it.

When the parents succeed with the pacifier, the baby may be free to use it until the age of about twelve months. Upon reaching this age, not only may the baby not be interested in a pacifier, but about three days after you throw the pacifier away or make it unavailable, he or she will not miss it at all.

CRADLE CAP (SEBORRHEA CAPITIS)

It is fairly common, mainly in babies. More commonly seen when the baby is two months old or about, and may progress to be a thick, greasy-looking layer covering the head. Quite often it covers much of the scalp, but more so only the top of the head. It can be either the dry type or the soft-and-greasy type. The latter you can spoon out with your fingernails. It is unsightly and bothers the loving parents a great deal.

What is it?

Cradle cap consists of an oily substance secreted by the scalp of the baby, usually becoming mixed with shedded scalp cells. It may be in the form of a thin layer, but if left unattended it may become ugly and fairly thick. The top of the head is its favorite area, though it may be seen in other areas of the scalp too.

In many cases you will see some shiny rash on the cheeks or even on the forehead.

Why the rash?

The rash is caused by the same phenomenon. It is called seborrheic rash, and individuals who get it often inherit this tendency from their parents or grandparents (see page 90).

The rash looks shiny, slightly greasy, pale pink, and occurs in a few tiny spots, mainly on the cheeks and forehead. You may see it behind the ears too. In more severe cases, the whole cheek may be covered with the rash, and when extensive, the armpits, elbows, groins, and other creases of the body become affected.

Shall I use baby oil for it?

No, it is better not to. Baby oil may make the cradle cap worse. You can use baby oil to soften the dry type of cradle cap. Most cases of cradle cap, however, are the greasy, moist ones. Even if you use baby oil, this will only prepare the area for treatment.

How shall I treat it, then?

If the cradle cap is mild and in the form of a thin layer, you may use special shampoos that can be of much help. Sebulex shampoo is good. It will "melt away" this form of cradle cap. However, if the cradle cap is in the form of a thick layer, such shampooing will be inadequate.

Thick cradle-cap may have to be spooned out with your fingernail. It is a tedious process and it may take half an hour or so for the whole head. The thick but soft cradle cap will come out in chunks, without hurting the baby, and the hair of the scalp will remain where it is. You can go in this manner for the whole scalp, not sparing the soft spot.

By the way, don't be afraid that you might injure or hurt the soft spot. Such a thing does not happen. Dig out the ugly cradle cap from the soft spot, and let the whole head look clean. This should be followed by combing the hair and getting out all the leftover small pieces of cradle cap. Even then, the scalp won't be completely clean. You may use Sebulex shampoo by now, and let the scalp look as nice as could be.

How many times do I have to do that?

Not often, perhaps once or twice. Shampooing the scalp with Sebulex or the like will do the rest, since cradle cap does not accumulate that fast. However, as long as a trace of cradle cap remains, you keep using these shampoos.

Most babies seem to outgrow this condition as they reach their first birthday, though a few stubborn cases will continue for many years to come. This is more true of the dry type of cradle cap.

How about the rash on his or her cheeks?

It is called seborrheic dermatitis. It is a shiny, greasy-looking, pale pink rash. Some babies show it at the age of one month, but it usually becomes more obvious at the age of two months. It tends to appear slowly, and in two or three weeks may cover the cheeks and/or forehead; then it seems to go away slowly over two or three weeks, just to appear again and repeat the cycle over and over again. In mild cases the baby has it once or twice before losing it for good, but the average cases may continue until age twelve to eighteen months.

It is good to wash the face once a day with Johnson's baby soap. This may keep the condition under control to some extent. For mild cases you may try a mild cortisone cream such as Cortaid 1/2 per cent (nonprescription). However, average cases will need the doctor's visit and advice. Quite often the doctor will use certain creams or lotions and in a few days the rash will go away. In two to three weeks the rash may show up again, and you will have to apply the cream again for a few days. The cream will have to be applied three to four times a day, but in tiny amounts. You must keep after the rash, and the longer the baby's cheeks are clear of this mess the better.

Some mothers are tempted to use baby oil. By so doing they make the condition worse. A greasy rash does not need oil, instead it needs soap and water along with the use of proper medicated cream.

TOOTH ERUPTION AND TEETHING

Usually around the age of five months, the local gums of the baby start reacting in preparation for the teeth to come through. They become round-edged and slightly swollen, and the baby seems to enjoy "biting" at them. Often there is an increase in drooling. The drooling may have started much earlier, even at the age of three to four months, but the degree seems to intensify during teething. Occasionally the baby may also become fussy, but not to the point that he or she becomes sick.

One morning, to your delight, the edge of the first tooth is there to behold. It may be in either the lower or upper jaw, and as the days pass by, the tooth will come to be quite noticeable. This will be followed by other teeth in the area, so that in a few weeks, the four front teeth will be in view.

Doesn't the baby become sick with teething?

Unfortunately there is an erroneous belief in the minds of many parents that teething leads to various forms of sicknesses. Teething is an innocuous natural process, and other than local reaction in the gums, there is no scientific evidence that it leads to any sickness, including fever, colds, and coughs. If the child happens to develop these symptoms while cutting teeth, then there is an incidental presence of infection, i.e. the baby has caught viruses at a time when he or she happened to be teething.

We have seen many cases of ear infections, respiratory infections, high fever, gastroenteritis, and even meningitis, that parents erroneously attributed to teething! Of course these assumptions are dangerous and are likely to lead to a lot of trouble if the baby is not treated promptly for these infections.

In some cases, the gums will react further locally where the tooth is to erupt, developing a nonpainful bluish swelling, quite noticeable. Given enough time, happily this will go away once the tip of the tooth comes through.

What shall we do about teething?

Since teething is an innocuous process, not much is to be done. With most babies, you simply enjoy observing their eruption. If unusual symptoms of fever, cough, or excessive crying happen to show up at the same time, you better see the doctor, since such symptoms are not related to teething at all.

For the local tenderness of the gums, a teething ring or similar object may be used. Rubbing the gums may be soothing to the baby. Some doctors use Chloraseptic gel, Orajel, Num Zit, or similar material (all nonprescription). This may numb the area slightly, but its value is certainly limited. Liquiprin, **Tempra** or Tylenol may reduce the fussiness, but still in most cases it is better to avoid medication.

Most babies get their first tooth around the age of six to seven months. However this timing is irregular, and a few babies may get them earlier, even by the age of three months or before. On the other hand, some babies are late teethers, and they may be nine to twelve months and beyond before the first tooth appears. Be patient, and the tooth will erupt eventually.

What are the "baby teeth"?

Baby teeth are of course the first set of teeth. They are twenty in number. It takes about two to two-and-one-half years before this dentition is completed. Usually the incisors or the front teeth are the first to appear. The order of their appearance is irregular; either the upper or lower incisors come first.

By the time all eight incisors have erupted, the baby may have reached his or her first birthday.

By this time the gums of the jaw bones will be preparing for the jaw teeth. Gradually these teeth will show up, and it may take two to three months before each side and each jaw has a jaw tooth. This is followed by the filling of the vacant spaces between the jaw teeth and the incisors by the canine teeth. From outside, the mouth will seem as if it is becoming full of teeth. The child by then is eighteen to twenty-four months old.

The final baby teeth to appear are the back jaw teeth. They will come in almost unnoticeably, making the set of twenty teeth complete. When this dentition is completed, the child is two to two and one half years old.

CARE OF THE TEETH

A few steps started early in life can prevent a good deal of expense and toothache. Your child can even grow up with no cavities whatever!

Parents should encourage children to brush their teeth at an early age. Do it for them if they allow you, even as early as around the age of twelve months. Some will be scared, so you may postpone the brushing until perhaps the age of eighteen months. Use a soft brush to begin with, and brush in the direction the teeth grow, i.e. up and down. Twice a day (after breakfast and before going to bed) is adequate.

When children are a few years old, they can do the job themselves, but the parents should stand by to help in case they fail to do it well. At this age and after, use a medium brush. Don't allow a glass of milk or anything to eat after the teeth have already been brushed at night, because you will be undoing all the good work the brushing is accomplishing. If you ignore this important principle, your child may end up with many cavities or even worse complications.

What toothpaste shall I use?

A toothpaste with fluoride is the best. You choose your favorite brand. The fluoride in the paste will cover the teeth and give them added protection. Yet this is still not enough.

What else do you need?

Fluoride in the drinking water will go a long way in helping to prevent cavities. Most of the big towns have this added convenience, but some small towns and rural areas do not. In such cases, fluorides can be taken on a daily basis, from birth until the age of ten years. They come in liquid form or in pill form, by themselves or in conjunction with vitamins; you will need a prescription, however.

In addition to all the above, the dentist may directly apply fluoride to the teeth once or twice a year as an added protection.

Will fluoride pose a danger to my child?

Not at all, if you have it in the usual safe range in the drinking water as usually provided. Actually in certain natural water supplies the fluoride level is several times higher than what is supplied in our drinking water.

By the way, when can my child visit a dentist?

In most cases at the age of two to three years, depending on his or her level of cooperation. Such visits will offer you the benefit of cleaning the teeth, detecting any potential problem, possibly applying fluoride, and performing good preventive medicine. An average of two visits a year is customary.

How about the Water-pic?

Water-pics are excellent if used correctly and if your child cooperates. They remove a goodly amount of the decaying food material that not only becomes imprisoned between the teeth but also acts as a focus for cavities. They also strengthen the edge of the gum and leave a fresh taste in the mouth. If you brush after using the pic, you stand a better chance for the toothpaste to reach the deeper grooves of the teeth.

Put the pressure of the Water-pic at low or moderate when you use it on your child, and on moderate if you use it for yourself. Use it once, mainly before bedtime. Don't overdo it with the amount of water you use; less than a fifth of a "tank" is enough.

Are there any rules to help reduce the chances for cavities?

Yes, pay attention to the following:

1. A bottle of milk, pop, orange juice, and the like, before going to bed can play havoc with teeth. The last thing to be done before going to bed is brushing the teeth; not giving milk or the bottle. The reason for that is that a film of milk, or whatever being given will cover the teeth all through the night, thus acting as an encouraging medium for the bacteria to keep growing. This may lead to a good chance for cavity formation.
2. Cookies, crackers, starchy foods, pies, and cakes can all accumulate between the teeth. If these foods are used excessively and if they are not followed by brushing or water-picking, there will be a good potential for cavities.
3. Contrary to the general belief, an occasional lollipop or chewing gum is perfectly safe. Cookies and crackers are far more dangerous than lollipops.
4. Regular visits to the dentist to clean the teeth and to fix potential trouble are most rewarding.
5. Fresh fruits such as apples will help maintain healthier teeth.

Regular and consistent care of the teeth, and observing the above rules, will offer the best chance for healthy white teeth.

MY BABY'S EYE KEEPS WATERING

The baby is only a few weeks old, you tell the doctor, and his or her eye is looking "wet" lately. Some tears seem to roll down the cheeks every once in a while, but they are not tears caused by crying. Things just don't look quite normal; what is it?

It is an "obstructed tear duct":

This is not an uncommon condition in babies. It usually affects one eye, but sometimes both eyes are involved. Usually the tears are clear, but occasionally infection sets in. When that happens, the discharge from the eye becomes "milky" or "pussy yellow." Quite often this keeps on and on for many weeks, if not months. Fortunately this is not a permanent condition. In the majority of cases the tear duct will open up by itself when the baby is six months old or older, and the eyes will clear up nicely.

You mean I have to wait that long?

No, not at all. You will massage the tear duct with the hope of opening it. Massaging the tear ducts will only be successful in a certain percentage of babies, but all parents of affected babies must still do it, to help as much as possible.

To massage the tear duct, use the small finger of your hand. Cut your finger nail closely. Place the tip of your small finger by the inner corner of the affected eye. Give it a firm but deep rolling massage movement. Keep doing this repeatedly, for a minute or so. You may see some pussy mucoid material suddenly collecting at the corner of the eye. This material has been pushed out of the tear sac by your massaging.

Do this massaging three times a day for one to two weeks. If you are successful, the eye will not "well" with tears any more. Even though your chance of success is not very high, it is worthwhile trying.

An alternative method is to use the tip of a Q-tip to do the massaging, instead of your finger tip. You roll the Q-tip firmly by the inner corner of the affected eye, back and forth, several times, three times a day.

And if I don't succeed?

Even if the massage fails, the odds are quite high that the tear duct will open up by itself if given long enough time. However, only rarely does the tear duct open spontaneously before the age of six months. Often, it opens up between the age of six to twelve months. The reason for the massaging, therefore, is to hurry up the process of opening the tear duct, thus avoiding the almost constant tearing of the eye and the chance for infection.

<u>What am I to do if it doesn't open up?</u>

If by the age of twelve months the baby continues with the same trouble, then you have to go to an eye doctor for "probing procedure." This operation is not a complicated procedure, but it does need the delicate hand of the ophthalmologist. When the operation is over, the eye will look perfectly normal.

TONGUE-TIE

Years ago, parents and doctors used to make a big issue out of tongue-tie. But things have changed for the better.

To understand the condition, lift your tongue in front of a mirror. You will see a sharp fold which holds the lower surface of the tongue to the floor of the mouth. This is called the frenulum, and it is pliable enough to allow the tip of the tongue to be protruded beyond the front teeth, the lip and beyond.

When the frenulum is too short, it will limit the tongue's mobility somewhat, mainly in its forward protrusion -tying it down so to speak.

<u>Is that why you call it tongue-tie?</u>

Yes, but there is a difference in the way it is interpreted now as compared to years ago. In the old days, if the frenulum seemed short when the baby's tongue was raised doctors would operate.

It was found out, however, that as a baby grows, the front part of the tongue is the main part to grow. Therefore, most of what appeared to be a tongue-tie in a baby was actually normal and the front part of the tongue would complete its growth with age.

<u>When shall we call it tongue-tie then?</u>

The condition is truly rare: over a period of twenty five years of pediatric practice, I have had only two or three cases of genuine tongue-tie that needed an operation.

At first we have to wait until the child is two to three years old or older. Then, we ask him or her to protrude the tongue forward. If the tip of the tongue goes beyond the front teeth and the lip, then the child is not tongue-tied. If the tip of the tongue cannot be protruded beyond the front teeth and the lip, then the child will have to have a small operation to relieve the tongue, because by then he or she can truly be classified as tongue-tied. The test is simple and straight forward, and you can do it to yourself or your child.

Will tounge-tie impede the function of the tongue?
As rare as tongue-tie is, when it is present it impedes to some extent the free mobility of the tongue. This impediment does not interfere with the child's eating or sense of taste, but it may create problems with pronunciation of some letters during speaking. However, by far most speech difficulties are not related to tongue-tie, and instead have to do with the child's use of the tongue, lips, palate, and related organs.

THRUSH

The baby has many tiny white spots, firmly attached to the lining of the mouth, be it the sides, the tongue, palate, or the gums. The baby acts fussy, unhappy and seems to cry easily. He or she does not take to nursing or to the bottle well. The baby tends to have some degree of constipation and perhaps gas.

Waiting a few days seems to have been of no help, and the baby's condition may have become worse.

What is it?
This is what is called thrush. The doctor upon checking the baby, will first make sure that it is thrush and not milk curds, and then will look for spots of rash in the diaper area. Milk curds and thrush look alike, but milk curds lay loosely on the mucous membrane of the mouth and can easily be removed by a Q-tip; not so with thrush. Thrush is caused by a special fungus (candida) which is present in the vagina of as many as one out of every three pregnant women. The baby picks up the fungus during birth, and it takes about two to three weeks before the thrush shows up.

Why look at the diaper area?

When the baby has thrush, the doctor looks for particular diaper rash too. This may sound funny, but there is a connection. The fungus often travels from the mouth down to the intestine, then infects the skin of the diaper area. In some cases the diaper area becomes infected to a fairly extensive degree. It will look sore, be "dry," and be fairly red in color, with satellite spots near the edge. Usually the baby seems unbothered, as if the bottom is not hurting (see page 102).

What can we do about it?

Once the doctor makes sure it is thrush, he will put the baby on a special medicine (Mycostatin suspension). You are told to shake the bottle, dip in three to four Q-tips, and touch every spot, be it the sides of the mouth, gums, tongue or palate. After that, fill the dropper to the level the doctor instructs, pour half of it on the right inside of the mouth, the other half on the left side, and let the baby swallow the medicine.

Repeat the procedure four times a day, for a total of two weeks, otherwise the fungus may grow back again.

Some doctors prefer to use a purple liquid medicine that looks like ink. It is effective but quite messy. It is now largely used when the other medication fails to produce a good result, which is not that often anyway.

Does thrush tend to come back?

In the majority of babies, when thrush is gone it is gone for good. When the infection is gone, the baby will stop being fussy, will eat better, and will move the bowels regularly again.

However, a small percentage may get reinfected a second or even a third time. If the thrush comes back, it will have to be treated again, but if it continually recurs, mother's vagina will have to be checked to see if it harbors this kind of fungus in profusion. Another reason for recurrent thrush is that the nipples of the bottles are not sterilized. Thus it is important to sterilize nipples and pacifiers especially for the first two weeks after discovering thrush.

CONSTIPATION IN BABIES

The baby grunts so much, passes some gas, seems to be in some discomfort, and the bowels haven't moved. This has been going on and off for the last two or three weeks. The bowels seem irregular and the parents are worried. The baby is only a few weeks old.

<u>What shall I do?</u>

Has the baby been checked? If yes, and the anus was found to be "tight," you will have to dilate the area. This usually leads to fast satisfactory results. See page 6.

If there is no "tightness," then take a look at the diet- though better be avoided during the first year of life, homogenized milk is quite a constipator. Formulas such as Similac, SMA, Enfamil, can lead to some degree of constipation but not as often as homogenized milk. Breast milk is, of course, the best. Rice cereal tends to bind too, while oatmeal cereal will do just the opposite. Bananas will also bind. Therefore, in such cases, you should avoid the foods that constipate, and try to use substitutions, e.g. different formulas, and foods that tend to loosen the bowels such as: oatmeal, plums, peaches, prunes, apricots, or prune-apple juice.

<u>Is there anything else I can do?</u>

Yes, of course. If the baby is suddenly constipated, one half of a baby glycerine suppository or Fleet Babylax enema (both nonprescription) usually works. If you want a mild nourishing laxative, mix Maltsupex (nonprescription) with the milk. One to three teaspoons in one day's formula will usually do. Start with one teaspoon and gradually increase it by one half teaspoon a day, until you reach the dose that will make the baby's bowel movements soft enough. Continue with the same dose every day for a few weeks.

<u>How about prune juice?</u>

Three to four ounces of prune juice, diluted half and half with water, can be successful enough, and it is worth a try. It may give some gas pains however. Prune-apple juice may be used too, and it will work just as well. If all the above measures don't work, give your doctor a call.

DIAPER RASH

The baby's bottom is red and sore-looking, but it doesn't seem to hurt. It may even look raw, yet sometimes home medications seem to do a good job in clearing it. At times the diapers and diaper area smell of ammonia, but at other times they don't.

What causes the ammonia smell?

There are several kinds of diaper rash. The commonest is the one caused by "maceration." This means that the tender bottom was in contact with wet, soggy diapers over a prolonged period. This wetness makes the skin macerated (soggy), and the urine is changed by bacteria into ammonia. The ammonia will "burn" the soggy skin and lead to the red, inflamed, irritated bottom. If the skin is untreated, bacterial infection is likely to take place, or shallow ulceration may show up, including the tip of the penis, or sides of the female genitalia. The smell of ammonia can be detected for a number of days, and at times it may be so strong that you must catch your breath.

How does this happen?

A baby will always wet diapers. Changing diapers is important, but it is not practical when everyone is asleep at night. Having wet diapers all night will make the skin soggy, especially when the urine cannot evaporate because of the plastic pants. The "imprisoned" urine is a good source for certain bacteria to grow and change it to ammonia. Prevention and cure can be had easily.

To prevent the ordinary diaper rash (ammoniacal diaper rash), prevent the constant wetness of the diaper area by frequent changes of the diapers, powdering with caldesene powder, or using protective ointments such as A & D, Desitin. The ointments may be used liberally to protect the skin from wetness. In severe cases you may have to see the doctor, since the baby may either be having complications, or need some internal medicine to acidify the urine.

What can I do about ammoniacal diaper rash?

1. For a few weeks use regular cloth diapers.
2. Double-diaper at night without using rubber pants.
3. Before you want to go to sleep, e.g. 11 pm, wake your baby up, double-diaper again. No rubber pants should be used this time either.
4. You may use rubber pants during daytime.
5. Make sure to change your baby often during daytime.
6. You may use A and D ointment, Desitin, or other ointments.
7. In persistent cases, your doctor may prescribe Pedameth to be put in the milk.
8. When the diaper rash is gone, go back to disposable diapers.

Occasionally your own diagnosis may not be correct, since the infant may prove to have a "fungus" diaper rash.

What is "fungus" diaper rash?

This is the second most common form of diaper rash. Suspicion should be aroused when treatment of the regular diaper rash seems to be going nowhere. It is caused by a special fungus called candida or monilia. The fungus happens to be in the diaper area, and tends to sneak in and establish itself when the area is weakened (devitalized). Often it shows up as dull red dry spots, slightly elevated, clustered in a fairly big diffuse patch with the spots at the periphery. These spots are called satellite lesions.

The whole thing grows slowly and gradually. The parents often treat it as ammoniacal diaper rash, mistakingly using the wrong medicine. The fungus rash is not itchy or irritating to the baby, and doesn't smell of ammonia. It is a persistent rash, and can be mean if left untreated; it may even spread up to the umbilicus. In spite of all this, the baby keeps on having a radiant smile! That is, unless he or she has thrush in addition (see page 98).

How will you treat it?

A special ointment will be given (Mycostatin), which you should use sparingly three to four times a day, not only on the rash but on the normal skin around the rash by about half an inch. The doctor will also tell you to use the ointment for a total of two weeks, though the rash may be gone in a few days. The reason for that is that the fungus does not get killed or immediately eradicated by the medicine, and may strike back if treatment is stopped too soon.

There is no need to use the same precautions as used in ammoniacal diaper rash. Also it is not unusual to see babies having such infections two or three times until they reach the age of toilet training, by which time diaper rashes become extinct because of the dryness of the bottom due to the use of training pants.

Are there other kinds of diaper rash?

Yes, there are, and they are less frequent than the above two. One of them is called seborrheic dermatitis see page 90, and it seems to like the crease of the groin. It looks moist, shiny pink, and may have a distinct edge. There may be similar spots in other areas, such as the armpits, behind the ears, the cheeks, and the neck. Once more, this is not itchy, doesn't seem to bother the baby, but parents will be concerned about it. For mild cases you may want to use 1/2% cortisone cream such as Cortaid (nonprescription). If after a few days the condition does not seem to improve, then a doctor's visit will become imperative. This condition tends to recur.

Another kind of diaper rash is caused by bacteria, (see page 148).

JAUNDICE

The baby's skin and face will have a yellowish hue, as will the white of the eyes.

Jaundice can show up at all ages, but it is more common at the newborn period. All kinds of children are likely to show it, Caucasian, Black or Oriental. There may also be other symptoms, depending on the cause of the jaundice.

What causes jaundice in babies?

Jaundice is fairly common in newborns, whether they are full-term or premature. Many mothers are Rh negative, and they may produce a baby who during pregnancy will react with her in such a way as to produce jaundice. This is called the Rh baby. Luckily the problem can be prevented to a great extent by using special shots given to the mother by the obstetrician soon after delivery of the baby.

There is another fairly common category that results when a mother with type "O" blood gives birth to a baby with a different blood type. This can lead to what is called "ABO incompatibility". Such cases are fairly common, and the jaundice may take a few days before it goes away. Occasionally certain forms of treatment might be needed for this type of jaundice.

Believe it or not, breast-feeding may lead to jaundice at times too.

How is that?

The jaundice of breast-fed babies is usually not severe enough to cause serious problems. It usually shows up when the baby is a few days old and may persist for a long time, even two to three weeks or longer- usually there is no other problem but the jaundice.

In such cases, after proper blood tests are done, the breast-feeding is discontinued for a few days, and the baby is put on the bottle. When blood tests are repeated daily, the level of the yellow substance known as bilirubin will gradually drop down to safe levels. When that happens, breast-feeding may be started again.

What kind of tests and what kind of treatment do you do?

It depends on what the doctor suspects. Bilirubin tests, however, are essential to monitor the level of bilirubin in all cases of jaundice, and they may have to be done once or twice a day or even more often. There are numerous other tests, (mainly blood tests) that might have to be done. This is because there are more than fifteen diseases in the newborn period that can cause jaundice. The most common, however, are the ones mentioned above.

A baby who is jaundiced may need what is called phototherapy. This means that he or she will be put under an apparatus with neon (ultraviolet) lights, and the bilirubin level will be tested carefully twice a day or more often. When under the light, a mask will also be placed on the baby's eyes for protection. This method has proved to be quite safe and effective if the jaundice of the baby happens to be mild and the bilirubin level not climbing fast. There are certain levels of bilirubin in the blood which can become dangerous to the baby's brain if we don't interfere.

What will the doctor do?
Depending on how fast the bilirubin level is climbing, along with many other factors, the doctor may decide to do exchange transfusion. This means exchanging the blood of the jaundiced baby with another. It usually takes one to one and one-half hours to perform, but the procedure, though fairly safe, may carry some risks.

Occasionally two or more exchange transfusions may have to be done. Luckily, there is certainly less need nowadays for these measures as there was in the past.

Can you have jaundice without yellowing of the eyes?
No. A few-months-old baby who develops yellowish skin, despite a clear white of the eyes, is said to have carotenemia (see page 27). This is a disease caused by eating too much carrots, beets and some other foods! There is an abnormal accumulation of a substance called carotene from these vegetables. Stop the above foods and the condition will disappear after a few weeks or months.

Can jaundice show up in infants?
Yes, jaundice can show up in babies other than newborns, though this is not so common. Jaundice in a few-months-old baby may mean certain obstructive diseases of the liver. It is very important to recognize this condition early, since there is a special operation for it, but this operation is more likely to succeed if it is done before the baby is three months old. This operation can correct a certain form of obstruction to the bile flow.

An older child can develop jaundice too, and it will most likely be caused by infectious hepatitis. Jaundice in such children is often associated with other symptoms, such as fever, severe nausea, vomiting, lethargy, dark urine, and clay-colored stools (see page 378).

A FEW TIPS ABOUT A CLEAN-UP JOB

A. <u>In case of a baby boy:</u>

Most boys are circumcised these days. Whether or not your baby boy is circumcised, part of the foreskin may lay covering the ridge behind the tip of the penis itself. If the baby is circumcised it is important that you pull the skin of the penis back until it is behind that ridge (called corona). You may see some smelly, cheesy, yellowish-white stuff (smegma) behind the corona. Please clean it with a Q-tip dipped in Vaseline or baby oil.

If the above is not done regularly after each bath, the odds are that the foreskin will stick to the glans of the penis. This would then require breaking the adhesions by the physician. It is easier, and certainly better to prevent these adhesions than have to break them; sometimes repeatedly.

In an uncircumcised baby, pull the foreskin back a little until you see the tip of the glans of the penis. This will stretch the opening of the foreskin and help prevent phimosis (see page 108).

B. <u>In case of a baby girl:</u>

The way the genitalia are shaped makes it easy for her to pick up some germs from the nearby rectum. This is especially true if you wipe off her bottom from behind to front. You may even see, in so doing, some of the material of the bowel movement gathering in the genitalia. The germs will find a "haven" for multiplying there and may be able to ascend to the bladder causing urinary tract infection.

Therefore, please observe the following:

1. Wipe away her bottom from the front to the back.
2. Carefully clean the genitalia of any bowel movement material accumulating there, using a ball of cotton dipped in water.

C. <u>In babies, for both sexes:</u>

1. Don't let your baby sit in the bowel movement too long. Not only will the smell repel you, but it is unhealthy for the baby.
2. Don't just smear the bowel movement on the bottom; wipe well, wash

the area if possible, and please don't forget to wash your hands. You would be surprised to see how many parents do forget such an elementary rule.

TO CIRCUMCISE OR NOT TO CIRCUMCISE

When a boy is born, his penis has a foreskin, which is a piece of thick skin that covers the glans of the penis to its tip and beyond. Some religions decree that this piece of tissue should be disposed of, but others don't care one way or the other. There are, however, a few medical points worth considering.

What if the boy is left uncircumcised?
The foreskin is lined with a certain kind of mucous membrane. This lining folds in on itself, (invaginates), to become continuous with the cover of the glans of the penis (the forepart of the penis). There are glands in that area which secrete the smelly, cheesy, white material called smegma. Often a baby's foreskin gets stuck or even glued to the glans of the penis.

Therefore, to have a healthy front of the penis, the parent will have to pull back the foreskin. To be successful, the foreskin has to be pulled back until its free edge goes behind the bulging edge (corona) of the glans of the penis. In babies this is difficult to do, not only because of the adhesions between the foreskin and the glans, but also because the opening of the foreskin is narrow and tight in most of them (see page 106).

Even so, the parent should persist every day in pulling back the foreskin. Usually by the age of one to two years, the foreskin may become pliable enough to be pulled back behind the corona of the penis. When this happens, the glans may be cleaned of smegma, the adhesions will have been broken, and the tight orifice of the foreskin will have been loosened.

Are there any problems besides?
An uncircumcised child may develop certain forms of infection (balanitis) in the area between the foreskin and the glans. The reason is that the area can lend itself to the growth of bacteria,

mainly if the foreskin cannot be pulled back as mentioned above. Infection with certain germs can also ascend through the penis to the bladder and other parts of the urinary system.

In some baby boys, irritation and infection of the opening of the foreskin, even with ulceration, can take place. This is more prevalent when there is the ammonia smell in the diapers associated with diaper rash. Even the opening in the glans (the meatus), can become red and irritated. When the condition subsides, some scarring may even take place. Not only that, but some mechanical problems can show up with the foreskin.

<u>Like what?</u>

In some children, the opening of the foreskin can be quite tight. This is called phimosis. Such a tight opening can hamper the passage of the urine to a slight extent, or even balloon the space between the foreskin and the glans penis. This conditon can present a problem to the doctor when it becomes infected.

Another mechanical condition is called paraphimosis. This happens when the foreskin is pulled back to beyond the corona of the glans. If the opening of the foreskin is too tight and pulled back to that position, it can cut off the circulation of the glans penis to some extent. This will lead to swelling and much pain of the area, and it becomes an emergency, making it necessary for a doctor or surgeon to intervene right away.

An uncircumcised adult may be a likely target for certain forms of infections, sexual or otherwise. It is also said that he may tend to ejaculate sooner during intercourse.

<u>How about circumcision?</u>

Most American boys are circumcised nowadays, and it is mainly done during the first few days of life.

This makes it easy, since the tissues of the penis will heal easily without the need of much assistance. No need to use ointment or anything on the newly circumcised, raw-looking penis, unless there is evidence of some infection, and this is rare indeed. The circumcised area usually heals in seven to ten days.

The length of foreskin to be removed during circumcision varies from one doctor to another. Some take out a good deal of the foreskin, others remove only a small part at the front. When the latter is done, some parents wonder if the boy has actually been circumcised. The important thing in this situation is to see if the remnant part of the foreskin is free and can be pulled back easily; if so, the condition can be regarded as satisfactory. But if adhesions develop they must be broken up.

How do you break these adhesions?

During the first year of life, some adhesions are likely to show up between the remnant of the foreskin in the circumcised boy and the back part of the glans. If left alone, they become firmly attached, and they may hold an increasing amount of smegma in the form of nodules. To prevent this, the doctor will usually break the adhesions and show the parents how to do it. There may be a slight amount of bleeding. The process may recur a few times, but the parents must keep after it as long as necessary.

To do so, put one of your thumbs at the glans, and the other thumb on the shaft of the penis. By pulling the thumbs apart, you will break the adhesions, leaving a wet, slightly glistening surface underneath, along with some smegma.

THE SORE BOTTOM

Sore bottom is fairly common, and it affects more girls than boys. She may pull at herself on and off, and may complain that it hurts some. There is hardly any discharge, if any. When you take a look, you will see a red irritated area, mainly around the genitalia, but it may be around the anus too.

What can be the cause of such a thing?

There are many causes for such a "sore bottom," and they depend upon whether the irritation is around the anus, or around the female genitalia.

If the irritation is around the anus, it may show up not only in girls but also in boys, and it is more common in younger children than the older ones. The reason is that it is related most often to the way these children clean themselves after having a bowel movement. At times, the skin becomes inflamed and irritated, tender and sore, red and slightly swollen, and perhaps even ulcerated.

Poor care after a movement is not the only cause of sore peri-anal area. The child may be sensitive to the chemical in the toilet paper, or to the roughness of the paper itself. Another cause is pinworms, because they produce intense itching in that area. Scratching leads to soreness.

What causes the problem in girls?

If the sore bottom is mainly around the female genitalia, a common cause is the delicate relationship between the low level of the female hormone in girls at this age and the mucous membrane of their genitalia. This can be easily controlled by the doctor with a special cream.

Aside from the above, there are other reasons that lead to the sore bottom in girls. Tight pants, particularly if made of non-cotton fiber, is an important cause. The crotch of such pants, especially when tightly fit, will rub against the area, leading to a good deal of irritation. Not only that, but the non-cotton pants don't absorb moisture, and they can be a means of incubating germs from around the anus and transferring them to the female organs.

Harsh soaps, sensitivity to the chemicals of some soaps, or over-zealous cleaning with soap, may all play a part in causing such irritation.

What can we do about irritation around the anus?

The obvious answer is to eliminate the cause. If it happens to be a need for a better cleaning technique, you have to stress this to the child. This is more so when he or she is four to seven years old.

If the toilet paper is suspected, use a different brand, which ought to be soft, and also white in color. Colored paper may be sensitizing because of the color's chemical.

If pinworms are the cause, then proper medication will take care of the problem.

On the irritated area itself, you may use Balneol lotion (nonprescription), once or twice a day for a week or so. This lotion is cleansing and soothing and will be welcomed by the child.

What do we do if the irritation is of and around the female genitals?

As mentioned before, a special cream (containing a small percentage of female hormone) will usually correct this cause of sore bottom in the female, i.e. that condition which needs an added level of female hormone. Such cases may also benefit from Vaseline, baby oil, Balneol lotion etc., but these prove to be of only temporary relief in most cases.

If the cause seems to be tight pants, simply switch her to loose pants, made of cotton fiber, changed once a day or so.

Avoid zealous use of soap, especially harsh ones. This is also true of bubble baths and/or detergents in some sensitive females.

In older females, mainly the adults, the frequent use of douches, the kind of douches used, and some of the feminine hygiene deodorants can be irritating and may be annoying causes of "sore bottom" until they are discovered as such and disposed of.

UMBILICAL HERNIA

An umbilical hernia is fairly common, and it is seen in many babies at the age of two or three months. As its name indicates, it is a hernia of the umbilicus itself. It can be of various sizes, from that of a pea to that of a walnut or larger. It is not at all painful. Usually it bulges when the baby cries or strains, such as upon having a bowel movement, since this increases the pressure inside the abdomen.

Usually an umbilical hernia increases in size over a period of two to three months from the time of its first appearance, and by the time the baby is about five months old the hernia will have reached its largest size.

When you gently press on it to reduce it, you may feel the gurgle of the intestine. You may also be able to feel the ring of the opening. This ring is important, since the smaller it is, the sooner the hernia will go away. Sometimes the ring is large enough to admit the tip of your finger, or even larger. If the ring is too large, as assessed by your doctor, the hernia may not go away by itself and a small operation will have to be done. Rarely is this needed however.

<u>You mean umbilical hernias can go away by themselves?</u>

Yes, the majority of them will go away if given enough time. The doctor will advise you to wait. A high percentage will go away by the age of one year, others by one and one half to two years; though rarely they linger longer even until the age of six or seven years. Therefore, much patience and observation is all that is needed. An umbilical hernia is an innocuous condition that rarely produces trouble, and though strangulation of the hernia can occur, this is the exception.

<u>What shall we do about it?</u>

People in the past used a half dollar or a quarter, wrapped it in cloth and taped it over the umbilical hernia after reducing it. This procedure proved to be useless. If for cosmetic reasons you want to hide the hernia, you may want to use the taping, but it is likely that the skin in contact with the tape will develop dermatitis. Therefore, it is best to leave the umbilical hernia alone and give it time to slowly go away by itself.

BRUISES

The little toddler who used to be such a nice, quiet baby is nothing but a bundle of energy by now. However, despite the activity and vigor, the coordination still leaves a lot to be desired; he or she seems to bump into so many things. To your surprise you notice a good many bruises, far more than seem normal. The bruises are mainly on the legs, especially in the area of the shinbones. But you can also see them on the arms, and sometimes even on the trunk.

<u>What causes such a nuisance?</u>

By far the majority are caused by a bump or a hit, be it against a coffee table, a tree, or something else in the way. A child who is quite vigorous is somehow always in a hurry, and is less likely to pay attention to obstacles.

However, there is a small number of diseases that can manifest themselves as bruises. These are blood diseases, some of which are quite serious in nature. It is because of these diseases that we should pay attention to frequent and incessant bruising. This is especially true if there seems to be little or no associated injury.

What does a bruise consist of?

A bruise is a result of ruptured capillaries. The capillaries are a very tiny network of vessels that get their blood from the arteries, and that drain into the veins. They are present almost everywhere in our bodies.

When these capillaries rupture, blood seeps into the tissues, causing the bruise. The color of the bruise at first may be dark red, but within a few days it will change to a yellowish brown, then to a greenish tinge, until it becomes a faint yellow before fading within a week or two.

A bruise may feel hard at the center, and it may be slightly tender too.

Shall I ignore these bruises?

It is better not to in some cases. Although most bruises mean nothing more than a simple trauma, there is a likelihood of blood disease. The disease may involve platelets, clotting factors or the blood cells themselves.

A child should see the doctor if the bruises are too frequent, if they affect areas less likely to be traumatized (such as the abdomen, chest, etc.), if they accompany severe nosebleeds, or if there are pinpoint "blood spots" under the skin (petechii). Of course, in addition to the above, if the child doesn't feel good, looks pale, has a decreased appetite, loses weight, or becomes feverish, he or she should see the doctor right away.

What will the doctor do?

The doctor will check the child, paying special attention to the character of the bruises and the size of the spleen, the liver, and the lymph nodes. He or she may find nothing significant, or may check the blood and do a number of tests. The decision depends completely on the findings. It is good to know that by far the majority of frequent bruising turns out to be a result of simple trauma only.

How common are these bruises?

Since it is very common to see active children, it is very common to see bruises. They are therefore more common in children three to seven years old, after which they gradually become less noticeable. Needless to say, bruises are usually seen far more frequently in boys than girls.

As for treating such bruises, there is little in the way of treatment that can make them disappear faster.

What about the blood diseases that cause easy bruising?

They are many, but fortunately they are not that common. With diseases like purpura, leukemia, hemophilia, etc., there may be other signs and symptoms besides the bruises. As mentioned before, occasionally bruises may be the earliest sign of any of these blood diseases. If the child starts running a fever, if the appetite deteriorates, if the color becomes pale, if the joints start hurting, etc., it will mean possible trouble, and an early visit to the doctor is highly recommended. The list of blood diseases can be quite long, and the diagnosis may demand a good many tests.

ACCIDENTS AND THEIR PREVENTION IN THE VERY YOUNG

Children may be very active or quiet, overly inquisitive or apathetic, but no matter what they are, they are likely to precipitate an accident. They may be hurt by it, but at the same time they will come out of it a little wiser. Very young children are in a stage of exploration and learning, and often must learn by making mistakes. They must have a feeling of pain so that they will not repeat the same mistake over and over again.

Because of their need for this kind of education, and because many accidents can prove serious and even devastating, they need understanding and patience from their parents, and a gentle guidance and protection. If they get it, they will shift from a need for protection 100 percent of the time, to a need for protection of only 10 percent of the time a few years later. The other 90 percent will be the education of experience.

How is that?

An infant who is less than one year of age is far too young and too immature to understand accidents. At such an age your protection will have to be in the range of 100 percent. Growing babies will have more leeway to experiment, and, whether we like it or not, will do whatever they want to do anyway.

Upon approaching the age of three to four years, a baby will have had a period of experimentation, and will have experienced different forms of accidents, small or large, mild or serious, painful or frustrating. He or she will have had a number of years for such experiences and at the same time will have grown up to understand what to avoid and what not to.

Will small infants have accidents?

Believe it or not, it is not at all rare for the small infants to have accidents. Most of them are easily preventable. Parents can do a good deal in that regard:

1. Don't put the baby on a table unattended. He or she may roll over unexpectedly and fall to the floor, and may end up with a fractured skull, a fractured collarbone, a concussion, or the like.
2. Don't leave a baby alone in a bathinette or a bathtub; drowning may easily occur. Always take the child out of the bathinette or bathtub before you do your chore, even if your chore takes a few seconds.
3. Keep a baby away from a stove or a hot pan, a hot cup of coffee, etc., thus preventing burn.
4. Never use lead-base paint on cribs or any other surface an infant may come into contact with. It may lead to lead poisoning; babies love to chew on the side railings of a bed.
5. Keep small objects away, such as pins, buttons, toy parts, etc. Infants can easily put these objects in their noses and mouths. Remember this is the put-in-the-mouth age.
6. Put guards on the stairways, to prevent your infant from falling down the steps.

How about when they are one to two years old?

This is the age of adventuring. They are active; walking, running, and constantly moving. They are likely to fall often, especially if there is a cluttered room. They lose balance easily and may hit something while in a hurry. Inspect the activity area and make it as accident-proof as possible.

They can climb and they love to do that, so watch the stairs and windows, and install screens. They can take things apart, so watch for frequent advances on the TV or hi-fi knobs, on electric appliances, on pots and pans, knives, etc.

At this age, they often open and close doors, and in this practice of ecstasy they may hurt themselves. Doors of cabinets are a special target, so beware of insecticides inside those closets, cleaning detergents, or medicines.

Also, be careful of them in the bathtub.

How about when they are two to three years old?

They love to hurry. They delight in going upstairs and downstairs, so make the stairs free of objects: a gate is very much worth using.

Discourage your baby from putting things in his or her mouth especially while running. Pay special attention to the construction of toys; they must be strongly built, have round rather than sharp edges, be sturdy, and have only a few knobs. Put toys away when not in use -a cluttered room is an invitation for a fall or some form of an accident.

Always teach and explain. This is a good age for reasoning. Teach your child about crossing streets, about handling sharp objects such as glass or knives. Keep an eye out while your child is learning to use the tricycle.

How about when they are three or four years old?

They are developing skills by now. Their self-education is such that they need less protection from you. Keep reasoning with your child but on a higher level.

Teach your youngster to ride the tricycle on sidewalks, and to beware of streets and nearby driveways. This is also a wandering age, so watch out! They love to climb, especially trees. Let your child do that, but in the correct way, and with the proper clothes. Allow ball-playing, but mainly in playgrounds and not in the street. Let your child learn to build, to share, to cooperate, but always with an accent on safety and avoiding accidents.

ABC'S OF CHILD SAFETY

Accidents come in different forms and severities. In a year's time, children from the age of one to fourteen years in this country are involved in an average of fifteen million accidents. This is a frightening number, but what is more frightening is that about fifteen thousand children lose their lives because of them.

This is mentioned to put you on the alert and to remind you that nine out of ten of all accidents are preventable.

There are interplaying factors that lead to accidents. Learning about these factors, foreseeing the possibilities for the accidents, and attempting to correct or bypass such factors, can go a long way to prevent them. It is true that no child can be absolutely safe, and it is also true that you cannot prevent all accidents, but preventing as many would-be accidents as you can is reasonable goal.

<u>What are these factors?</u>

To be involved in an accident, generally three factors are to be considered: (1) the child himself or herself, (2) the environment of the accident, and (3) the circumstances leading to the accident.

Briefly said, a child is in a constant learning process. To learn, a child has to explore and experiment. Thus, long before the first birthday and all through childhood, a child is likely to precipitate accidents, and in the process will learn what hurts and what doesn't. Safety education is a gradual process.

Remember please, the younger the child, the more he or she will need supervision and protection: one hundred percent before the child becomes one year old, until about only ten percent when he or she is past the age of five years. How fast the child is allowed to be trusted alone depends on his or her accumulated experience, "maturity," capability, and level of activity.

The second factor is the environment of the accident. An accident takes place only if a child does something "troublesome" to something already present; e.g. closing a door on the hand, falling from a table, putting the hand on a hot pan, falling from a bicycle, putting a finger in an electric outlet.

The third major factor is the circumstances that lead to or influence an accident. A child who is fatigued or in a rage is more likely to precipitate an accident; so is a child who is a busybody, or inquisitive, or a live wire. Other circumstances include times when the whole family is tired and fatigued (4-6 pm), or when there is discord, or when there is a decrease in or lack of supervision. Still other circumstances occur at school or outside. Since ninety percent of accidents are preventable, it would be silly not to try to prevent them. Therefore, this should be a point of challenge to us. Any child is likely to precipitate or be involved in an accident.

How can we prevent some of these accidents?

Prevention will naturally depend on the nature of the accident, the age of the child, etc. However, there are certain points that apply to many would-be accidents. These are general rules, many of which require no more than common sense and some degree of foresight.

1. Make sure the toddler is well rested and well supervised.
2. Take care of problem areas at home e.g. cluttered areas with toys, stairs without a gate.
3. Keep medicines, cleaning agents, pesticides, and the like inaccessible and locked up.
4. Emphasize safety rules in swimming, bicycle and car riding, tree climbing, use of matches, etc.

By and large, accidents in children under the age of five years are somewhat different than those in later years (see page 114).

ACCIDENTAL POISONING

By taking a simple look around your house, you will be amazed at the multitude and varieties of chemicals. Roughly speaking, these chemicals come in the following categories:

1. Medicines: aspirin, antibiotics, birth-control pills, cough remedies, tranquilizers, vitamins, pain killers.
2. Household cleaners and polishes: ammonia, lye, bleach, detergents, polishes, soaps.
3. Lotions and cosmetics: perfumes, creams, wood alcohol, rubbing alcohol, hand lotions, and nail polish and its removers.
4. Pesticides: liquids, powders, or sprays; weed killers, bug killers.
5. Petroleum products: gasoline, kerosene, paint thinners.

Each of these chemicals carries a certain amount of risk if swallowed by a child. Each of these chemicals is likely to produce some specific symptoms that can be dangerous or grave.

This year about 500,000 children in this country will swallow some of these chemicals, and better than nine out of ten of these cases will have been preventable.

It is worthy to note too, that nine out of ten of such cases involve children under the age of five years; young people who are fast, fearless, and curious.

How can I prevent such accidents?

The "crawlers" (those who are eight to twelve months old) will tend to explore "low places" such as areas on the floor, or low cabinets. Cabinets can contain paints, pesticides, kerosene, turpentine, lotions, cleaning equipment, etc. Such bright colors and pleasant odors are quite irresistible to babies. Therefore, store such items in their proper places, away from the reach of the baby, or lock the closet consistently.

The "toddlers" (those who are one to two years old) will be able to reach some kitchen counters, desks, and tables. Many of them are more likely to reach for anything left on top of these areas, things like cleaners, polishes, bleaches, lye, etc. Children at this age have the highest accident rate of any age group. Keep these chemicals stored properly, not within reach, and in their original containers.

The "busy climbers" (those who are two to five years old) can easily reach "safe" places, making them unsafe for themselves. Places such as cabinets, shelves, and medicine chests are of special attraction. At such an age, various medicines and drugs are the most troublesome cause for accidental poisoning. To do a good act of prevention, keep medicine chests locked, don't call medicines "candy," keep medicines in their original containers, make bottles tamperproof (child resistant containers with safety caps), and give medicines with care -and only to the person for whom they are prescribed.

What shall I do if my child has taken the stuff?

Call the doctor first; if not able to get in touch, call the hospital or its poison control center, or even the police. Save the container and the rest of its contents to take to the doctor or poison control center. To dilute the stomach content, give milk or water, as much and as often as you can.

IF A PETROLEUM PRODUCT SUCH AS GASOLINE OR KEROSENE OR A CORROSIVE SUCH AS LYE HAS BEEN TAKEN OR IS SUSPECTED TO HAVE BEEN TAKEN, DON'T TRY TO MAKE THE CHILD VOMIT. TAKE THE CHILD TO THE DOCTOR OR TO THE EMERGENCY ROOM OF A NEARBY HOSPITAL

If the child has taken a medicine or a chemical other than a corrosive or petroleum product, then induce vomiting by:

1. (the most effective way) Giving the child one tablespoon (not teaspoon) of syrup of Ipecac. No prescription is needed. If you don't have this at home, take a tablespoon, a bucket, and the child with you and drive to the nearest drugstore. Buy the syrup of Ipecac. Let the child take one tablespoon of it and drink a glass of water. As you drive back home or to the doctor's office, the child will probably vomit; hence the bucket. Eighty to eighty-five percent of the cases will vomit in about fifteen to twenty minutes after taking the syrup, or
2. Tickling the throat with your finger, and/or
3. Giving the child a glass of warm water with one teaspoon of baking soda or powdered mustard in it.

Even if the child has vomited, the doctor ought to be informed; he or she may want to check the child in addition.

CONTUSIONS

Contusions usually show up after a fall or a hit. There may be one, two or more contusions, depending on the type of fall or injury. A laceration may or may not be there.

Contusions are usually injuries to the tissue under the skin, though the muscles and other tissues might be involved too.

How will the contusion manifest itself?

The area having the contusion reacts by producing local tenderness with some degree of pain; there will also be a variable amount of swelling depending on the extent and location of injury. The area will also look somewhat red at first, but as the days pass by the color will change to reddish brown, then yellow then faint yellowish green before disappearing in two to three weeks' time. The swelling and tenderness will subside before the color has faded.

How do contusions vary in different areas?

If the area involved is near the eye, there will be a likelihood for a "black eye" to develop. A black eye is nothing but a contusion of the soft tissues near the eye, but because of the loose connective tissue near the eye, there will be more swelling than there would be in other areas, and a more dramatic change in color (see page 192).

Similarly, if the contusion is of the foot or hand, the swelling will be especially pronounced, out of proportion to the degree of other signs and symptoms. The reason for that is that the soft tissues of the back of the feet and hands are fairly loose, thus more prone to swelling. Contusions near the shinbone or hipbones can be fairly painful and tender; they may become hard and develop a "soft" center.

The above are but a few examples of the various forms of contusions. It is important to make sure that there are no serious injuries associated with the contusions.

Can you give us some examples of associated injuries?

A contusion is only one manifestation of an injury, and if the injury is severe enough, it may lead to further damage. Contusions near the eye can be associated with concussions, skull fractures, or injured eyes. Contusions of the extremities can be associated with fractures or damage to the joints, or damage to the muscles or blood vessels. Contusions of the chest or abdomen may be associated with internal injuries to the spleen, lungs, or other organs.

What shall we do about these contusions?

If it is a simple contusion without associated trouble, you may apply some cold packs or ice to the area. This is helpful during the first half-hour or so of the appearance of the contusion. The ice or cold applications help reduce the size of the swelling and to numb the pain to some extent.

After this is done, apply heat. This may be in the form of a hot-water bottle, warm compresses, dry heat, etc. This will help in the healing process after the cold has helped reduce the swelling. The heat should be applied for about twenty minutes, three or four times a day, for two to three days. Aspirin may help to some extent and it may be used to relieve the pain.

Of course the area is to be kept from too much movement, mainly if the contusion is near a joint. Application of Ben Gay or a similar substance is of no value.

The treatment of contusions is variable, depending on the location, the size and the degree, and many other factors.

CUTS AND LACERATIONS

The sight of blood will upset both the child and you. Only when the child calms down some, and when you clean the area, can you assess the damage to any meaningful extent. When the area cleaned shows only a small cut or laceration, the child will calm down considerably knowing that he or she was scared by the sight of the blood.

How can we assess the laceration?

Once you have cleared the area of the blood, see whether the cut has gone through the full depth of the skin. Also look to see if the laceration has a jagged irregular edge, is at an angle, or is curved, and of course try to estimate the length of the cut, and the degree of separation of the edges.

All the above are important points to help your doctor when you call him or her to decide whether or not stitches will be needed.

Naturally the location of the laceration is very important, and so is whether or not it is contaminated or soiled.

How does the location affect treatment of the laceration?

Lacerations in some important locations do require special care and attention. Good examples are cuts on the face, especially near the eyes, nose, and mouth. For such lacerations, a plastic surgeon is often called upon so that the outcome will be more acceptable.

Lacerations of the scalp can lead to a great deal of bleeding because of the rich blood supply there, yet the scar left will be well-covered with hair.

Lacerations that involve the nails or are deep enough in the fingers or hands may need a hand surgeon or a plastic surgeon. The reason for that is that some of the tendons or their sheaths may have been cut, or the bed of the nail may have been involved if the cut is nearby.

What shall I do when the child is cut?

To allay the fear at the sight of blood, try to calm the child (and yourself) as best as you can; clean the area around the wound of all the blood. The blood on the laceration will clot in most cases. Profuse bleeding (such as occurs in laceratins of the scalp) might require some pressure application. If this is the case, try to put pressure with your finger on the area adjacent to the cut (not on the cut itself, otherwise you may infect or devitalize it).

Have a good look, assess the laceration as described earlier, and try to determine whether or not there was an associated injury, like a broken bone, a joint injury, a contusion of the deep tissues, etc. Call the doctor then and give all this information.

What will the doctor do?

The doctor may refer you to the emergency room of the nearest hospital, or to a surgeon, plastic surgeon, or a hand surgeon, depending on the laceration. Some doctors do the stitching themselves.

Of course the doctor will check the child's record for the tetanus shot. If the child has had a tetanus shot within the past five to ten years depending on age, the immunity will be solid enough to preclude the need for any tetanus booster shots; if not, the booster will be given.

If it is not possible to check on the records for the tetanus right away, and if you don't remember the approximate date the child had the last tetanus shot, it may be wise to follow one of the two steps below:

1. Have the laceration sutured in the emergency room of a nearby hospital, but wait for the tetanus shot until the next day; ask your doctor to check the record to see if the child will need it. If needed, let it be given (You have a period of seventy two hours from the time of the laceration during which a tetanus shot can be given). This is the preferred method.
2. Let the tetanus shot be given once the laceration is sutured. This may lead to an unnecessary extra shot; however, if the cut is contaminated, it is better to take this precaution.

When shall the stitches be removed?

In most cases it takes an average of a week before the stitches are removed. This is a reasonable number of days for the scar to form and solidify. However, in special situations (such as cuts of the palms of the hands or soles of the feet), it may take longer.

If you see swelling and redness near the sutured laceration or at its edges, or if beads of pus come out upon mild pressure, call the doctor, since this indicates infection. It is also good to remember to protect the stitched laceration from futher insults; avoid hitting it or making it dirty, wet, or contaminated. Even after removing the stitches, keep it from becoming wet for about three days, and help protect it from opening again via another fall or hit.

CHAPTER FIVE

FEVER AND INFECTIOUS DISEASES

fever and infections
to bring a high temperature down
febrile convulsions
viruses, bacteria and fungi
viral infections
flu
why the culture
the strep germ
the staph germ
pneumococcus
antibiotics, use and abuse
roseola
scarlatina
chickenpox
measles
rubella
mumps
rheumatic fever
infectious mono
fifth disease
rocky mountain spotterd fever

FEVER AND INFECTIONS

<u>My child's temperature is up,</u>

And in addition, the child has a headache, looks flushed, is achy and irritable, may refuse to eat and even is nauseated. He or she wants to sleep or prefer to be left alone, and not be as full of energy as usual.

<u>Is this caused by a sore throat?</u>

Not necessarily. Fever is a symptom of a good many diseases. Fever is only a symptom, and sore throat or pharyngitis is only one of the causes of fever. Usually fever indicates some kind of infection-viral, bacterial or otherwise. Other signs beside the fever help in directing us towards the correct diagnosis. An earache with fever makes you suspect ear trouble, a cough with fever makes you suspect an upper respiratory infection.

To reach a correct knowledge of the cause of fever, often a doctor's examination is essential.

<u>Do I have to see a doctor every time the child is feverish?</u>

Not at all. If the temperature is not too high, and if it lasts for only a day or so and the child seems to be okay afterwards, then you can relax. That kind of fever is more likely to be caused by a virus than anything else.

But make sure to see the doctor:

1. If the temperature has gone way up, say to around 104 degrees F within the last twenty-four hours.
2. If the temperature has persisted for longer than few days, even if it is low-grade, i.e. around 100 degrees F.
3. If there are other symptoms with the fever, such as vomiting, cough, stiff neck, rash, etc.
4. If the child looks very sick to you.
5. If you feel at ease to have the child seen by a doctor.

But the temperature always shoots up at night:
That is true to some extent. Usually our temperature is higher in the evening and the fever is at its all-time high in the evening. This doesn't mean it cannot wait until next morning. Actually, it is more advisable to wait until next morning to see the doctor.

Why wait?
Because you give the body more time to be stimulated by the virus, bacteria, or whatever the cause of the fever. By so doing, a better resistance will build up. Another important point is that by waiting, other signs of the disease will show up better, thus making it easier for the doctor to diagnose the sickness.

What shall I do in the meantime?
Don't stew, just approach the whole subject intelligently. Fever is a symptom of something wrong. So

1. Use the proper dose of an antipyretic: aspirin, Tylenol, Liquiprin, or similar medications, every four hours, if the temperature is high enough (see page 132).
2. Don't overdress the child. Too much clothing is likely to keep the temperature up. Pajamas are adequate. In case the child is shivering, cover him or her with a blanket.
3. Don't feed a feverish child regular meals. Instead, offer liquids such as colas, soups with toast or crackers, jello, pudding, applesauce and other forms of a soft diet. A soft diet is easier on a fussy stomach.
4. Don't let the child go to school until the temperature has been normal for twenty-four hours.
5. Limit the child's activity. Being indoors, resting, watching TV if so desired, is far better.
6. In addition to the above steps, use any medication your doctor gives you.

How often should I take the child's temperature?
If the child feels hot to you by feeling the stomach or forehead, then it is time to take the temperature. If he or she is slightly

warm, don't bother to take the temperature, just keep an eye on the child. Don't be a "thermometer-addict", give the toddler's mouth or rectum a break.

I'm worried, though:

It is understandable; here is a guide to determine how much worry is warranted.

A temperature under 102 degrees F is regarded as low-grade; for such a level, bothering about a thermometer is extra effort that can be spared. You may not even need to use Tylenol or aspirin if the temperature is 101 degrees F or under. If the temperature is higher than 102 degrees F, especially around 102 to 104 degrees F, then it is worth being concerned. The more the temperature is near 104 degrees F the more you should do to fight it. In such cases, you will take the temperature more often, give the Tylenol or aspirin more regularly, perhaps even administer a cool bath (see page 132).

And if it is a low-grade temperature?

You can relax a bit. Don't be that worried. Use the above treatment for a day or two. If the low-grade temperature persists, then take the baby to the doctor. But do remember, temperatures tend to be lower in the morning than the evening, so if the child has been having fever for two to three days, don't be fooled with a normal temperature in the morning, especially if there are associated symptoms.

Can teething be the villain?

Teething doesn't cause fever. A teething child who develops fever is having some other disease. Teething causing fever and other symptoms used to be the notion many years back. It had since proven to be wrong (see page 91). Teething is an innocuous natural phenomenon, calling for a tooth fairy.

Will having a fever benefit my child?

Of course. Fever serves several purposes: it lets you know that there is something wrong, it mobilizes the defenses of the child, and the high temperature is one means of killing the virus your child may be sick with.

Don't infections always lead to fever?

No, infections don't always lead to fever. A good many infections can lead to other signs and symptoms without any rise of temperature. Fever can be an important symptom of infection but it is not always present. Many infections do exist without the presence of any fever.

What is a dangerous fever?

A very high temperature (i.e. 105 to 106 degrees F), especially persisting, can be dangerous. You should call the doctor right away and discuss the line of action.

Please put the following schedule for antipyretics in a place where you can refer to it easily. The medication listed below can be bought without a prescription.

It is better for you to stick to one medication and have it available all the time. And remember:

KEEP ALL MEDICATIONS OUT OF REACH OF CHILDREN

ANTIPYRETICS

AGE	BABY ASPIRIN tablets	TYLENOL syrup	TYLENOL drops	TEMPRA drops	HOW OFTEN: every
6 mos.	1/2 tablet	1/4 tsp.	0.4 ml	0.3 ml	4 hrs.
12 mons.	1 tablet	1/2 tsp.	0.8 ml	0.6 ml	4 hrs.
18 mons.	* 1 to 1 1/2	1/2 to 3/4	0.8 to 1.2	0.6 to 0.9	4 hrs.
2 yrs.	* 1 1/2 to 2	3/4 to 1	1.2 to 1.6	0.9 to 1.2	4 hrs.
2 1/2 yrs.	2 tablets	1 tsp.	1.6	1.2	4 hrs.
3 yrs.	* 2 to 3	1 to 1 1/2	LESS LIKELY TO USE		4 hrs.
3 1/2 yrs.	3 tablets	1 1/2	THE DROPS AFTER		4 hrs.
4 yrs.	* 3 to 4	1 1/2 to 2	THE ABOVE AGE		4 hrs.
5 yrs.	4 tablets or 1 adult tablet	2 tsp. or 1 adult tablet			4 hrs.
10 yrs.	2 adult tablets	2 adult tablets			4 hrs.

* above means dose depends on the size of the child.

Baby aspirin tablets can be chewed and so are the chewable Tylenol tablets. There are many preparations similar to Tylenol, such as Tempra syrup. Remember not to overuse the above medications. Use your medications only when needed.

TO BRING A HIGH TEMPERATURE DOWN

It is rare to go through the experience of rearing children without being confronted with a sudden steep rise in temperature that can make parents shake in their boots.

So often, the little one who seems so happy and at ease, becomes irritable and fussy, looks flushed, and seems to be burning up. The parents rush to the thermometer and insert it; to their amazement, the temperature registers 104 degrees F, or even higher.

<u>What do I do in such a situation?</u>

There are three ways of dealing with a situation like this:

1. COOL WATER BATH: This is effective if it is done right, and it is preferred by most doctors. The water in the bathtub should be up to the level of the navel of the sitting child, and should be lukewarm to begin with. Turn on the faucett of cold water slowly, and it will gradually cool the water. In this manner, the child will take the tub experience better.
The child may fuss and fume and try to come out of the bathtub, but keep him or her in it and pour some of the water over back and chest. In a few minutes the child will accept the predicament and may even like it. Twenty-five to thirty minutes should be spent in the tub; diligently time this with your watch. Remember that dipping the child in and out of the water is useless, since it doesn't give enough time for the water in the bathtub to absorb the heat from the skin.
Once you are done with this procedure, you will see that the high temperature may have come down a few degrees (to 100 to 102 degrees F) and remained so for a number of hours.

2. SPONGING: This is done by mixing some rubbing alcohol with water, soaking a wash towel in it, wringing the washtowel, then spreading it on the child's bare chest or abdomen. When the towel warms up, you put it back in the bowl of alcohol with water and repeat the procedure, this time on the bare back, the thighs, or another big surface area of the skin. The child must remain in the nude, and

may fight you, cry, and shiver. You will persist in sponging for twenty-five to thirty minutes, and you will see that the temperature will have dropped down to 100 to 102 degrees F in most cases.
Some parents and only a few doctors prefer this method to the cool water bath, and by far the majority of doctors side with the bathtub. Sponging works because the rubbing alcohol on the skin evaporates gradually. When the alcohol evaporates it absorbs the heat from the child, thus lowering the temperature to a reasonable level.

3. COLD WATER ENEMA: Although this method also helps bring down the child's high temperature, it is in disfavor, and is rarely used. To do it, you add one teaspoon of table salt to one pint of cold water and offer it in the form of an enema. The cold water will absorb the heat from inside and whether the child expels or retains it, his or her temperature will start dropping down to a more reasonable level in a matter of one-half to one hour. Remember, when given, the enema is to absorb the heat from the child's colon, not solely to move his or her bowels.
Any of the three above methods is messy and makes the child struggle and resist, yet each helps bring the temperature down effectively in most cases.
Of course, you should also continue to use an antipyretic such as aspirin or an equivalent, every four hours.

What if I don't treat the fever?

If the temperature is that high (especially above 104 degrees F) and you don't try to bring it down, there is a chance:

1. That the temperature will have peaked up, and it may start coming down by itself or with an antipyretic such as aspirin or Tylenol.
2. That the temperature might climb higher, say to 105 or 106 degrees F level. At this level, complications in the central nervous system may result if the temperature remains high for a long time. This can be disasterous.
3. That a febrile convulsion may develop in children who are likely to have this kind of trouble.

Remember please, most children shoot their high temperature in the evening. A child who has had a temperature of 101 to 102 degrees F during daytime, is likely to have a much higher temperature in the evening or midnight. If such a child is checked by his doctor earlier that day and put on the proper medication, you are more likely to avoid much of the trouble high temperature gives.

Another point worth repeating here, is that overclothing the feverish child tends to keep the temperature high. Therefore avoid this tendency. Also don't forget to give the child cold liquids, such as coke, crushed ice and similar things, since this helps absorb the heat as well as replace the fluid loss caused by the fever.

FEBRILE CONVULSIONS

It is the most common form of convulsions in children. It scares anybody -the poor child's temperature shoots up, he or she starts to twitch; arms, legs, and the whole body seem to twitch mercilessly. Parents have the urge to hold the child still to stop those blasted twitches, but the helpless child is oblivious to the world around, clenching the fists and teeth, frothing at the mouth, usually twitching and turning the face to one side, and breathing with difficulty. The child's color may even turn blue.

The parents will have a sinking sensation inside; they are so alarmed and feel so helpless.

What shall we do?

The immediate thing is to clear the breathing passages and to stop the child from biting his or her tongue. A convulsing child is likely to "drown in his or her own saliva" and/or bite the tongue severely. Therefore, a parent ought to turn the head to one side, get hold of an object with a round edge, such as the handle of a knife, and put it (not force it) between the child's upper and lower jaw teeth. Make sure to cover the handle of the knife with a piece of cloth so that the child's teeth can be protected. Do not put fingers in the mouth because you may end up with a terrible bite.

Separating the jaws will prevent biting of the tongue, and

turning of the head towards one side will help drain the saliva and open the respiratory tract. If the child is left on his or her back facing the ceiling, the tongue might obstruct the respiratory tract and choke the child.

In most cases the convulsion lasts for only a few minutes. This may seem like hours. Of course call the doctor right away, or let someone else call if you are busy with the convulsing child.

Why does my child get febrile convulsions?

Some children have this tendency, but it is good to know that most of them usually outgrow it when they become six years old or older. Whatever its cause, in some children the sudden rise of temperature can lead to a special response of the brain that signals a convulsion.

Usually the tendency runs in the family and you may find a relative who had suffered from it during his or her childhood.

Do these convulsions tend to come back?

Unfortunately, most children who get the febrile convulsion tend to have a recurrence, although some lucky ones may get only one. The majority, however, may show febrile convulsions of various severity, some being mild and lasting a few seconds, others being severe, prolonged and lasting even as long as half an hour or more.

When would you investigate the case?

If it is a mild convulsion happening for the first time, lasting only a few minutes, your doctor may elect not to investigate.

If the convulsion is prolonged, if it is severe, if it affects only half of the body or only one limb, if it is not associated with high enough fever, or if it is repeated, then it is worth the investigation.

A spinal tap, X-ray of the skull, EEG, blood tests, etc., are worth doing, even if we suspect that they will turn out to be normal. Each case, however, has to be considered according to its own merits.

Can we prevent them?

Most authorities agree that giving phenobarbital (prescription) will prevent these febrile convulsions. Some authorities feel that phenobarbital should be given only when the child develops the fever, and it should be accompanied by an antipyretic such as aspirin or Tylenol. Often this method fails, since the temperature shoots up so fast that the phenobarbital absorption is not fast enough to stop it -a high enough level of phenobarbital in the blood takes some time to build (two to three days).

Most authorities suggest putting the child on phenobarbital every day, whether sick or not, until the age of about five to six years. This is to be done if the child has experienced a few mild febrile convulsions, or one or two severe ones.

Given in the above way, the phenobarbital is not habit-forming, it helps prevent many would-be febrile convulsions (but not all), and it is safe to give if the proper dose is used.

Will my child be likely to have epilepsy?

The majority of children who have the experience of febrile convulsions outgrow them by around the age of five to six years or after. Only a very small percentage of children may show a tendency towards epilepsy.

VIRUSES, BACTERIA, AND FUNGI

Viruses, bacteria, and fungi are the main cause of diseases, the major source of misery and morbidity to all ages. They are present in the environment almost everywhere, but in various degrees of concentration. The troublesome group of these agents form only a small percentage of the family of germs at large. The majority, however, serve a very useful role in the execution of beneficial functions in nature.

They are microscopic in size, though the viruses are often smaller than that. They vary in shape, constitution, and reactions, and can thus be classified into families, groups, and subgroups.

What are the viruses?

The viruses are the smallest and tiniest of these living things. Some can be seen with the aid of an ordinary microscope, but many require larger magnification to be seen. There are many viruses, some can cause mild diseases, others can cause dreadful if not deadly diseases. Some can infect the respiratory system, others the gastrointestinal system, while others produce generalized infections.

Antibiotics are useless in their confrontation with viruses, and medical science has to find other ways to combat them. Research is constant towards that endeavor and only a minor degree of success is at hand at the present time.

How about bacteria?

Bacteria are larger than viruses, though not always so. Bacteria can easily be seen under the ordinary microscope, once the slide is prepared and stained properly. They vary in shape from globular, to rod-like, to spiral-shaped, among other forms. They may form a chain and look beaded (e.g. streptococcus), or group themselves like a bunch of grapes (staphylococcus), or thay may be paired (pneumococcus or gonococcus).

Some bacteria have tiny tentacles called cilia, others have a capsule, and still others develop "spores"; each of these characteristics will help doctors study these germs and develop means of identifying them and fighting them.

Bacteria prefer certain circumstances and certain media before they can do their dirty work. Some of them prefer the tonsils and pharynx, others prefer the lungs, yet others prefer the intestines; the list goes on and on. Bacteria also vary in their degree of disease production.

How is that?

Some bacteria are notorious for the trouble they give- such as meningococcus, which produces meningitis; but others lead to less dangerous diseases. Cases like pneumonia, tuberculosis, tonsillitis, inflamed ears, boils, impetigo, and shigella diarrhea, are only a few examples.

Although some bacteria produce only one disease (such as TB, typhoid, etc.) others can produce multiple diseases. For example, the pneumococcus, which causes pneumonia and respiratory infections, can also cause ear infections and even meningitis. The "strep" germ can produce tonsillitis, lymphadenitis, scarlatina, impetigo, lymphangitis, etc. Another example is "staph", which can produce boils, abscesses, impetigo, osteomyelitis of the bones, sinusitis, etc.

Antibiotics are not the absolute answer in getting rid of the germs, since the body's resistance and the mobilization of its defences are the essential elements of fighting disease. Before the era of antibiotics, though, the toll of suffering, complications, morbidity, and mortality was quite high. With the availability of the antibiotics, a wonderful aid to the body's resistance was discovered, and the result has been less suffering and better control of disease.

How about the fungi?

A fungus is a form of germ with special mode of behavior in its growth, requirements, and forms of infection.

Most fungi infect the skin, producing various forms of ringworm (of the body or scalp), athlete's foot, or even diaper rash and thrush as is the case with candida. If they enter the circulation they can be devastating, especially in the debilitated.

Fungi produce slowly spreading diseases, which often are annoying because they can go on for a long time. Fortunately, many medications have appeared in the market that can easily conquer these diseases, but you will still have to use such agents for about two weeks or so. In case of fungus infection of the scalp or the nail, often medicines must be taken internally, and this may have to be done for a few months.

Fungus infections often spread in a slow manner from one person to another and some of the infections come from infected animals, such as dogs and cats.

VIRAL INFECTIONS

Viruses are probably the commonest cause of diseases. They are easily transmissible from one person to another, and the reservoir of infected people seems to be constantly there. It is amazing that as tiny and as insignificant-looking as they are, they can produce so much misery and trouble to people. Viruses have no respect for age, beauty, wealth or royalty! They simply do their nasty work to everyone who is exposed to them and who has not built a resistance towards them.

Are there many kinds of viruses?
Yes there are. Although there are many useful viruses, our concern here is about disease-producing viruses. There are many families of such viruses and each is divided into groups and subgroups.

Some viruses tend to prefer the respiratory system, particularly that of infants and young children; examples are the syncytial viruses and the parainfluenza viruses. The influenza virus, and the adenoviruses tend to infect the respiratory system of the children and older people. Other viruses, prefer the stomach and intestine and they produce gastroenteritis. Some others, such as the rotavirus and echovirus, prefer the stomach and intestine and they produce gastroenteritis. Some viruses prefer the skin; an example is the herpesvirus which produces fever blisters or infection in the genitalia. Another virus is the cause of warts.

Coxsackievirus is one which prefers the throat, producing herpangina, and at times can spread and produce severe problems to the unfortunate victim.

Each group of these viruses usually subdivides into many, and each of these subgroups can infect, thus we remain liable to pick up many infections from the same group depending on our exposure.

What kind of respiratory infection do viruses produce?
The most common is the common cold, which is caused by various rhinoviruses and others. The familiar upper respiratory infections, leading to bronchitis, pneumonia, etc., are quite common, and hardly a child can escape having one or two of them a winter. About eighty-five percent of these infections are caused by viruses, be it the syncytial, para-influenza, adeno, influenza, or others.

It is not that rare for some bacteria to take advantage of the situation and impose themselves on the virally infected area. This leads to many complications, from the infected postnasal drip, to tonsillitis or infected ears, to others that are more rare.

As suspected, most such infections are common during wintertime, and they spread through coughing, sneezing, kissing or other forms of close contact.

How about the ones causing gastrointestinal problems?

Most cases of gastroenteritis are caused by viruses, though the ones discovered so far can be counted on the fingers. Rotavirus may be common during wintertime especially in children and babies, and it can lead to troublesome, sometimes hard-to-control vomiting and diarrhea. Echovirus is another but less troublesome virus that often produces gastroenteritis, more during summertime than wintertime.

Similar symptoms can be produced by bacteria but this is rare, especially in the U.S. Unlike the case with the respiratory system, bacteria are unlikely to impose themselves after a viral gastroenteritis. All such gastrointestinal problems, be they viral or bacterial, can spread by close contact and through contaminated hands, from handling the bottom and the diaper area.

How about the viruses infecting the skin?

Viruses causing fever blisters (herpesvirus type I) are common, as you may suspect. Though this condition is common and often of little significance, it may occasionally cause real trouble to the newborn or to someone with eczema.

A very common slow virus leads to the production of warts. Most children will show up with a wart or two or a crop of them, and many by the time of their adolescence will be able to get rid of the warts by having developed a high level of resistance. Other viruses can cause some special skin diseases but they are not that common.

Do viruses infect other areas?

Yes they do, and they may cause real trouble. Some cause generalized disease such as infectious mononucleosis, measles, mumps, german measles, chicken pox, smallpox, etc. Some viruses can cause meningitis or some other dreadful diseases, such as polio. Fortunately some of the viral diseases are disappearing from the scene as they come under control.

How are viruses controlled?

With the advances in medical science, preventive measures are becoming more and more available. Smallpox has practically disappeared from the world, and polio, measles, mumps, and German measles (rubella) can be fully prevented if every child gets immunizations against them. But the number of viruses is large, and the hope for the future is to have an ever-increasing number of preventive vaccines.

Prevention of some viral infections is much easier than treatment of them. Antibiotics are useless for either preventing or treating viral diseases. The case is different with bacteria.

There are only very few agents that can be used in treating certain viral infections, and even so they are difficult to use and need special expertise. For practical purposes, however, we can safely say that there are no specific modes of treating viral infections. We have to depend on the resistance of the body in fighting such infections, and the treatment remains symptomatic, i.e. treating the symptoms as they show up and hope for the best.

FLU

The child may have a high temperature and achiness all over; the child may be hardly able to drag his or her body around, looking like a ghost with deep circles under the eyes, and eating practically nothing.

Another child in the same family may have some vomiting and/or diarrhea, with severe cramps in the stomach, cramps that may even cause doubling over.

Yet, a third child may have completely different symptoms. His or her nose may be stuffy, the cough may be barking, painful, and frequent, the temperature quite high, and the energy level sunken down to zero.

These are the different faces of the flu. Each of the above children has suffered in a different way from the same disease.

Does flu always affect the whole family?

Flu is highly contagious, and it is not encouraging to know that it is far more likely than not to cause the whole family suffering. During an epidemic the schools have a good number of absent students and teachers. Occasionally it may even be necessary to close the school for a few days. The whole community may come under the heavy invasion of the flu virus for as long as several weeks. You will read about it in the papers, or hear about it on the radio or TV; but count your blessings if you escape it completely.

How often should we expect this unpleasant situation?

Generally speaking, small, relatively insignificant epidemics of flu show up almost every year during the cold season. Then, every four years or so, a big epidemic may show up, making everyone suffer miserably for some time.

What causes the flu?

A mean virus is the cause. This virus tends to change its antigenicity every so often, making it very difficult to produce a specific vaccine to that particular strain of virus.

Do you mean the flu vaccine is useless?

No, not necessarily. Flu vaccine may be of some help if the flu of the year is caused by a virus to which a vaccine has already been synthesized. That is, in some years, the flu vaccine may work and in other years it may not, depending on what changes the virus had decided to undergo. Thus not everyone needs the vaccine.

When, then, should we use the flu vaccine?

For your child, you may use it in case the child suffers from asthma, cystic fibrosis, congenital heart disease, diabetes or any other disease that may make having the flu a heavy burden, with more chances of complications.

Children who seem healthy usually don't need the flu vaccine.

If we are to get the flu shots, how often should we get them?

In general, you may need two flu shots, two months apart or so and that is in case you have never had the flu shots before, or had them more than five years ago.

After getting the initial series, you have to get the flu booster shot once a year. Autumn is the best time; it is too late to get the shots during the flu epidemic.

Do I have to see the doctor in case my child has the flu?

By and large, yes. The child will be examined, to make sure there are no bacterial complications. If the child is diagnosed as having only the flu, the treatment is simply symptomatic, i.e. treatment of the symptoms: physical rest, Tylenol (for fever and achiness), cough syrup (see page 303), and humidifier for the cough (see page 290).

CAUTION: Don't use aspirin in cases of the flu, use Tylenol or an equivalent instead.

How about an antibiotic?

You certainly don't need an antibiotic unless, in addition to the flu, there is bacterial infection present, such as an ear infection, tonsillitis, etc. This is one of the important reasons your doctor should see the child with the flu.

Is there any other reason he should see my child?

Yes, and it is an important one. The flu symptoms can mimic many diseases. You will not be able to differentiate between flu with respiratory symptoms, and pneumonia; or between vomiting caused by flu, and appendicitis; or between fever and headache of the flu, and meningitis. Such dreaded examples do appear in every pediatrician's office. Therefore, don't be lulled into the belief that since the flu is hitting everybody, your child has nothing but the flu. Your child's symptoms may quite well be something completely different.

WHY THE CULTURE

Taking a culture is not a new innovation, but its use in the office is an advance in the science of delivering medicine. Cultures have been in use for a long time, but mainly in the hospitals. The office use of cultures has become practical only recently and it has helped pinpoint the diagnoses. Its use has proved so important that without it the office can be called obsolete.

What do throat cultures tell us?

Infection of the throat can result from viruses or bacteria. One of these bacteria is the strep (see page 145), and information that indicates whether or not strep exists can be found in throat cultures taken on some patients who have respiratory infections, postnasal drip, tonsillitis, pharyngitis, etc.

We also take cultures of any pussy matter or discharge. We gain a good deal of information from such cultures. A culture taken from a child who has pussy discharge from a "blocked" nose, or from a child with matter coming from a pink eye, may give us many surprises, and the treatment may have to be adjusted depending on what the culture shows. This is also true of a discharge from the ear or the vagina.

Do you do cultures of the skin too?

In certain skin diseases it is mandatory. An example is impetigo; if the culture of the impetigo shows staph, you may want to treat it only with an ointment and an internal medicine for a few days, but if the impetigo culture shows strep, then you will have to treat it with internal medication for ten days.

A boil, an abscess, a stye, or a pussy blister will each have to be cultured when it is opened. Although staph germ is the usual villain, surprises do happen.

There are also specialized skin cultures for fungus, but these are usually taken care of by the dermatologist.

How about urine cultures?

These are essential whenever we suspect urinary tract infection. Such a urine culture can be done in the office, from a urine specimen in a sterilized container. Such a culture is somewhat more complicated to do than throat culture and it requires four culture media. A colony count should also be done (see page 413). If the culture is positive and the colony count is big enough, then we have to do what is called a sensitivity test. This is a test that also requires twenty-four hours before we can read it, and it shows what kind of medicine the germ is most sensitive to.

If this battery of testing is done correctly, we will know what kind of germ has caused the urinary tract infection and what medicine can be most effective in killing it.

A screening urine culture is found to be a valuable addition to the other tests children ought to have. It is done on females coming for their yearly checkup (see page 413).

What is the screening urine culture?

It is a culture to be done on the urine of females at least every year, sometimes in addition to the urinalysis. That is because some girls can have urinary tract infection without showing any symptoms and without having any pus cells in the urine. It is estimated that around five girls with such an infection can be discovered in a year's time in a pediatrics' office. Such girls have no trouble urinating i.e. there is no burning on urinating, they don't go too often to the bathroom, they have no stomachache or other symptoms. They feel perfectly normal, yet when their urine is cultured, the culture turns out to be positive. This means that such patients have silent infection (infection without symptoms), and early treatment of such infection can prevent trouble in the future.

Boys are not prone to such an ordeal, and they don't have to have the screening urine culture.

Aren't these cultures expensive?

Yes, the cost adds up. We as pediatricians, are just as concerned. But the medical value of these cultures is so unquestionable, and the surprising results we get at times are such that they easily justify the expense and more. They help greatly in pin-pointing the cause of the suspected infection and in the treatment as well.

THE STREP GERM
Streptococcus

Strep (streptococcus) is a colorful germ, mean at times, dangerous at other times, and tends to infect various parts of the body, giving rise to different diseases. Most of us have heard of strep throat, tonsillitis, pharyngitis, scarlatina, blood poisoning, impetigo, etc. Many such diseases are caused by the strep, some exclusively so.

There are almost 200 varieties of streptococcus. Therefore the chance for reinfection is great. The mode of infection is such as to make the strep an easy germ to spread. Not only that, but a strep infection, if not treated, is likely to lead to some serious immediate disease, or later aftermaths.

How is that?

The immediate diseases usually consist of strep pharyngitis, acute tonsillitis, scarlatina, infected lymph nodes, nasal infections, blood poisoning (lymphangitis), and impetigo. There are many other diseases caused by strep, but they are not that common.

If these diseases are left untreated, in three to five percent the body will somehow develop certain conditions, leading to rheumatic fever (see page 166) or glomerulonephritis (see page 418). These diseases are dangerous, debilitating at times, and may even lead to fatality. These diseases are preventable simply by discovering the strep and treating it immediately.

How can we discover the strep?

When the acute strep infections (diseases mentioned above) show up in the child, take the child to the doctor right away. Once checked, and after a culture is taken, medication is to be used. A course of ten days of penicillin (or equivalent in case of penicillin allergy) will be given.

Why a ten-days' course of penicillin?

Once the child is put on medication, he will respond within twelve to twenty-four hours. However, the medicine has to be used for the ten days. Though the patient will feel good and you will wonder why you should keep administering the medicine, the medicine has to be used for that long to completely eradicate the strep.

Even when used for ten days, medications still won't eradicate the strep in one out of every ten patients. That is the reason we repeat the culture after the course of medication has been finished. If this culture proves negative, everyone will feel at ease, but if it is still positive, a second course of medication is to be used, again a ten-day course, but usually with a medicine other than penicillin.

This course is to be followed by another culture. This culture usually proves to be negative; if not, other measures will have to be taken.

Why insist on eradicating the strep?

If the strep is not eradicated, it may lead to further infections, repeatedly. The child will keep getting sick, and become a source of strep infection in the family whereby many members of the family will keep getting infected and pass the infection to each other. It is not rare to see a pediatrician having two to three such families every winter.

Is it that contagious?

Strep infection is fairly contagious. A family whose child has strep infection stands a ten to forty percent chance of picking up the infection, depending on how close the members of this family are. Therefore when a child comes down with the strep infection, often we take throat cultures of every member in the family, even if everyone in the family feels good and has no sore throat or any other symptoms. In this way, we can see who has picked up the strep, and treat such person accordingly.

Is it worth all this trouble?

Going through this nice "ordeal" of culturing has paid a great dividend in recent history. Because of this approach, the infections that used to jump through families from one member to the other like ping-pong balls, have been reduced to a great extent.

Besides that, rheumatic fever and glomerulonephritis have become rare, and rheumatic heart diseases have been disappearing from the scene. Rheumatic fever and glomerulonephritis are well rid of; they are serious diseases, associated with much suffering if not crippling effect.

Will you then do a culture on everyone suspected of strep?

Yes. Identifying any germs is very important, be it in the throat, skin or any discharge. This is more so when there is suspicion that strep may be there.

Only exceptionally do we see strep cases where treatment won't be able to eradicate the germ, no matter how persistent and vigorous this treatment is. In such a situation, the tonsils and adenoids will have to be removed since the strep may be hiding deep inside "pus pockets" in the tonsils. This is rare indeed.

THE GERM CALLED "STAPH"
STAPHYLOCOCCUS

The staph germ (staphylococcus) can be distressing in its own way, and it may lead to various types of infection, some merely a nuisance, others quite dangerous. It may strike different organs, like the skin, lungs, bones, nasal passages, and others.

If it hits the skin, it can lead to impetigo, boils, abscesses, carbuncles, styes, etc. When it hits the respiratory tract, it may infect the sinuses, the ears, the lymph nodes under the angle of the jaw, or even the lungs (especially in babies). Staph infection of the bones (osteomyelitis) used to be quite troublesome and still is.

<u>What will the skin look like?</u>

If there is impetigo, the lesions are dull red, small but variable in size, slowly spreading, but hardly itchy; they may have a yellow crust on top, and in general, they are ugly-looking.

If the staph infection is deeper, it can lead to a slightly swollen "gouched" lesion, called echthyma, that is likely to stay in for a long time (months).

Boils are familiar to most people and they tend to come out every once in a while, sometimes two or three at a time. They are the ones with cores.

An abscess is bigger than a boil; more advanced, so to speak. Of course, a carbuncle is the big abscess with many "eyes", (they are "tunnels" full of pus). The styes are like boils, but affect the eyelids; an eyelash juts out from the center of the stye.

<u>What else can the staph do?</u>

As mentioned before, it can infect the ears. Such an ear infection, however, is quite rare compared to those caused by other offending germs.

If staph shows in a throat culture, it is usually meaningless, since it is regarded as no more than a parasite over there. A throat culture showing staph is considered a normal culture and no treatment is needed for the throat.

However, staph can be nasty in the sinuses, which mainly affect older children and adults. The sinuses can suffer for weeks; pussy yellowish-green mucus can come out, and can lead to postnasal drip. Though a person with an allergic constitution is more likely to get sinus trouble, staph or other germs can come on top of the allergy and put the sinuses in a miserable shape.

Another trouble the staph germ gives is infection of the nodes at the angle of the jaw. These will be easily seen if you ask the child to raise his or her head and look at the ceiling. By so doing, the bumps will show as big as a walnut or bigger, and may be tender to the touch. They may even become abscessed if left untreated for long enough.

Staph can lead to staph pneumonia, which is extremely dangerous, especially in small babies. Fortunately this is rare.

PNEUMOCOCCUS

Pneumococcus is a germ that is more likely to invade the respiratory tract than anything else. It is sneaky, often lying still without causing any trouble. Every once in a while, however, it can be quite troublesome, and it may give rise to a variety of different diseases. As said above, most such diseases are of the respiratory tract.

What are some examples?

A good example is pneumonia. Such a disease used to be the dread of everyone in the days when antibiotics were not available. Nowadays it can easily be controlled, although pneumonia can still be classified as a troublesome disease. Pneumococcus can also cause bronchitis of various types and severity; it can also cause some complications of the common cold. In such cases, when the cold is over, the child may start to have yellowish-green thick discharge from the nose.

In older children and adults, sinusitis and sinus trouble may be the result of pneumococcus infection too, and this can play havoc with the rest and comfort of the patient.

Does pneumococcus cause any other kinds of infections?

It is one of the germs that can cause ear infections, and it can also be one of the causes of pink eye.

In rare cases it can cause pleurisy, and even meningitis, among other diseases.

Are there any ways to prevent getting this bug?

Unfortunately, so far there are no shots or medicines that can make us immune to all varieties of this germ. There is a shot that can prevent only certain types of this germ. So we are at the mercy of our degree of exposure to it, our condition of resistance, our body's fighting capacity and many many other parameters.

Pneumococcus vaccine is available, but it is given to some rare select patients with certain conditions such as in patients who had their spleen removed.

What can you do for it?

Thankfully, pneumococcus can easily be killed by antibiotics if they are properly chosen and if they are given for a long enough time. Many drugs can easily get rid of this germ, especially penicillins.

Even though pneumococcus produces pneumonia, bronchitis, or upper respiratory infection, culture of the throat may not help at all. Antibiotics are usually prescribed in these cases.

How easily can pneumococcus spread?

As stated before, this germ is sneaky. It might be present in the respiratory tract as a parasite, not causing any trouble, yet waiting for the proper moment to strike. In such cases we don't even bother to eradicate it. But when there are diseases indicating the pneumococcus as a cause or effect, then it is time for treatment.

Happily it is not that contagious, at least not as contagious as strep. For pneumococcus to be contagious, there has to be close contact, such as coughing at a close distance, or kissing.

It is not rare to see a few members of a family suffering from a variety of infections caused by this germ. Fortunately, treating with the proper antibiotics will set things right again.

ANTIBIOTICS: USE AND ABUSE

Will you call me some penicillin, please?

So the parent pleads over the phone. After all, the child is having a fever and is feeling sick, and an antibiotic is a cure for all.

What is wrong with that?

To call for an antibiotic blindly is not right; it is not fair to your child nor to yourself. Even though it seems to you that the fever is caused by some "infection", you have to know more about the condition of the child before you can give the proper medicine.

In other words, the kind of antibiotic to be used depends on:

1. where the infection is,
2. what kind of infection it is,
3. how severe the infection is,
4. how old the child is, and
5. a good many other factors the doctor must consider.

Doctors are in the dark when a parent says the child has some form of infection and may need an antibiotic. If the child proves to have a virus, an antibiotic will be useless. Conditions such as gastroenteritis, flu, colds, or upper respiratory infections, are mostly viral infections and don't need any antibiotic, and they may even become worse with the use of an antibiotic.

Besides, the doctor who prescribes a medicine over the phone will be legally responsible, and if it happens to be the wrong medicine prescribed (since the doctor hasn't seen the child), then legal trouble can arise.

What is the harm in using antibiotics if they don't hurt?

Don't say antibiotics can't hurt. Antibiotics can be mischievous at times; tetracyclines can make the teeth an unsightly yellow for life, if they are used in children before the age of 8 to 10 years. Some antibiotics can produce photosensitivity and rash. Overuse of an antibiotic can help fungus to invade the mouth, and the area of the underpants.

Some antibiotics may prove allergenic, such as penicillin, and others can irritate the intestine, leading to diarrhea.

Does this mean you want to be stingy in using antibiotics?

No, not at all. When an antibiotic is needed, be it penicillin, ampicillin, sulfa or others, it should be used wisely and carefully according to type, severity, and location of infection; and it must suit the proper age of the child. To use it haphazardly will give you a haphazard result.

How long should an antibiotic be used?

The length of treatment is just as important as the type and dose of the antibiotic you choose. For ear infections, that length is ten days. This is also true of strep infections.

But in case of certain urinary tract infections, you may have the ungodly mess of using the medicine for at least two weeks and up to six months or longer, depending on the type and chronicity of the infection. Infections such as bronchitis or pneumonia require antibiotics for variable periods depending on many special factors of their own.

How about antibiotic injections?

On certain occasions such shots may be needed. Penicillin and bicillin are very useful, when used properly and conservatively. Some other severe infections may respond better to shots of specific antibiotics.

However, too many shots of one antibiotic are likely to be quite sensitizing; the child may become allergic to them, and will be deprived from their benefit in the future.

To make a pincushion of the poor child's buttocks is a disservice to the child and to the art of medicine.

How about giving two antibiotics to get
rid of the bug once and for all?

That is a form of abuse of the antibiotics. For most patients seen in the office, one antibiotic is enough. If it hasn't worked after a few days, then take another look:

1. Is there a complication?
2. Was the infection a virus, therefore not needing an antibiotic?
3. Was the germ resistant to that special antibiotic.
4. Were there some other reasons?

Don't be hung up on antibiotics; cooperation with nature and using antibiotics only when nature needs help is best. Your child will be much healthier that way, and will benefit in the long run.

ROSEOLA

Their temperatures shoot up all of a sudden; the mercury keeps going up and down, not unusually up to 104 degrees F and higher. They are fussy, their color tends to be flushed and nothing seems to please them. They eat as usual, though occasionally their appetites seem to suffer. An antipyretic such as aspirin or Tylenol seems to be of only temporary help.

This state of affairs continues for as long as three days. Then, and only then, their temperatures drop down to normal and you give a sigh of relief. But to your surprise, they become covered with rash. The rash is rosy pink and in small spots, and it covers them all over, including their faces. During this period of rash they continue to be fussy, but act normal otherwise. These are babies with roseola.

Why did you use the term "babies"?

Roseola affects babies most frequently. Rarely at all does it appear before the age of six months or so. It shows up most commonly between the ages of six and twelve months. After the age of one year it shows up less frequently, and it is very rare indeed after the age of two years.

How long does the rash last?

In most cases, the rash lasts for three days. Only rarely does it last for less or more than three days. The rash shows up in most cases after the temperature has dropped down to normal. In rare cases it may show up a few hours or more after the temperature has come down to normal. The rash is not itchy, bothersome, nor blistery. If the rash shows up while the baby is still feverish, then it is not a case of roseola.

Is roseola contagious?

Roseola is not that contagious, but you may not have to worry about that anyway, since it affects mainly babies and not older children.

It is a disease entity by itself, caused by a virus, and is not a form of measles.

How can we prevent it?

In most cases the baby breaks out with roseola as if from nowhere, without any known exposure. So far there is no known way to prevent this disease.

The disease is innocent enough, though on rare occasions it may cause trouble.

What do you mean by that?

In most cases of roseola, the baby will have a high temperature for three days, and this will be followed by the rash for three days, then the condition ends and the baby is as happy as could be.

In a few cases, however, as the baby's temperature shoots up, he or she will develop a generalized convulsion. The convulsion can be quite nasty and prolonged at times and difficult to stop. These convulsions cause the most concern about roseola. Fortunately, they do not mean that the baby is going to have a convulsion with each and every rise of temperature.

Can you diagnose roseola easily?

Every baby with a high temperature, especially for longer than twenty-four hours, ought to be checked by the doctor. If the feverish baby comes to the office before the rash appears, the doctor will see a slightly red throat and may identify the problem as a virus. He or she may take an educated guess and warn the parents to look for the possibility of roseola. In other words, there is no sure way to diagnose roseola until the temperature has come down to normal by the third day, and has been followed by the rash. Fortunately roseola shows up only once in a lifetime.

What is the treatment for roseola?
 Since roseola is a viral infection, all you can do is use an antipyretic such as aspirin or Tylenol, tub-bath when needed (see page 136) and count your blessings when the roseola is over. Antibiotics are not needed for such a disease, nor are any other medicines. It is good to know that complications don't show up in most cases of roseola.

SCARLATINA

Their bodies are covered with rash, but not their faces. The rash consists of bright red pinpoints, and causes no itching. Their faces are quite pale around the lips, yet they have rosy cheeks. Their temperatures are usually high, their throats are quite sore, and even their talk has a twang in it as if their throats are lumpy and sore. They look sick, and feel sick, but when the doctor asks "How are you?" they answer, "Fine!"
 These are children with scarlatina.

What is scarlatina?
 Scarlatina is the Latin term for scarlet fever; it is not, as some parents think, merely a mild form of scarlet fever.

What causes scarlatina, and what happens if it is untreated?
 Scarlatina is caused by the strep germ, be it in the throat or somewhere else. The strep can cause trouble when not treated. If not treated or treated too late, glomerulonephritis of the kidneys or rheumatic fever may be the result, or a string of other complications in the ears, throat or other areas (see page 145).

We hope that all cases of scarlatina are treated promptly, since it can be a serious disease. If it is untreated, the rash will slowly go away, the temperature will gradually come down and the child will look slightly better, even though the complications are only beginning to set in, and may do so for weeks! So don't let the appearance of well-being lure you.

What will the doctor do for it?

A throat culture is a must. A ten-day course of penicillin medication will be given (or a bicillin shot), and that will depend on how severe the scarlatina is and who is treating it. Prompt treatment is essential.

Usually the culture will be read by the next morning; if it is positive, then a culture on everyone in the family will have to be taken. About ten to forty percent of the exposed family members stand a chance of having picked up the germ, depending on how close they had been with the patient, and how long. (Kissing the patient is a good way of picking up the infection.) Family members who have picked up the germ will have to be treated too.

How about quarantining?

In the "good" old days, they used to quarantine the family for a certain period of time. Antibiotics were not heard of in those days, so the treatment used to be to wait, and pray that no complications would show up.

But now, with specific treatment readily available, you don't have to go through that.

How about school?

On being diagnosed as having scarlatina, the child should be kept at home, and away from contact with sisters and brothers, etc., for a period of one to two days. By then, the medicine will have eradicated enough of the strep to make it safe for the child to mix with others.

The child can also go to school a few days after the symptoms have come under control, but on condition that he or she continues with the medication.

How about a repeat culture?

A repeat throat culture, two or three days after the course of treatment is finished, is a good thing to do. The reason is that the strep is not eradicated by the treatment of about ten percent. Some doctors even recommend a urinalysis afterwards, to make sure the kidneys haven't been involved.

A few tidbits about scarlatina:

1. My child had fever that is going down now, but he or she is covered with a rash. What is going on?
   You better see the doctor for the correct diagnosis. Scarlatina can be sneaky sometimes and appear in unusual forms. Don't take chances.
2. I had scarlatina when I was a child, can I pick it up again?
   Yes, you may pick up a strep infection; you are not as immune as you think.
3. The child's sibling doesn't have tonsils, can he or she pick up the strep?
   Yes, it is possible, tonsils or not.
4. The child's sibling is allergic to penicillin. What will you do if he or she picks up the germ?
   Other medicines are available, and they are good substitutes.
5. If the child gets it once, can it occur again?
   Yes, it is possible, especially if the scarlatina is treated so early that the body hasn't had the chance to build immunity to it yet.

CHICKENPOX

So many watery blisters are popping up; each is about the size of a lentil or split pea, has a red base, and causes a good deal of itching that can drive the child crazy. These blisters appear in successive crops, usually on the chest, back, and abdomen, then gradually spread all over, in a matter of a few days.

Fever may be there (but not necessarily) and so are other symptoms. Some attacks can be quite severe, and the blisters will cover the child all over, yet in mild cases of chickenpox, the blisters are relatively few, but scattered here and there and don't amount to anything significant.

Is it a cousin of smallpox?

Smallpox may look like chickenpox to the untrained eye, but it is a vastly different disease. Smallpox is a tremendous public health hazard. We hope not to see smallpox anymore in our time; it has probably been eradicated completely.

Are there any vaccines against the chickenpox?

Yes, but not for general use as of this writing. Chickenpox is more or less a mild disease. Though it can lead to complications, these complications are so uncommon and mild, that so far the vaccine has not been recommended for the general public.

What can you do for the chickenpox?

Not much, other than let it take its course. For the partial relief of the itching, however, a medicine can be prescribed. This medicine, Periactin or Atarax or the like (prescription), will work internally and is much better than local application of Calamine or other lotions. It is also better than giving the child a baking soda bath.

When the itching is mild, however, Calamine lotion or baking soda will do. Let the child soak in a bathtub of lukewarm water to which one cup of baking soda has been added for fifteen to twenty minutes.

What will happen to the rash?

The rash will gradually dry up, leaving a scab which will take a long time to fall off, perhaps three to four weeks. Chickenpox is highly contagious. The child shouldn't be sent to school during the blistery stage, i.e. for a period of about one week. If the child has too many scabs on the face, forearms, and legs, keep him or her a little longer until some of the scabs have fallen off.

Will there be any scars left?

Usually not, but in some cases there are. If the blistery lesions are itchy and the child scratches often, then the lesions can rupture, get infected, become deeper, and lead to a deep scab followed by a scar. To avoid scars on the child's face, parents should try to help stop the scratching medically, verbally or by other means.

Does the chickenpox affect areas other than the skin?

Yes, it can cause a sore throat, with or without bacterial complications. If it affects the eyes, you have to be very much on the vigil. If it affects the ear canal, the canal will swell painfully. If it affects the genitalia, it can disturb the child's tranquility.

Besides the above, there are other complications, some quite serious. Fortunately they are rare. Herpes zoster (shingles) is caused by a dormant chickenpox virus.

Does this mean I have to see the doctor for any case of chickenpox?

No, not at all. If the case is mild, then you treat it at home; wait patiently, discourage the scratching, administer Tylenol (don't use aspirin in chickenpox) for the fever, give baking soda baths, etc.

If there is a possibility that the child is having a complication, and that his or her chickenpox is severe, affecting the eyes, ears, or female genitalia, then invest in an office visit and be on the safe side.

Occasionally, impetigo or other diseases look like chickenpox. So if you are not sure, please consult your doctor about your diagnosis.

How many times will the child get the chickenpox?

Only once in a lifetime, for practically all people.

Can a baby get chickenpox?

Some babies, even at age two months or so pick it up. Chickenpox immunity is not effectively transferred from mother to baby during pregnancy.

The incubation period for chickenpox is fourteen days plus or minus a few days.

MEASLES

To a greater or lesser degree, in this country measles has become a disease of the past, though every year we have a small outbreak here or there. The memory of the massive outbreaks of the times past, however, continue to linger in the minds of many.

What does a measles case look like?
The young child usually starts with what looks like a runny nose, hacky cough, congested and runny eyes sensitive to light, fever, loss of appetite, and, in a few days a rash. The rash is dull red in color, blotchy, starting on the face and neck and descending to the trunk and extremities in a few days. In about a week's time the symptoms will have eased off and the child will recover in a gradual manner.

By so doing, such a child will have built a lifelong immunity.

If that is all to measles, why all the fuss about it?
We fuss about measles mainly because of its complications. Even if a child develops measles without any complications there is no reason why we should not spare him or her the morbidity of measles and spare ourselves the worries about the child's chances to develop complications.

What are the possible complications of measles?
Measles can lead to many many complications. Some of these complications are mild and insignificant, others are troublesome and may even be dangerous. Some rare complications can even be fatal.

Pneumonia, bronchopneumonia, tracheobrochitis, tonsillitis, pharyngitis, and ear infections, are common complications of measles. Most such complications are treatable with antibiotics though some of them may need a fairly extensive course of treatment.

Measles can lead to a certain form of encephalitis, and this is a big worry to a good many pediatricians. Not only that, but there is a disease known as subacute sclerosing panencephalitis that may show up several years after the measles had come and gone. Such complications can lead to convulsive disorders, mental retardation, and even death.

There are a good many other complications not listed here, but it suffices to say that by simply preventing measles we can prevent them all, and avoid the worry and expense that they entail.

How can we prevent measles?

All that needs to be done is to give the child one shot of the live measles vaccine after or around the age of fifteen months. If it is given before the age of twelve months, some children will not develop immunity because of the immune material they received from their mother when they were in the uterus. If the child has had the measles shot before the first birthday, then it will be wise to give a second measles shot sometime later.

It is gratifying to know that one measles shot can be enough to probably give lifelong immunity. Although less than 100 percent of the children develop immunity this way, by far the great majority do.

What reactions are there to the measles shot?

Most children who receive the live measles shot by itself or in conjunction with others (rubella and/or mumps) will develop no reaction whatsoever. However, there are some who will. Such reactions usually show up about a week or so after the shot has been given, and vary from child to child in degree and severity. Possible reactions include a runny nose, cough, rash, fever (usually not that high, but occasionally up to 103 to 104 degrees F or even higher). These symptoms are not contagious. The happy news is that severe reactions to the measles shot are fairly rare.

What shall I do when my child is exposed to measles?

If the child has had the live measles shot, you have little to worry about. In such cases there is only a two to five percent chance the child will catch it after exposure. In case your child has not had the measles shot and is then exposed to a case of measles, call the doctor right away. In such a case, a shot of gamma globulin given early enough will either make the measles less severe or prevent it completely.

If all children get their measles vaccine at the proper age, measles as a disease will disappear altogether.

RUBELLA (GERMAN MEASLES)

Yes indeed, slowly but surely rubella is becoming a controlled disease too and it is hoped that one day it may become extinct. It used to show up in epidemics every few years, and it used to leave its mark on thousands and thousands of babies born following those epidemics.

What kind of disease is it?

Rubella (or three-day measles) is caused by a virus, and it is quite contagious. More often than not, it comes in epidemic forms. A child with this disease will have a pale pink rash all over, and this will usually last for about three days. Some aches and pains, a rise in temperature, and/or slight enlargement of the lymph nodes may show up too. The rash is difficult to ascertain, even sometimes to the trained eyes. That is why it is worth doing a special blood test to see if the patient has immunity to the disease.

Why all the fuss about rubella?

This disease is very innocuous in appearance, but it can be devastating in certain situations. If a pregnant woman develops this disease, especially in the first few months of pregnancy, the chances are high that the baby will be born with many defects. Some of the defects are very serious: blindness, deafness, mental retardation, congenital heart disease, etc. Some babies may even be miscarried or stillborn; having been riddled with abnormalities. Others may be born extremely sick and in need of immediate or extensive care. However, there are some who will have but a few less life-threatening abnormalities, such as deafness in one ear or a minor abnormality of the heart.

If rubella is that severe, can we prevent it?

Thankfully, yes. A vaccine has been developed and it has earned its good reputation. This vaccine is given by most doctors after the child has reached the age of fifteen months, often in the same shot along with measles and mumps. Other doctors may prefer to give separate shots for each of these three preventable diseases.

On the other hand, there are some doctors who prefer to wait on the rubella vaccine until the child is in the second decade of life. In such cases, the males are not given the vaccine, but the females are usually tested (HI test), and if they still prove to be susceptible, they will be given the rubella vaccine. This is often the case in Europe.

Which way is better, and how good is the immunity?

The timing of the shot and the way of its delivery depends on the doctor and his or her conviction. It is easier to give one shot that will confer immunity to these three diseases (measles, mumps, and rubella) all at the same time.

So far the immunity to the shot has proved to be very good, and it is claimed that better than 90 per cent will have developed this immunity with only one shot. No boosters are recommended so far, since the level of immunity has continued to be good ever since rubella shots were first given.

Any reactions to the shots?

If the shot is given to young children, there is only a very small chance for pains in some joints, along with some tenderness and swelling of a joint or two. This is quite rare in the young, but if the child is not vaccinated until later, the chance for such reactions will be bigger. In teenagers, the percentage of such reactions can be uncomfortably high, and it is said that some of them might even develop some arthritis or arthritic changes.

To my mind, giving the rubella vaccine between the ages of one and two years makes the most sense, especially if it is given in conjunction with the measles and mumps vaccine.

How will rubella spread to children who haven't been vaccinated?

If the rubella vaccine is not given, the child will of course be susceptible, and sooner or later may get the disease from others. Most children, especially the young ones, will catch this disease and by so doing they will develope life-long immunity.

However, some children will grow to be teenagers without having contracted this disease. If this is true of a female, and if she develops the disease during her pregnancy (mainly in the early months of pregnancy) then the unborn baby will be in real trouble. In such cases, the rubella virus will cross over to the fetus and infect it. This will not only lead to a baby full of abnormalities, but the baby itself will continue to carry the rubella virus for a long time after it is born. To help stop such problems and prevent rubella epidemics, rubella shots should be given. It is wise to make sure that girls are immune to this disease before their child-bearing age, either through proper immunization or through blood tests.

MUMPS

Since the advent of immunization against mumps, this disease is slowly becoming one of the rare diseases too. In itself mumps is a mild and innocuous disease, but it can lead to some complications which may prove devastating. It is a disease that affects a person only once, after which there will be a lifelong immunity.

Like measles and rubella, mumps is contagious, though not to the same extent. It is more a disease of childhood, although some children will escape catching it, and in doing so they will continue to be susceptible to it through adulthood until they do catch it.

Of course, if mumps vaccine is given to the child at the proper age, the child will develop immunity against mumps and will avoid not only the disease, but all its would-be complications too.

What does mumps look like?

Mumps is a viral disease that affects the salivary glands. It usually affects the parotid salivary glands, sometimes the right and left at the same time, at other times only one gland. When these glands are affected, there will be a swelling that starts in front of the ear lobe, and sweeps underneath and to the back of it. The swelling does not usually have a distinct border, making the area quite puffy. This area may be tender to the touch and somewhat painful, and even more so upon eating something sour. The swelling may be tense at first and with little change in color if any. It is not unusual to have a rise in temperature at the same time, often not that high, though on rare occasions it may be high enough to cause worry.

How long does it last and how contagious is it?

Mumps usually takes about a week or more before it is gone. The swelling will slowly and gradually become less noticeable, and by seven to ten days it will have disappeared. But it is not unusual for mumps to show up in the other parotid or in other salivary glands a few days later and the poor child will have to go through this trouble all over again.

Mumps is usually contagious as long as the swelling of the salivary gland is noticeable and even a few days before. Mumps should not be confused with infected lymph nodes under the angle of the jaw (see page 265), or with some rare diseases that mimic it.

What kind of complications do we have to worry about?

Mumps can affect one testicle or both testicles in the male teenager or adult, and when this happens the testicle will become quite inflamed and painful. When the inflammation subsides, it will unfortunately leave the testicle functionless, and if both testicles are affected the person will become sterile. This complication shows up in a fairly high percentage of teenagers and beyond (thirty to forty-five percent), but not in young children.

Other complications can be in the meninges and brain, the pancreas, the thyroid gland, the ovaries, etc. Although on rare occasions these complications can be dangerous, none of them is as devastating as that affecting the testicles in the male.

Can we prevent it?

Very easily, with one mumps shot. The mumps shot (vaccine) can confer long-lasting immunity, probably for life. Most doctors give one combined shot (MMR) that will be good enough not only for preventing mumps but also measles and rubella. Some doctors prefer to give separate shots for each of these diseases.

There is hardly any reaction, if any, to the mumps shot, and it can be given anytime after the fifteenth month of age. It is worth giving to every child, male or female, not only to prevent the morbidity of the disease, but also to prevent the possible absence from school because of it. Children with the mumps should be confined indoors away from all others.

How can we treat it?

There is no treatment. Mumps must take its course; in the meantime you may apply hot or cold compresses to the tender swollen area, depending on which one will give the child the most comfort. You may also use an antipyretic such as aspirin or Tylenol to help control the temperature and help the tenderness and pain of the affected area.

RHEUMATIC FEVER

Thank goodness, we don't see it that often anymore. It used to be fairly common, quite troublesome, and it has always led to a good deal of related sickness. It prefers children more than adults.

Why children?

Rheumatic fever is an aftermath of a strep infection that had missed being treated. The strep "sensitizes" the body in a special manner, leading to this trouble. Children are more likely to pick up the strep, be it in the school, church, or other crowded areas.

If a child's strep throat is left untreated or treated too late, there will be a three to five percent chance that he or she will develop rheumatic fever.

What will happen then?

The big joints will hurt a good deal. They will also become swollen and painful to move. After a joint has seemed to improve in a few days, another big joint will start all over again.

A good example is a child who had a sore throat two weeks or so before. His or her shoulder joint will become sore, painful to move, and will swell to some extent. After a few days (usually two to three), this shoulder joint will feel and look almost normal. However, a new joint will be affected, be it the knee, ankle, wrist, or elbow. If not halted, the disease will affect the child for a number of weeks if not months.

If the condition is left untreated, the child will feel quite sick for a long time. It is said that rheumatic fever licks the joints, but bites the heart. The heart may become inflamed; its valves often become affected, and this will seriously disturb the flow of blood through the heart chambers. When this happens, the child will become crippled for life, unless the defect is corrected. The correction is usually heart surgery.

Is there a way to prevent rheumatic fever?

Once the child develops rheumatic fever, his or her system will have become sensitized to any future strep infection. Therefore, any subsequent strep infection is likely to ignite more episodes of rheumatic fever, with the possibility of more heart involvement and chance for more heart damage.

That is why we try to prevent rheumatic fever by detecting and treating strep infection early. If rheumatic fever shows up, our next goal will be to prevent any future strep infection in that child.

How will you prevent strep?

Once the child develops rheumatic fever (whether or not the heart has been affected), we put the child on penicillin twice a day every year up to adulthood, i.e. twenty to twenty-five years old. This is to be used day in and day out, summer and winter, vacation or no vacation. This may sound drastic but it is the only means at hand at the present time to prevent further strep infection. (Some authorities have even advocated using penicillin for life!)

How will you diagnose rheumatic fever?

Of course the child will have to be checked thoroughly, then some blood tests and cultures will have to be done once or repeated several times. An EKG may also have to be done.

Many diseases may mimic rheumatic fever, and we have to do such tests to prove or disprove the real villain.

Is rheumatic fever catching?

No, not in itself; rather, the strep infection that leads to rheumatic fever is the contagious element, so we must be cautious.

How will you treat rheumatic fever?

Once the diagnosis is confirmed, the line of treatment will depend on the severity of the case. Mild cases of rheumatic fever can easily be checked with prolonged courses of aspirin (not Tylenol), yet there are cases when steroids (cortisone medicine) have to be given for some time; some severe afflictions have to be treated promptly and energetically. Much depends on the degree and severity of the heart involvement.

Rest, and a subsequent gradual increase of activity to normal levels, are important factors. Several visits to the doctor are necessary and the details of treatment will have to be left in his or her hands.

INFECTIOUS MONONUCLEOSIS

The child's throat is very sore, the temperature may be only slightly elevated or it may be shooting up and down to a noticeable extent. When the child looks at the ceiling you may see that there is a lump under the jaw. There often is a complaint of a headache and fatigue. You will suspect that there is nothing but a nasty sore throat.

You take the child to the doctor and the doctor may take a throat culture because the throat not only looks red, but may have a layer of pus on it. Even though the culture is negative, the symptoms seem to be persisting if not becoming worse.

Does this mean that the child has infectious mono?

Infectious mono is multifacetted, and it comes in with so many different signs and symptoms. At times, the little one has low-grade fever for a number of days with little else, or the child may have a rash that looks like scarlatina or other diseases.

One or two checkups later may reveal that the spleen has become enlarged along with or without enlargement of the liver. At rare occasions even jaundice shows up.

How will you be certain that it is infectious mono?

Certain blood tests have to be done to prove or disprove the suspicion. The catch to these tests is that they may have to be done more than once before determining whether the condition is mono or not. If the tests at first turn out to be negative and the suspicion of the disease is strong, then a repeat testing may prove to be positive.

Does infectious mono affect children often?

Infectious mono is more common than most people assume. This is also true in children. The susceptible time is usually when the child is of school age and beyond. Infectious mono may also come in small "epidemic" forms in the spring and fall. Fortunately it is not as severe in these children as it tends to be in college-age people and adults.

What is the difference?

In children of school age and younger, it may last only two weeks, give or take one week. Most such cases can be treated at home, are fairly mild, and the child can come out of it with flying colors.

In adults and teenagers, infectious mono can often be quite nasty. The famous "fatigue" symptom can go on and on, especially if the person does not take the necessary rest. The spleen may remain enlarged for a good many weeks, and rupture of the spleen has been known to occur.

Can infectious mono be dangerous?

Like most diseases, most cases of infectious mono turn out to be mild, especially in children. It is a bothersome disease that has to take its course. Every once in a while, however, infectious mono may lead to acute or chronic complications. Fortunately, this happens only rarely.

What can you do about it?

As you probably know, not much can be done. The most important factor in the treatment is prolonged rest. If the child resumes normal activity too soon, his or her fatigue may go on and on and on.

This is particularly true for older persons who have a fairly heavy dose of the disease.

A light diet, with an emphasis on easily digestible meats (protein), is important too, along with some extra vitamins.

But there is no antibiotic or other medicine that can truly cure it. The disease may be exasperating at times, but with proper rest and given time, the disease will indeed disappear eventually.

Is infectious mono contagious?

It is contagious enough. It earned itself the title of "kissing disease," and many people think that infectious mono is purely a disease that affects the college population. In fact, any close contact with the patient, may make a susceptible person a target for the virus.

Does it tend to recur?

Once a child has developed the disease, he or she will have built a good and a permanent immunity. The chances of a second attack will therefore be exceptionally small.

FIFTH DISEASE

The child's cheeks look flushed for a few days, and the area of redness on each cheek may seem to join across the nose. As a matter of fact, when you look at the child from a distance, the flushed area will have a "butterfly" distribution on the face.

Just as that rash seems to go away, a new rash will start showing up. It will be mainly on the outer -more exposed- surface of the arms and legs. This rash will take a few days to become quite prominent, and it will assume an irregular "map-like" shape, with jagged edges. It may also involve the trunk, but that is not too common. The rash may fade and then grow prominent at times. It is not itchy in most cases, yet the looks of it may scare you. This is fifth disease.

Are there other symptoms?

It is rare to have a rise of temperature or cough. The rash, the disease's looks, and its behavior are usually the only symptoms. The child doesn't act or feel sick.

The butterfly rash on the face will usually last only a few days. However, the rash on the arms and legs may last for as long as one to two weeks. Sometimes, though rarely so, the rash may take a period of three weeks before going away.

What will influence the rash?

You may be surprised to notice that the rash seems to fade and grow at different times. The rash in this disease is a "moody" rash; it tends to look angry red at times and pale pink at other times, quite prominent now, not so later on, depending on certain factors. A good example is when a child with this disease becomes exposed to sunlight or a cold breeze, or when he or she takes a hot bath. Such irritating factors and a few others do tend to produce fluctuations in the intensity of the rash by making it look worse.

How contagious is fifth disease?

It is not that contagious. Although people in close contact are likely to get it, others are not so likely to do so. Brothers and sisters, or children who live and play together constantly, are the main ones to pick up this disease from one another.

In other words, it will be O.K. for your child to go to school even at the height of the rash.

What dangers will this disease pose to my child?

In most cases your child will not be in any danger. It is a mild, innocuous disease that hardly leads to any complications, and is presumably caused by a virus.

When the rash goes away, the child will have developed a lasting immunity, and you will not have to worry about recurrences.

The catch to this disease is the diagnosis. You, the parent, are not expected to be able to diagnose it. When the child gets this strange rash, please go to the doctor for proper diagnosis and advice.

Will it affect a certain age more than others?

Yes, fifth disease affects mostly children of school age. It is quite rare in preschoolers, and it is also very rare beyond the teenage level.

It shows up mostly in springtime and early summer, and for some reason it fades away during the rest of the year. It is not a common disease, but it is good to be alerted to it. There are other diseases that look like it, and it takes the trained eye of the doctor to pick up the right diagnosis.

Will antibiotics help in this disease?

Since fifth disease is a viral infection, the use of antibiotics is not helpful at all. The child doesn't act sick anyway, and usually doesn't need any medication. The best treatment for this disease is to know its course and be patient that it will go away by itself if it is given long enough time.

ROCKY MOUNTAIN SPOTTED FEVER

I have just removed a tick from my child, and today:

1. The child has been having a high temperature and a pretty nasty headache, or
2. The child has been having fever for two to three days, and has broken out in a rash. The rash is somewhat blotchy but not itchy; some is on the face and chest and some is on the arms and legs, or
3. The child's temperature has been rising, and he or she is having a pretty severe stomachache, as well as some headache. The child has vomited a few times too, or
4. The child has a funny looking rash all over, fever, headache, stomachache, and some vomiting.

Do you think this is Rocky Mountain spotted fever?

In answer to these questions, the above child probably does not have Rocky Mountain spotted fever but has something else. For such symptoms, he or she may prove to have a viral infection, scarlet fever, or some other disease. Either way, the child ought to be seen by the doctor. Whether it can "wait until tomorrow" or not depends on the child's condition.

I have just removed a tick from the child, and I'm scared:

You have done well to remove the tick, but this does not mean that the tick is always a carrier of the germ (Rickettsia). Even if it is, it can take up to fourteen days before any symptoms of Rocky Mountain spotted fever show up. It is also true that there are two kinds of ticks that may carry the agent that causes the disease: wood ticks and dog ticks. Both are prevalent in many states, especially the wood tick.

How prevalent is Rocky Mountain spotted fever?

Fortunately it is not as prevalent as the newspapers lead us to believe. In fact, it is quite rare.

If it is rare, why do we have to worry about it?

Although the disease is not as perilous as it used to be in the past, it is still serious. We have potent antibiotics and good ways of treatment at the present time, and it will help the doctor's diagnosis if you keep in mind the date you had removed a tick, especially if the tick was attached to the skin.

What symptoms will show up?

It is good to remember that only about half the cases of this disease are preceded by a tick bite that you know of. The other half are cases where the tick seems to have slipped your notice, and to have disappeared somehow.

Usually the child is quite sick: high temperature, pale skin, flushed cheeks, a tendency to talk out of his or her head, loss of appetite, severe headache, achiness all over, and maybe some stomachache and vomiting- and then some fine rash appears, starting on the hands and feet and marching toward the center of the body. The degree of the child's sickness depends on how severely he or she is infected with the agent.

As you can surmise, any of the above symptoms can also be easily caused by some disease other than Rocky Mountain spotted fever. Do not neglect to ask immediately for medical help when your child has these symptoms, following removal of a tick.

What is the easiest way to remove a tick?

There are many ways for that, such as applying baby oil or alcohol, burning the tick, etc., but one of the easiest ways is as follows:

Saturate a piece of cotton with acetone. (If you don't have acetone you may use fingernail-polish remover instead.) Put the wet cotton on the tick. This will immobilize the tick. Have a pair of tweezers and slip one jaw of the tweezers under the tick, to where its head has sunken into the skin. Press on the tweezers and pull the tick with a jerk. This will remove the tick plus some skin tissue.

Is there a way to prevent Rocky Mountain spotted fever?

There is a vaccine that can be used to "immunize" the child against the disease. However, because the disease is not common and because of many other factors, most doctors don't recommend using the vaccine, except in special cases: a person who walks in the woods, for example, is far more exposed to the attacks of ticks than other people. However, not allowing your child to play in the woods may be an extreme measure to prevent the chance for this disease!

CHAPTER SIX

THE EYES

the eyes
eye checkup
eye drops and ointments
the eyes are crossed
styes and chalazions
Conjunctivitis (pink eye)
black eye
the swollen eye lid
subconjunctival hemorrhage
eye accidents

THE EYES

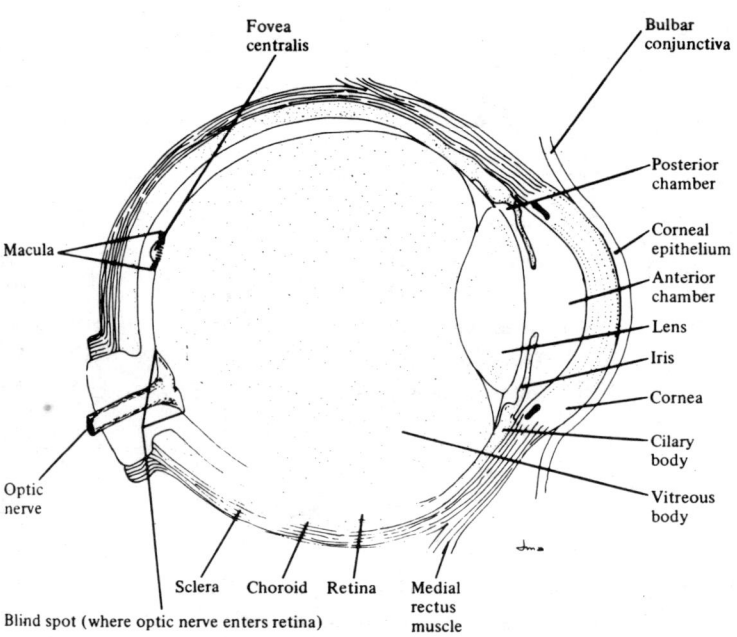

Courtesy Alexander & Brown
from Pediatric History Taking & Physical Diagnosis for nurses, fig 6-3
Written permission from the publisher McGrow-Hill Book Co.

THE EYES

They are precious and they are beautiful, and their structure is quite complicated. Likewise, their diseases can be just as complicated and bewildering.

When you take a look at a normal eye, you will see the pupil at the center of the iris. The pupil looks dark, and it varies in size (contracts and dilates) depending on the amount of light it is exposed to; therefore, you may see it as a pinpoint in strong light and quite wide in the dark. Such a principle is imitated by camera designers whereby the variable size of the aperture controls the amount of light falling on the film.

The pupils are circular and equal in size; they react simultaneously, and their size is controlled by the iris.

What is the iris?

The iris is the colored part of the eye. It may be dark brown or honey-colored in darker people, and blue, bluish grey, or greenish in light-skinned people.

Whatever the color of the iris, it gives distinction to the eye and to the person. The color of the eyes is genetically determined, and it becomes the permanent color of the eyes when a baby reaches the age of only a few weeks. Before that, the slightly greyish color may slowly change its hue until the permanent color sets in.

The iris lies behind the cornea, and the space between the cornea in front and the iris and lens behind is called the anterior or front chamber of the eye.

What is the cornea?

The cornea is the crystal-clear part of the eye that allows light to go through it and through the pupil to the visual spot in the back of the eye (called fovea). The cornea must be crystal-clear to allow the rays of light to pass through, and any trouble or spots in it (in the pathway of the light passing through) can cause considerable trouble in seeing clearly.

The cornea is a very sensitive part of the eye, and even slight damage (such as mild scratches) can cause the eye considerable pain and watering, thus making it necessary to seek the help of a doctor immediately.

At the periphery of the cornea, the sclera will continue to make the eye look semi-spherical from outside.

What is the sclera?

The sclera is the white part of the eye. It is a coating of the eye, with few tiny blood vessels visible on the surface. Sometimes the sclera shows brown spots, especially in Blacks and other very dark-skinned people. This is normal in most cases. The sclera is likely to show specks of "blood" spots on its surface as a result of mild injuries, such as in some cases of "black eye." These hemorrhages are called subconjunctival hemorrhages, and need to be checked by the doctor to make sure no serious trouble is in store.

The sclera is covered by a coating of conjunctiva.

What is conjunctiva?

The conjunctiva is a very thin covering that protects the sclera. It also lines the upper and lower eyelids. It is a clear covering and is well supplied with tiny blood vessels. It is the part of the eye that most frequently becomes inflamed, hence the term conjunctivitis (or pink eye). It is frequently involved in allergic reactions of the eye and other diseases. Since the conjunctiva is loosely held against the sclera, swelling of the space between these two layers can make the conjunctiva bulge –and can scare the daylights out of you! This is seen in patients with a good deal of allergic conjunctivitis.

How about the eyelids?

The eyelids contain certain glands within their structures, and they are lined by the conjunctiva on the inside, and covered by very thin skin on the outside. On their edges are the eyelashes, which have oil glands near their bases. When these oil glands become infected, they form the styes that are so familiar to all. When the glands inside the eyelids are inflamed, they form what is called chalazion.

The tear glands are situated deep to the out edge of the bony orbit of the eye. When the tears are secreted, they wet the eye to keep it healthy and lubricated, and to have a mild anti-infectious effect. The tears drain to the inside of the nose through an intricate drainage system.

What about the area behind the lens of the eye?

The lens of the eye is held in a unique way to the area around. Behind it, the eye is lined on the sides and back by specialized layers of tissue such as the retina and choroid. This part is filled with a gel-like, crystal-clear material, while the front chamber is filled with a clear, watery liquid.

Each part of the eye is likely to develop certain diseases, and each disease has its own characteristics and forms of treatment. This even includes the six muscles that control the movement of the eyes simultaneously and in synchrony with each other, and also includes the nerve pathway that takes the vision impulses to the back of the brain which is the part that sees.

EYE CHECKUPS

Eyesight is a precious gift. Many a child may be having a problem with eyesight completely unknown to the parent. Some of these problems can be traced to early infancy, and a good deal can be done to help prevent them.

How can we suspect it in infancy?

In most cases, the problem is not as difficult to pick up as you may think. Even as early as the age of a few weeks, a baby will be able to see a big moving "figure" such as father or mother. The infant's eyes will slowly follow the moving figure from one side to another. If this doesn't happen by the age of six to seven weeks, bring it to the attention of the doctor.

Far more frequent however, are cases of infants whose eyes seem to be crossed. The appearance of the baby's eyes may be deceptive, since the degree of crossing can occasionally be intermittent. Not only that, but a baby with a low bridge of the nose may also show a sharp fold under each eye. The baby may look cross-eyed, but tests show normal eyes. This is called "false crossing of the eyes".

How do you test the baby?

Simply shine a flashlight at about two feet away from the bridge of the baby's nose. Look at the reflection of the light in the baby's eyes. If the reflection of the flashlight is at the center of both pupils at the same time, you have nothing to worry about: the eyes are O.K. If the reflection is at the center of one pupil, and at the periphery of the pupil of the other eye or completely out of that pupil, then take the baby to the doctor for confirmation of your finding and treatment.

What happens if we don't?

If you wait a long time, months or (God forbid) years , the child will develop amblyopia, the partial or complete loss of eyesight in one eye. The stakes are high for not detecting and treating this easily-diagnosed problem early enough.

How can I suspect eyesight trouble with my child?

Older children may squint, trying the best way they can to put the subject into focus. This will happen to various extents depending on how weak the eyes are. This may be especially true when they try to see something at a distance.

Some children will not be able to see the blackboard well, and you or the teacher may begin to suspect that there are some eyesight problems brewing. Some children may become unable to read street signs clearly, and the severity of this problem will depend on how shortsighted they happen to be. Checking the eyesight in school or at doctor's office will pick up many unsuspected cases.

By the way, headache is not a common manifestation of eyesight trouble, and neither is holding the book too close to the eyes.

How often do you think it is worth checking the eyesight?

Some doctors will do screening tests for eyesight starting at the age of three to four years. There are special cards with common pictures on them and the three to four-year-old is required to recognize the picture from a certain distance.

Eyesight screening tests are done with special charts or by special machines, and they are available for different ages. Such screening tests are quite valuable, and they are good for shortsightedness, farsightedness and muscle balance; however, they won't help with astigmatism (unequal curvature of the cornea). It is worth screening for eyesight every two to three years, but if you suspect trouble, it is better to do it every year. As the child reaches adolescence, there is more of a chance for him or her to need glasses. Therefore, yearly eyesight screenings tend to be more fruitful.

What happens if I don't have the screening tests done?

If the child's eyesight is O.K., you will have lost nothing. If the child's eyesight is in the process of developing problems, however, and you had decided to bypass such tests, the eyesight will become progressively worse. The eyesight may become quite weak and the glasses (when they are finally prescribed) may be quite thick. Amblyopia, of course, can also be the result.

As you easily see, eye screening tests are worth doing regularly, and they are a sound investment in your child's well-being; they are a form of good preventive medicine.

Most doctors have the equipment to perform these tests in their offices. If they find out that the child has problems with the sight of one or both eyes, they will of course refer the child to an eye doctor. Eye screening is less expensive than full eye checkups by an eye doctor, and by knowing that, it will be an incentive to have these tests done regularly.

EYEDROPS AND OINTMENTS

Infection is the commonest trouble affecting the eyes of children. It comes in various degrees of severity and in various forms. To treat and correct such infections, a doctor usually prescribes eyedrops or ointments, of appropriate strength, and the parent is told to use this treatment a certain number of times a day.

Can we use (nonprescription) medications without seeing the doctor?

Yes, this is possible. Generally speaking, however, you better do that in mild cases only, and only for a few days. If the infection does not seem to be clearing up, you should call the doctor and seek his or her help.

If the child has a mild conjunctivitis (pink eye), you may want to try boric acid solution (nonprescription). You can use this as an eyewash or as eyedrops. Be careful to use it as instructed on the bottle.

If there is only a slight eye irritation, Visine eyedrops may also be used. Remember, though; use this material for the very mild infections or irritations, and do not take chances with eye infections of greater severity.

What will the doctor do?

If the eye infection is not that mild, the child's eyes will not only be red and bothersome, but there may be yellow sticky material that will make the eyelids "matted" together upon waking up in the morning. Or there may be pain, swelling of the conjunctiva, inability to open the eyes comfortably when facing light, etc.

Upon examination and diagnosing the problem, the doctor will give the appropriate eyedrops and/or ointments for the condition, and will suggest using them in a manner that may make the applications easier for you and the child.

How shall we instill eyedrops?

Because the tear glands secrete almost constantly, the eyes are perpetually in a constant "bath", and the tears drain down constantly, though in minute amounts, to the nasal cavity.

When the eyedrops are used, three points have to be remembered:

1. The constant wetness of the eyes will dilute the eye medication to a good extent.
2. The eyedrops will not be in contact with the eyes for more than a minute or two before the drops are washed away.
3. The child will be too scared to let you use the eyedrops, and will therefore tend to tightly close his or her eyes and fight your efforts to put the drops in.

To counteract all the above points, it is much easier to instruct the child to be on his or her back with closed eyes. Upon doing that, put two or three of the eyedrops in the "well" between the eye and the bridge of the nose. Then tell the child to open the eyes and look at the ceiling. By so doing, the eyedrops will go into the eye. Don't try to wipe the eye right away; instead, steady the head to let the drops be in contact with the eye for as long as is practical. This method will let the medication work for a longer time than any other method will.

Another popular method is to gently pull down the lower eyelid and to instill the eyedrops in the "cup" which is formed. This means that the eyedrops will fall at the inside of the pulled lower eyelid, near its junction with the eyeball. Make sure the dropper does not fall on or be too close as to pose a danger for scratching the eye.

It is fairly common for a doctor to instruct you to use the eyedrops every hour or two for the first day of treating conjunctivitis, to be followed by using them four times a day for four to five days. The reason for using them that often during the first day is that the antimicrobial effect of the eyedrops will exert its beneficial influence more frequently against the agents of infection, thus producing a faster recovery.

How about eye ointments?

Eye ointments may be even better than eyedrops against infections in the eyes of children. This is because the ointment dissolves slowly in the tears of eyes, thus the medication will be in contact with the eye for much longer than the eyedrops.

It is true that the eye ointment will be sticky and it may make the child react with disgust, but the good effect is certainly something to be welcomed. Not only that, but you may not have to use the eye ointments as often as the eyedrops, thus relieving the burden of these frequent chores.

How can we administer the eye ointment?

To do it efficiently, the child has to be on his or her back; someone should hold the child's hands down. Have the tube of ointment in your hand. With your free hand, open the eyelids apart, then put a line of the ointment along the inside of the lower eyelid. Eye ointments are meant to be applied to the inside of the eyelid and not to the outside except in certain diseases.

The child may or may not react by closing the eyelids tightly, but either way the eye becomes sticky or "greasy" for a minute or two, while the ointment dissolves in the tears of the eye. If there is infection of the edge of the eyelids or the eyelid itself, you may want to put a small amount of the eye ointment on the skin of the eyelid too, in an attempt to reach the infection from inside and outside.

THE EYES ARE CROSSED

The baby looks at you but the eyes don't seem to be straight. You will gaze at him or her trying to discover anything unusual, and you will see that the eyes are not in good alignment. You become concerned and wonder if something has to be done about it.

Crossing of the eyes is fairly common, and it can be either an internal crossing or an external crossing.

<u>What is that?</u>

When the eyes are crossed internally, it means that one of the eyes will turn more towards the side of the nose, while the other eye is fixed seeing an object. On the other hand, an externally crossed eye shifts to the outside while the other eye is fixed on an object.

It is more common to see the "internal crossing," and it can be seen in babies as well as older children. In babies, however, the folds at the base of the nose can give a false appearance as if the eyes are crossed and this can confuse you (see page 181).

<u>Then, how can I find out?</u>

There is a simple test that you can do, and it is described on page 182.

It is much easier to correct crossing of the eyes in the early stages, especially in babies. Sometimes crossing of the eyes is transient and will go away by itself as the baby grows to be a few months old. In such cases we ought not to raise our dander about it, just give it time.

What causes the crossing of the eyes?

In many children it may mean that there is trouble with the eyesight of one or both eyes, and in others it may mean that one or more of the external eye muscles have become weak. So, if your suspicions are confirmed by your doctor, he will usually make arrangement for you to see an eye doctor.

An ophthalmologist (eye doctor) will try to find the cause and degree of the crossing of the eye. He or she may choose to wait and see, i.e. to check on the eyes in a few months to see if there has been any further change.

Or the eye doctor may find it necessary to patch one eye. This is done to give the other eye a chance to see and "exercise" itself. The doctor may even use certain kinds of eyedrops in one eye to be used for a period of time, or may prescribe certain eye exercises.

In other cases, an eye doctor may find it nesessary to prescribe eyeglasses of the proper strength. Even in such cases the doctor may find it necessary to patch one side of the glasses.

In more severe cases, the eye doctor may find it necessary to operate on the eye.

What kind of operation?

It is a delicate operation to adjust the "length" of the weak muscle of the eye. In many cases one such operation will do. However, sometimes two or more operations are needed.

In all cases of crossing of the eyes, the eye doctor will have to be the surveiling guardian and will have to check the child at regular intervals.

Does the trouble run in the family?

Usually not. Although a cross-eyed child is usually the only one in the family, occasionally it happens to two children in one family. A child with this problem will need prolonged follow-up, but thank heavens it is something that can be corrected easily.

Can I ignore intermittent crossing of the eyes?

It is better to pay attention to all forms of crossing of the eyes, including the intermittent type. Actually it is the intermittent type of crossed eyes that can fool you and give you a sense of false security. It can lead to trouble with eyesight if you let it go too long.

STYES AND CHALAZIONS

Styes are fairly common, to most people. The edge of the eyelid looks sore, red, and somewhat swollen. If you look carefully you may see that the swelling is coming to a head and an eyelash may be jutting out of it.

A stye is an infection of an eyelash follicle and it can make the eye look and feel sore.

What causes it?

Most styes, if not all of them, are caused by the staph germ. For some reason, this germ will zoom to the eyelash follicle, leading to inflammation and even a tiny abscess of the area. At times, there might not be one stye but two or even three, either at the same time or in succession.

It may show up in one eye, and then jump to the other eye. Usually it is the child himself who transfers the infection by rubbing the sore eye, thus infecting the fingers. By rubbing the other eye with the now-infected finger, the infection will have been transferred.

Occasionally the whole eyelid looks swollen, red, and painful, nevertheless everything seems to be okay with the eyeball itself.

Do styes tend to recur?

Yes, this tends to happen in some children, though it is not that common. Only rarely do they become stubborn and keep coming back. This usually means that the germ has not been eradicated with treatment, or that there is a source of staph infection somewhere in the child or his close surroundings.

Are styes catching?

Close contact among children may become a source of spreading styes, but this is not common. It is more common to see styes spreading from one eye to the other in a child than from a child to a friend. You can help prevent their spread simply by urging the child to wash his or her hands often, especially after touching the stye, and by preventing him from tinkering with his infected eyelid. Remember that the infected eyelid is swarming with the ugly germs, and that they can go on the finger tips and become a source of reinfection in case you or the child play with the area but manage to forget washing the hands afterwards.

How do you treat styes?

If the child has one stye that doesn't seem to be too bad, you may want to treat it at home. Apply wet heat if possible, for about fifteen minutes at a time, three to four times a day, prevent the child from playing with the area, and see if the stye will gradually melt away in a few days.

Make sure to see the doctor if: (1) the stye looks bad, (2) there is a pussy discharge, (3) there is more than one stye, (4) your treatment has failed, (5) the eyelid is swollen, (6) or if both eyes are affected. He or she will prescribe the specific eyedrops or ointments. Some of the styes may even have to be opened surgically, though this is not often the case!

What is "chalazion"?

Chalazion usually is an infection, also by the staph germ, that affects certain glands deep inside the eyelid. These glands lie along the length of the upper and lower eyelids. When they get infected, a small swelling will develop, almost as big as a split pea. It is not as painful as you think, but it makes the eyelid somewhat unattractive. The surrounding area may become slightly red, and the swelling will seem to stay put without signs of going away.

Is chalazion catching too?

Fortunately most chalazions are not catching, and they don't behave the same way as styes do, though the staph germ is the offending agent. They are not as easy to get rid of as styes are, however.

What do you do for treatment, then?

After checking the chalazion, your doctor will prescribe certain kinds of eyedrops or eye ointment. You must keep using the medication for three to four weeks in most cases, but at times even as long as three months.

The swelling will gradually dissolve and you may be tempted to stop the treatment, but it is wise to continue the treatment for seven to ten days after the swelling has gone away completely.

In rare occasions, a small operation may have to be done to open the chalazion and evacuate the pus, and we certainly hope this doesn't happen to your child.

CONJUNCTIVITIS (PINK EYE)

The child rubs the eyes and complains "they feel funny." You notice that the eyes are red, the eye lids perhaps engorged, and there may be some yellow matter at the corner. The yellow matter varies in amount, usually accumulating at the inner corner of the eye. In more severe cases, the material may cake, making the eyes "matted-shut" in the morning. A rise of temperature, sore throat, running nose , and some cough may also be present, though not necessarily so. The child may be fussy and irritable.

What does it mean?

Conjunctivitis is an infection of the conjunctiva, which is the lining of the eyelids and also the cover of much of the eyeball (see page 180). Conjunctivitis is fairly common, especially in the young child. It may affect one eye or both, and can be mild or severe. When severe, the condition can be troublesome, leading to marked swelling of the eyelids, and shutting the eye completely.

Usually it is caused by a viral infection, although bacteria can cause it too, making culturing of the eye desirable. It is contagious, and can go from one child to the other through contaminated fingers.

Many a time such infections are precipitated by the child himself. This happens when the child wipes his or her nose with the hand, then rubs the eyes with the contaminated fingers. Thus a good dose of the virus or germ is transferred directly to the eye, causing a conjunctivitis.

A parent who wipes the child's runny nose, only to wipe the child's eyes with the same contaminated kleenex, will also transfer the virus or bacteria to the eye, leading to conjunctivitis.

What shall I do about it?

If conjunctivitis is mild, you may want to treat it at home. If the eye is not too congested, if the pussy matter is small in amount and not enough to make the eye matted shut in the morning, or if the child does not seem that sick, you may try treating it by yourself. Use boric acid solution or drops (nonprescription). Use it four times a day for a few days, and watch the eye for improvement. If there is improvement, continue with your treatment, but if you seem to be getting nowhere or the infection is getting worse, then visit the doctor.

What will the doctor do?

Having assessed the degree and severity of the conjunctivitis, the doctor may take a culture of the pussy matter of the eye, and prescribe eyedrops or eye ointments. In severe cases an antibiotic may have to be given internally.

Eyedrops are good for an older, cooperative child. Using them for five to seven days is necessary, though sometimes the conjunctivitis goes away in a day or two from the start of the treatment. If the child is not of the cooperating age, eye ointments may be used instead. They are to be put on the inside of the lower eyelid (see page 158), and the tears will in turn diffuse the medication all over the eye. Five to seven days of treatment is usually necessary.

How can we prevent pink eye?

To prevent pink eye, do not let your child play with a child who has pink eye. Within the circle of your family, keep the child with the pink eye away from others. If this measure fails and your other children pick up the infection, you can use the same eyedrops or ointment the doctor gave you for your infected child.

Children who wipe their runny noses with their hands (usually the thumb side), then rub their eyes with the contaminated hand, should be discouraged from doing so if at all possible. The same applies to using a facial tissue contaminated with secretions of the nose; if used to wipe the eye, it will almost surely infect it.

Does the eye become pink from other causes?

Yes, from many of them, but certain causes stand out. Slight redness of the eye with a lot of watering and bagginess often means allergy of the conjunctiva. This is more common during springtime when the pollen count is fairly high in the air. Itching is more pronounced, and the child often sneezes, rubs the nose, and seems to be fairly uncomfortable. Allergic conjunctivitis is fairly common, mainly in allergic children, and is quite variable in its severity. For mild cases, antihistamines are worth a try. Novahistine, Naldecon, Dimetane and the like (nonprescription) may be tried (see page 305).

The eyes may also look red after being irritated. This can happen in the swimming pool (from chlorine), or from other forms of irritation. Visine may also be of help in such cases and it is worth giving it a try. No prescription is needed.

BLACK EYE

Black eye is a common thing and I am sure you are familiar with it. The child comes crying to you after an injury near the eyes, and not too long afterwards the black eye will develop. Usually only one eye is involved but occasionally the two are affected.

What causes black eyes?

The soft tissues around the eyeball are very loose. Since they are very soft, they are likely to swell easily, out of proportion to the trouble causing it. When the injury takes place around the eye, this swelling affects the soft tissues around the eyeball, and the exuding blood cells will give it the peculiar color.

Is it dangerous?

In most cases the injury is mild and so is the reaction. It will take its course and in due time the black eye will disappear.

In rare situations the reaction has to be taken seriously and dealt with promptly. This usually happens when the injury is severe and might lead to other manifestations (such as car accidents leading to fractures, concussion, etc.)

Watch out for black eye with the following symptoms:

1. Watering eye,
2. Pain in the eye,
3. Inability to open the eye,
4. The tendency of light to hurt the eye,
5. Inability to move the eye,
6. Bloodiness in the white of the eye,
7. Concussion,
8. Any associated injury besides the black eye.

In any of the above cases, ask your doctor to have a look.

What kind of trouble can an eye receive?

It all depends on the kind of injury and the cause of the injury. The cornea of the eye may show an abrasion or a superficial cut, the conjunctiva might develop a bleeding spot, the front (anterior) chamber of the eye may hemorrhage, and laceration of the iris or other scary damages can happen. Most such lesions will need immediate attention by an expert eye doctor.

What will the doctor do?

The doctor will have to evaluate the child, and check the kind of injury, its severity, and which tissue it has affected. The treatment depends on the diagnosis. Your doctor might have to refer you to an eye doctor right away. Injuries to the eyeball itself can occur along with the black eye. You will not want to be the one to evaluate such a delicate thing, and it is always better to be on the safe side.

And if it is a plain black eye?
An average ordinary black eye will undergo certain color changes over a period of two to three weeks. Slowly, you will see that the dark color will fade, to be replaced with various hues of brown, yellowish-green, and a yellow tinge, before it disappears.

Should we do anything about it?
If the black eye is plain and without complications (see above), leave it alone. You may want to apply an ice pack to the area if the injury is fresh, and you may do that for about thirty minutes every three to four hours for two to three times. This may prevent the swelling from growing. You may follow the ice packs with application of heat (moist heat is preferable) for twenty to thirty minutes too. However, it is somewhat questionable if the above is as useful as we hope for.

THE SWOLLEN EYELID

Not every swelling of the eye lid is the same, although they may all look the same to you. There are many subtle differences in their appearances, each a result of various causes. Some of these diseases are of major significance; others may be taken lightly or even treated at home.

You may notice that either the lower or the upper eyelid is swollen, or both; the lid may look red, there may be matter in the eye, the swelling may be limited to a small spot or involve the whole lid. One eye may be affected or both.

What are the major diseases that cause swollen eyelids?
If you see puffiness of both eyelids, especially the lower eyelids, there will be a chance for nephrosis or glomerulonephritis. Both are specific diseases of the kidneys, and they should be treated promptly and properly. Both diseases can be serious, and both require prompt attention.

Similar swelling can also result from bee stings or insect bites, but often you will be able to recognize a sting, because the swelling will occur around the specific area of the sting (usually the bridge of the nose).

Certain forms of allergies, e.g. to food, may cause this kind of swelling too, but in addition to the swelling there may be hives, hoarse voice, some swelling of the lips, or other allergy manifestations. Either way, a visit to the doctor is mandatory.

A swelling of the eyelids, which resembles a bruise "black eye" is familiar to most people. It follows accidents involving the forehead or the vicinity of the eyes (see page 192).

How about infection?

Infections of the eyelids or conjunctiva present themselves in a different manner. In case of a stye or chalazion of the eyelid, quite often the swelling is localized, and it may be pea-sized, may be coming to a head, painful to some extent, and red in color. Occasionally one whole eyelid becomes red and swollen, but the other eyelid of the same eye looks normal (see page 188).

If there is blepharitis, which is acute inflammation of the whole eyelid, the eyelid will be tender, painful angry-looking, red in color and the child will complain and complain. Occasionally there may be matter in the eye, but the conjunctiva usually looks normal.

What if the conjunctiva is infected?

When there is severe conjunctivitis, not only will the white of the eye be very red, but the eyelid may also become slightly red and swollen. The usual case of conjunctivitis will be associated with pussy discharge, but rarely with swelling of the eyelids (see page 190).

The same applies to allergy of the conjunctiva.

How about allergic conjunctivitis?

Allergy of the conjunctiva shows up as swelling of the tissues under the conjunctiva, usually crystal-clear, as if there is blister underneath. There is hardly any redness of the eyes, but there may be a runny nose, sneezing, and other signs of allergies.

When allergic conjunctivitis shows up, both eyes are involved. Usually in such cases there is no swelling of the eyelids themselves, since the trouble is mainly in the lining of the eyelids.

Are there any other causes of troubled eyelids?

Yes there are. Some are rare and it is better not to mention them here. One , however, is fairly frequent. This is called seborrheic blepharitis.

This is a disease of the skin, and it shows up in babies as cradle cap and/or seborrhea of the cheeks. When these babies grow up, the nature of the skin is such that the eyelids may become affected, thus producing seborrheic blepharitis. In this disease the edge of the eyelids becomes crusty, and the eyelashes look unhealthy and sparse. The edges of both eyelids may look red, slightly swollen and indurated (slightly hard to the touch). It may show up on and off for years if not for life, and it often improves for a while just to become worse once again.

The treatment is tenuous and not so satisfactory, and an eye doctor is often needed. It can lead to complications, such as a smoldering low-grade infection.

SUBCONJUNCTIVAL HEMORRHAGE

You notice your child's eye, and when you look closer, you discover a red spot on the white of the eye. The spot may assume various shapes and will usually be small or tiny, but occasionally it may be quite big and even cover the whole white of the eye.

This shows up in cases of black eye too, as if it is part and parcel of the whole thing. The child will say that the eye doesn't hurt, and often you will not be able to detect any discomfort, vision trouble, or sensitivity to light. There will also be no tearing of the eye, or noticeable swelling of the conjunctiva.

Should I do anything about it?

That depends. Many if not most cases of subconjunctival hemorrhage are mild and go away by themselves. However, in a small percentage there may be an injury to the wall of the eye, and this may lead to a heap of trouble. Once I saw a child with a small subconjunctival hemorrhage, which upon careful examination showed a tiny area of ulceration at its center. I sent the child to an eye doctor who was able to remove a tiny splinter that was imbedded inside the eyelid and adjacent to the ulceration. The splinter was so imbedded in the eyelid that it was invisible except for a minute tip! This is mentioned to bring to your attention that such crazy things can happen.

Subconjunctival hemorrhages are usually the result of some injury, and they may be associated with injury to the internal structure of the eye itself. Therefore it should be checked by your doctor.

What will the doctor do if he or she sees it?

The important thing is that the doctor will examine the eye to make sure there is no injury to the eye structure itself. He or she will check the two chambers and the various structures of the eye, and will assess the extent of the injury. If the doctor rules out trouble, you will be reassured; otherwise, the child will be sent to an eye doctor. The eye doctor will have to deal with the specific problem.

What will happen to the hemorrhage when left alone?

If the subconjunctival hemorrhage is not associated with other injuries, you simply give it time. The redness will slowly resolve, and as it does, it will assume different colors and hues. The redness will slowly give way to brownish discoloration, then a greenish hue, until it slowly fades to yellow and disappears.

These changes take about two to three weeks or longer before they disappear. More severe subconjunctival hemorrhages take longer before they go away completely.

Some of these subconjunctival hemorrhages have a notorious way of showing up.

How do they show up?

Most cases of subconjunctival hemorrhages show up clearly in the white of the eye which is exposed when the eye is open. Every once in a while, however, the hemorrhagic spot will appear in the hidden white of the eye, e.g. in the white of the eye covered by an eyelid. Therefore, when you suspect such a condition, instruct the child to look to the extreme left and right, and to the extreme down and up while you hold the eyelids apart. By so doing, you will have full view of the entire white of the eye (sclera); you will thus be able to confirm the extent of the hemorrhage or rule it out completely.

Do we need any eyedrops or ointment?

No, you don't need them in practically all such cases. The reason is that most cases don't become infected. This is also true of using eye patches or keeping the eye closed for a few days; there is no need for such drastic measures unless there is a concomitant problem, then the eye doctor will advice.

Can subconjunctival hemorrhage show up in babies?

Believe it or not, it is fairly common to see a newborn with a subconjunctival hemorrhage. This often alarms the parents, especially those not familiar with the condition. Such hemorrhages are of various sizes and shapes, and show up more often in one eye than in both. Mostly they are discovered during the first day of life.

Generally speaking, the baby looks perfectly content and happy, although the eyelid may be slightly puffy and bruised looking, and so may be the cheek.

What causes this condition in a baby?

The cause is usually the process of birth. Though most babies born will not develop subconjunctival hemorrhage, some others whose birth is slightly more difficult, will end up with this condition. What it usually means is that one of the small capillaries (microscopic blood vessels) will have ruptured, and a minute amount of blood has oozed under the conjunctiva. Give enough time, it will disappear spontaneously.

EYE ACCIDENTS

The child comes running to you, closing one eye, complaining excitedly that it hurts. The child keeps the eye shut, and the eye may water a good deal. If he or she tries to open the eye, it will only be for a short while- the child will quickly close it again, saying it hurts. Upon further questioning, the little one may give you the story that some foreign object had lodged in the eye, something had hit it, or perhaps something had scratched it.

You may try to take a look, but to your untrained eye, the injured eye looks normal except for the tearing.

Why does it tear so much?

This is a reflex action. The eye will tear excessively in an attempt to wash away the cause of injury. This will help if there happens to be dirt in the eye, but it won't help that much if the injury is a scratch or some foreign body embedded in the eye. Keeping the eye closed is also a reflex action by the eye in an attempt to protect itself.

What is to be done?

If there is a tiny insect or some dirt in the eye, i.e. something that can easily be washed away with water, wash it with water, sit tight and observe. In such situations, see if the eye will feel normal to the child and look normal to you afterwards; make sure that it tears no more, and that the child doesn't keep it closed. If on the other hand the child keeps the eye shut or the eye keeps watering, let the doctor have a look.

Anytime the child has an injury to the eye beyond what is mentioned above, call the doctor, and if the doctor is not available, take the child to the emergency room of the nearest hospital.

Any eye injury is potentially dangerous. Therefore, a child who comes with the possible story of an eye injury often has to see the doctor.

Why should it be checked?

If a doctor doesn't check the child's eye, and if the child happens to have a scratch in the cornea left untreated, a scar may form. If the scar happens to be in front of the pupil, it will interfere with the eyesight to variable degrees.

If the child happens to have a foreign body in the eye, and if this foreign body is embedded into the tissue of the eye, it may penetrate the wall of the eye and lead to serious trouble.

With some accidents, the doctor has to determine whether there has been bleeding in the chambers of the eye or whether any internal injury has taken place to the eye structure itself. Such injuries often prove to be serious.

What other kinds of eye accidents can take place?

Some chemicals such as household detergents may accidentally come in contact with the eye, which is not as rare as you think. Although many chemicals are mild, some are quite strong and destructive. Some can damage the whole eye in a short period of time. The degree of harm depends on the kind of chemical, its strength, the manner in which it comes in contact with the eye and other factors.

What will happen then?

The child will scream in fear and pain, and will keep the eye closed reflexly. The eye will water a good deal, and the white of the eye may become red and congested after a short while. You will be justifiably excited, but you must set to work right away.

What shall I do?

Wash the eye thoroughly with cold water from the faucet as soon as possible. The water will wash the chemical away and prevent it from doing more damage to the covering tissue of the eye. When that is done and finished, call the doctor.

Better still, an attempt to prevent such accidents can go a long way in saving you and the child the potential trouble and worry. Keep chemicals away from the child, don't let him or her play with them or work with them unless necessary, caution repeatedly about these chemicals and the possible dangers they pose, and educate the child in the art of self-protection.

What will the doctor do?

The doctor will check the eye carefully, and try to assess any damages on the outside or inside. If there is a small foreign body the doctor may try to remove it, or send the child to an eye doctor. If there is any other damage that is more than he can manage, he will send the child to an eye doctor too.

A good many accidents to the eyes are manageable in the doctor's office. The doctor may elect to use eyedrops or eye ointments, may put a patch covering the injured eye for a few days, and may want to check the eye again in a few days to see if the eye looks normal again.

   Prevention of accidents to the eye is something that is hard to do and is easier said than done. The naturally fast reflexes of the eye are usually sufficient in themselves, but accidents do take place and I hope that they don't happen to your child.

CHAPTER SEVEN

THE EARS

the ears
hearing
earache
the inflamed middle ear
the gluey ear
discharge from the ear
diseases of the outer ear (auricle)
the inflamed ear canal (swimmer's ear)
ear drops
foreign body in the ear
ear wax

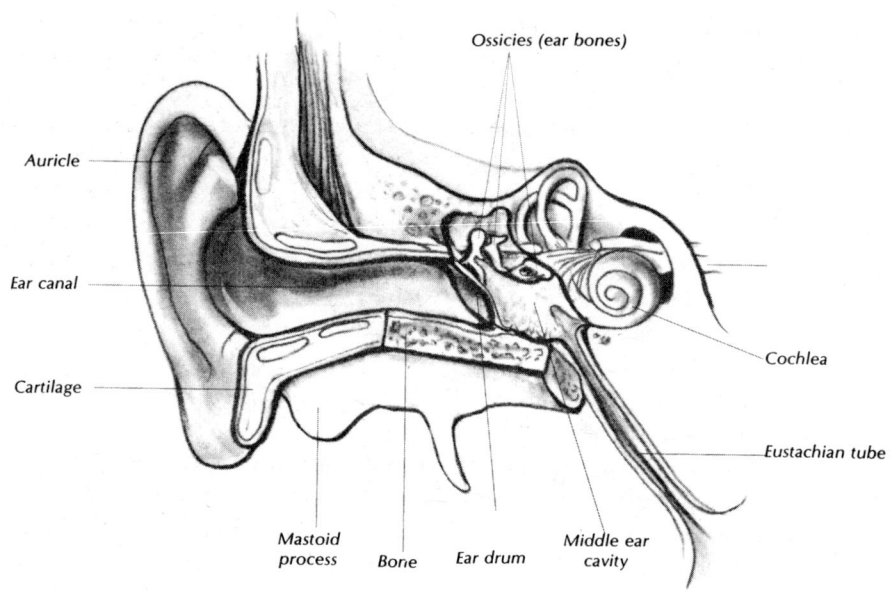

Courtesy Barbara Bates, M.D.
from a Guide to Physical Examination, p 58
Written permission from the publisher, J. B. Lippincott Co.

THE EARS

The ears are the gateway to speech. The child must first hear before he or she learns to speak. Although all of us are familiar with the external appearance of the ears, the rest of the structure of the ear needs to be explained.

The part we see is called the auricle and it leads to a canal, or a tunnel called the external canal or auditory canal. Together they form the external ear or outer ear. The auditory canal is where the ear wax forms. When this canal is inflamed, it is called "swimmer's ear" by many doctors. The canal is closed on its inner side by the eardrum. The drum can be clearly seen by the doctor using an otoscope when the ear canal is devoid of wax. The eardrum separates the outer ear from the middle ear.

What is the middle ear?

The middle ear is a small cavity, having air inside. On the outside the eardrum separates it from the external ear canal. The eardrum vibrates as a reaction to the sound waves coming from outside. The vibrations of the ear drum will be transmitted to each of the three tiny bones of the middle ear, one after the other. The third bone inside the middle ear is attached to the inner ear in a delicate way, and its vibrations will be passed to the fluid that is inside the inner ear (cochlea), and the fluid will then move fine hair-like tentacles. These tentacles on their part will stimulate the nerve of the ear, which transmits the impulses to the brain, where hearing takes place.

The middle ear also communicates with the mastoid bone which lies behind the ear.

How come there is air in the middle ear?

A healthy middle ear has to have air. The cavity of the middle ear is connected to the back of the throat with a special tube called the eustachian tube. Air from the throat goes through this very important tube to the ear every time a person swallows. This causes the distinctive click you sometimes feel upon swallowing. Better still, pinch your nose and then swallow, and you will hear and feel the air going to the ear.

Certain problems with the eustachian tube are some of the major factors that lead to frequent infections of the middle ear, or the accumulation of fluid to replace the air inside the middle ear, something called "gluey ear" by some doctors.

What is the inner ear?

The inner ear is snugly lodged in the bones of the skull. It consists of two parts, the hearing part or the cochlea, and the balancing part or the three semicircular canals.

To the naked eye the cochlea looks like the spiral of a snail. It is connected to the third bone of the middle ear in a delicate manner. The inside of the cochlea is lined with special cells from which tentacles project. These tentacles bathe in fluid. The fluid will develop waves as the tiny bones of the middle ear move back and forth in response to the sound waves. When the fluid moves, the tentacles pick up the movement and stimulate the hearing nerve. The nerve will then transmit the impulse to the hearing part of the brain, thus you will be able to hear. The whole thing is just as miraculous as the mechanism of seeing!

The balancing part of the inner ear consists of specially located semicircular canals, whose function is to keep us well-balanced and aware of our position and posture.

Fortunately, diseases of the inner ear are very rare. The commonest ear diseases are those of the middle ear, especially in preadolescent children.

Why do children get middle ear infections?

Infections of the middle ear (see page 211) are quite common in small children. It is unusual to have a family whose children have not experienced one or more middle ear infections, accompanied by crying episodes in the evening or middle of the night.

The reason is that the eustachian tube is such in a child that it can very easily transmit infections from the throat up and through to the middle ear (see page 295). Besides that, colds and sore throats are quite common in young children until they develop a good enough level of resistance. Also some children seem to be unusually prone to ear infections especially if they happen to have an allergic constitution.

Accumulation of thick, sticky fluid in the middle ear is quite a problem too. In most cases it is a result of middle-ear infection, and if it does not go away it will interfere with hearing and lead to a good deal of problems for the developing child.

Infections of the middle ear are the commonest of ear problems, but this doesn't mean that the external ear can be free from disease. The external ear has its own share of infections and other problems too, but hardly as often as the middle ear. Infection of the external canal is fairly common during summer time because of swimming, since water may enter the ear canal. That is why it is so aptly called swimmer's ear. Foreign bodies in the ear canal, boils, wax accumulation, and other problems are fairly common too.

HEARING

Hearing is a vital function to everyone. Hearing difficulty and partial hearing loss are unwanted guests. In children, however, such a problem is even more ominous.

Difficulties can arise early in childhood, even among some newborns. Fortunately, temporary hearing difficulty arises mainly from ear trouble that can be treated with relative ease.

What happens if a baby has this trouble?

If the baby cannot hear well, he or she will have great difficulty learning how to speak. In early babyhood this may pass unnoticed, but later on the speech may not be clear, and the child's power to communicate may suffer. It is usually at this point when your suspicion or your doctor's suspicion may be aroused.

In milder cases, the child's speech might be "passable," but his or her behavior might suffer. After all, the poor child is frustrated with the predicament, and this may even be reflected in below-par schoolwork and other accomplishments.

What causes such problems in a baby?

There are many causes, but certain ones stand out. Good examples are babies born to a mother who had German measles (rubella), certain viral diseases, or some other diseases during early pregnancy.

Babies who are (a) very tiny at birth (prematures), (b) or who had difficulty during birth, (c) or who were jaundiced to a certain degree in the first few days after birth, (d) or who had extensive hospital treatment after birth, may prove to be the victims too. All such babies ought to be observed carefully, and if you or the doctor suspect a hearing problem, the child must be treated properly as early as possible. Early treatment will go a long way in correcting the situation.

More so than other childhood problems, hearing trouble is likely to cause the parent concern, because of the effect on the baby's behavior.

How about older children?

Hearing difficulty in older children can have many causes too. The main cause, though, is an infected middle ear, which will often develop into the "gluey ear" (or serous otitis media), in spite of good and conscientious treatment. The doctor is usually the one who discovers such a condition, and will assess the degree of hearing loss.

What will the doctor do for it?

The doctor will probably refer the child to an ENT doctor (ear, nose, and throat specialist), who will most likely observe the condition over a period of time, while administering some medicines. In some cases, the doctor may have to operate, putting tubes in the eardrums, and may remove the adenoids in such instances.

If the doctor operates, the hearing usually comes back to normal right away. The hearing loss in such cases is easily curable.

Is it worth testing the hearing on all children?

It is said that of all cases of permanent hearing loss, fifty percent are inherited and twenty percent are related to birthing conditions. Furthermore, about one out of every one hundred children has a substantial degree of hearing loss acuity, and that two to three out of every one hundred children have a mild degree of hearing difficulty. Therefore, testing the hearing accuity every two to three years can produce a rich dividend.

EARACHE

Sooner or later, one of your children will have an earache. When mild, the ear may hurt only occasionally and the child will mention it in passing; or it may hurt a little yet the pain becomes persistent for a few days; but at times the pain may be severe, making the child feel miserable and cry. Sometimes it is only an earache and no more, yet at other times the earache is associated with fever, runny nose, sore throat, cough, and other symptoms.

The earache may also be quite bad at one time, yet next morning the child feels and acts happy and cheerful.

What causes earache?

As mentioned before, we have three ears on each side of us: the outer ear, the middle ear, and the inner ear.

Most earaches are caused by inflammation of the middle ear. When mild, there may be pain without fever, cold, or other symptoms, and this pain may be "in" at one time and "out" a few hours later. But when the infection of the middle ear is severe, there will be a fairly severe pain, more or less persistent, with or without other symptoms, be it fever, sore throat, or cough.

If the infection is truly severe, the earache can be very bad indeed; the child will cry uncontrollably if not persistently and may also suffer high temperature and other symptoms. In a small baby, constant crying may be the only symptom present, and it may be your only clue to ear infection (see page 78).

Can the middle ear give pain without infection?

In many cases, the eardrum can become "retracted." In such a condition, there is no infection, but the tube that connects the middle ear to the throat (the eustachian tube) can become blocked by swelling, mucus, large adenoids, or some other causes. In such cases, the eardrum will retract because of the difference of pressure between the two sides of it.

The pain is usually dull, but it may give the feeling of a click or a blocked ear. The same feeling can also be generated when you ascend a significant height in a car or an airplane.

How about the inner ear?

It is very rare to have trouble with the inner ear and pain caused by inner ear trouble is practically non-existent.

How about the outer ear?

Pain caused by the outer ear is usually due to inflammation of the ear canal itself. This is the case in swimmer's ear or similar conditions. In such cases the canal becomes swollen and tender and there may be some pain. You will know about such a condition if you cause the child a lot of pain by moving his outer ear, or if you push at the ear canal from behind the ear.

An abscess in the ear canal is much more painful than a foreign body in the same place. An abscess, or boil in the ear canal can lead to even excruciating pain. Boils may have to be opened and drained of pus, thus relieving the pain. A foreign body in the canal usually causes irritation and discomfort though occasionally there may be some pain. At times you will not be aware of the pressure of a foreign body in the canal, but the substance will be discovered by the doctor during a routine exam.

What is best to temporarily relieve the earache?

It all depends on what is causing the earache. In most cases of earache, it will be wise to visit the doctor the same day or the next morning, and not to take chances.

Eardrops will temporarily take the pain away but they give a feeling of false security, because they don't treat the cause of the pain. A good example is Auralgan (prescription), or warmed up sweet oil (olive oil). Three to four drops of these every three hours or so can help calm the earache until next morning when you make your visit to the doctor. Applying heat and giving aspirin may also help.

Why should earache be treated promptly?

Since treatment of the disease causing earache is so variable, and because it is so successful if given early, it is important to offer the advantage of early treatment.

If you delay your visit, especially for more than a day or so, your child may end up with pus draining from a ruptured eardrum, or a loss of hearing which will consequently need prolonged and complicated treatment (see page 215). At times the infection shows up in both the middle- and outer-ear simultaneously, thus making it necessary to use several medicines at the same time.

THE INFLAMED MIDDLE EAR
OTITIS MEDIA

The earache may be quite severe and they may cry for hours; if they are old enough, they may scream, complaining that their ear hurts, and may put their hand on it as if to protect it. Yet, in others the pain may be mild, or even to the point that there is nothing to complain about.

They may have other symptoms with it, the main one being fever of varying degrees, from low-grade to as high as 104 degrees F or more. In some the fever may not show up at all. Sore throat, signs of a cold, and respiratory infection may also show up, simultaneously with the earache or precede it.

Middle-ear infection is quite common, especially in young children and in infants, and most parents are quite familiar with it.

How does the infection happen?

The infection travels to the middle ear usually by way of the eustachian tube, a tube that connects the throat with the ear. In babies and young children, infection of the throat and the respiratory tract is quite common, and the middle-ear infection is often an "extension" of such an infection.

Some babies and children are prone to such an infection, much more than others. The reasons for the tendency to infection lie in the peculiarities of the eustachian tube; it can be floppy, narrow, or slightly obstructed by some enlargement of the adenoids or by some degree of allergy.

What shall I do about it?

Every child who has an earache should be seen by the doctor. This ought to be done within a day or so, depending on the severity of the pain and other symptoms. You can never be sure of how severe the inflammation is until the doctor checks the child up and has a look at the ear (see page 209).

To relieve the pain until next morning, you may use sweet oil (or olive oil) that has been warmed up, four to five drops every two to three hours, or you may use Auralgan (prescription) or some similar drops to help ease the pain. Aspirin and heat application may help ease the pain too.

What will the doctor do?

Upon checking the child, the doctor may or may not confirm the suspicion of the middle-ear infection. He or she will assess the degree of the inflammation if there is one, determine if it is mild or a moderate infection and check if the middle ear is abscessed and if the eardrum is ruptured.

The treatment will depend on the degree of inflammation and some other factors. Quite often he will take a certain type of throat culture (called nasopharyngeal culture), and in case of ruptured eardrum with pus coming out of the canal, will take a culture of that pus.

The child will be put on an antibiotic for ten days, or be given a shot for that. Some doctors prefer to give eardrops (see page 222), nosedrops (see page 274), and/or antihistamines (see page 305) in addition.

It is important to know that the antibiotic should be given regularly for the full length of the course of treatment, otherwise the infection may not go away as hoped for. Please don't compromise with the treatment of middle ear infection.

How do I know that the infection is over?

When the pain subsides and the symptoms seem to go away, you may think the trouble is over. This may or may not be true, especially in the case of an abscessed ear or ruptured eardrum.

For such cases it is best to see the doctor again when the course of treatment is over. He or she will check to see if the eardrums look normal or not, if all the pus has been absorbed, and if the child needs a hearing test to make sure the hearing is okay. This is one way to prevent the gluey ear.

Can I prevent some middle-ear infections?
Yes you can if you observe the following:

1. When your child has a respiratory infection or a sore throat, have it treated without much delay. Often these can lead to ear infections.
2. Some children may develop this kind of infection after swimming, and in susceptible children, nose pinchers may be of help.
3. Some children's allergies may make them more likely to develop this infection; therefore, controlling the allergy will help.
4. On rare occasions, diseased and enlarged adenoids may have to be removed to help towards this goal.
5. Don't offer a bottle to the baby while he or she is flat on the back.

By the way, during winter months, putting a hat on the child's head will not prevent middle ear infection (sorry grandma!) this is an old disproved theory.

THE GLUEY EAR

This has nothing to do with glue in the ear. In medical circles we call it serous otitis media, but it becomes easier to explain if we call it the gluey ear.

Gluey ear often results from an inflamed middle ear that has not been treated with antibiotics, or has been treated too late. The pus in the ear will become sterilized if the antibiotic is used, but the remaining fluid in the middle ear becomes thick, almost like gel. When the fluid becomes thick, it would rather stay put in the middle ear than drain down the eustachian tube to the throat.

Is gluey ear dangerous?

Gluey ear can lead to a lot of trouble. The fluid is thick and viscid, and its presence will impair the movement of the eardrum. As a result, this will lead to a degree of hearing loss that can lead to poor school performance.

If the condition is left untreated for a long time, it can lead to further complications, and such complications can cost us a lot in worries and in finance.

What will the doctor do about this mess?

When the gluey ear has progressed to "maturity," and especially if the child seems to have lost some degree of hearing, the little one has to visit an "ENT" doctor.

The ear, nose and throat specialist will confirm the diagnosis, and will recommend surgery which is usually done in the hospital. The fluid will be suctioned and a tiny plastic tube (one type looks like a tiny bobbin) will be put through the eardrum. The tube will be left in place for several months. Sometimes removal of the adenoids may have to be done at the same time.

The child's hearing will become normal almost immediately, and both he and the parents will be in ecstasy again.

While the tube is in the ear drum, swimming should be discouraged, as well as any means whereby water is likely to enter the ear, e.g. during taking a bath.

In occasional cases a tube may not have to be put in; instead, opening the eardrum (myringotomy) will suffice, thus draining the fluid from the ear. This is done if the fluid is thin.

Will my child be okay after the tube is out?

In the majority the tube will fall out by itself and the ear will be all right afterwards, though in a few instances the tube may have to be removed. In a few cases the fluid may accumulate again and the tube may have to be inserted a second time. If this troublesome situation persists, and the tube has to be put in for even a third time, then allergy will be suspected.

Why is that?

Children who need to have the tube for a third time usually show a strong evidence of allergy. If such is the case with your child, allergy tests and allergy shots will have to be instituted. Fortunately, this is rare.

Can I prevent gluey ears?

Since gluey ears are more related to infection of the middle ear especially if it is not treated or only partially treated, the answer to such a question becomes obvious, i.e. prompt and complete treatment is the best assurance. This is more so of children with allergies.

If the ear infection is fairly bad, a second visit to the doctor after a course of treatment becomes mandatory. The child may prove to have thin residual fluid that will need treatment, and a hearing test and a special procedure (pneumatic otoscopy) may have to be done.

One other point should not skip our attention. A small percentage of children are non-complainers and they may develop ear infections without crying or complaining much of earaches. In such cases the parents may slough off the child's complaint of an earache, and they may leave the condition untreated. It is here that the biggest challenge lies.

How can I tell if my child has gluey ear?

This diagnosis can be made only by the doctor. You may suspect such a condition in case the child seems to have trouble hearing after an ear infection.

A child with allergy tendency who gets many ear infections is more prone to gluey ears, so parents of these children have to be particularly careful if the children seem to have trouble hearing.

Gluey ears are not that common, thank God, and in a year's time a busy pediatrician may not see more that two to four cases, if that many at all.

DISCHARGE FROM THE EAR

The child may complain of earache, or the pain may cause the child to cry persistently with hand on ear, and this may go on for hours. To your surprise, all of a sudden the pain seems to go away and a thin yellowish-brown discharge will come out of the ear canal for quite some time. You may take a sigh of relief and so will your child, but you wonder if the trouble is over.

Is the trouble over?

No, unfortunately it is not. You see, in such cases the child has had a severe middle ear infection, and this is the reason for all the earache. The pus in the middle ear had accumulated, not only causing all this severe pain but also causing the eardrum to bulge. Finally, when the eardrum could bulge no more, it gave way and let the pus drain from a small hole that had formed in the drum itself. In other words, the eardrum had ruptured or perforated.

The reason why the pain goes away is that the pus in the middle ear is no longer under pressure, since it is draining to the outside.

What shall I do?

When earache develops, see the doctor soon. This is a good preventive measure. A doctor tries to treat ear infections energetically to help get rid of the infection, and to prevent the ears from "abscessing," or ending with a ruptured eardrum. Remember too, if such drainage is not treated promptly, it is quite likely to become chronic, and this in itself may lead to other problems.

Will ruptured eardrums affect the child's hearing?

When a ruptured eardrum heals, it will heal by forming a very thin layer of tissue that will close the hole. Some people call this a scar. Usually the hearing will not be affected by having one, two, or even a few more such "scars." But what we worry about are other complications that may take place, some of which can be dangerous or difficult to treat. This is the reason why with an ear infection a second visit to the doctor is mandatory, so that the doctor can check the hearing, the mobility of the eardrums, and the disappearance of infection among other things.

What else causes the ear discharge?

There are some common conditions that lead to discharge from the ear.

Many a time, a parent confuses a fairly thin drainage of wax from the ear canal for a pus discharge. In such cases, if there has been no earache at all, and if the drainage of this wax does not look bloody or pussy, you may simply clean the wax on the outside and worry not.

On the other hand, if along with the drainage there is pain when you move the outer ear, or there is pain and tenderness when you press in front of or behind the ear, then there will be a possibility of outer ear infection.

Occasionally, a child will have a bloody discharge from the ear, and this may or may not be preceded by pain. Of course, such cases ought to go to the doctor since some of them mean a ruptured eardrum, while others may prove to be a boil in the ear canal or even a foreign body introduced into the ear canal by the child. The treatment depends on the cause of the bloody discharge.

If there is a boil in the ear canal, the pain may be severe, and you may even be able to see externally the swelling caused by the boil inside. Once the boil ruptures by itself or once it is lanced, the pain will usually cease spontaneously after the boil has discharged its contents. The discharge is often bloody, or it may be pussy with a tinge of blood.

Can we do anything to prevent such problems?

Yes, in most cases. A good example is a child who has an earache that then seems to ease off. This might lull you into false security, thinking incorrectly that the infection has gone away by itself. However, such a child should be taken to the doctor for an early treatment to prevent a ruptured eardrum.

Discharge from the ear should never be ignored, and any child with such a problem should see the doctor, even if the child has stopped complaining of any pain.

You also ought to discourage the child from putting things in the ears, trying to scratch the inside of the ear with anything sharp, since these may lead to cuts of the ear canal, which can lead to subsequent infection.

DISEASES OF THE OUTER EAR (auricle)

The outer ear consists of the visible part (auricle) that all of us are familiar with, and a canal that goes from the outside to the eardrum. The eardrum separates the outer from the middle ear.

The visible part consists of cartilage (gristle) covered by skin that sits on a thin layer of soft tissue. Because of the peculiarities of these structures, we sometimes see diseases in this area that are worth mentioning.

What kind of diseases are they?

They are usually diseases of the skin in that area. Often a baby will develop various degrees of seborrheic dermatitis (see page 90) and will continue to be susceptible to this condition for a number of months if not years.

The condition will look like sore skin, may become wet with secretions (oozy), and will show up behind the outer ear, from the earlobe and up. You have to turn the outer ear forward to see the troubled skin. Sometimes the oozy material cakes on the ear into crumbly yellowish granules. It is not itchy and the baby seems not to mind it unless you monkey around with it. It is not unusual for this condition to resist treatment to some extent. You may use mild cortisone cream such as Cortaid (nonprescription) four times a day for a few days. It is worth mentioning that this condition is often associated with similar lesions on the cheeks, forehead, neck, underarms, and other creases.

Any other diseases of the outer ear?

Children may develop poison ivy of the outer ear, or occasionally impetigo.

Since the skin is more likely to be firmly attached to some parts of the cartilage of the ear than to other areas, little swelling may develop in those areas. If poison ivy affects these areas, they will of course be very itchy, but besides that they will show some redness, blistering, and much discomfort. The distress can be pronounced.

If poison ivy affects other areas (the edge of the outer ear), a painful swelling will show up. This is also true if an insect bites this area. When these happen, the swollen red outer ear will look as if it has doubled its size, and the area will feel warm and tender to the touch. You may use calamine lotion (nonprescription), but with limited success. The looks of the ear will usually cause you to rush to the doctor anyway, and this is the wise thing to do in most cases.

How about impetigo?

Occasionally impetigo of the outer ear can look messy. It won't be too different from other areas with impetigo, but the whole ear with the impetigo will not look at all inviting. A culture of the impetigo should be done at the doctor's office, and treatment with an internal antibiotic along with ointment application are often necessary (see page 441).

Any other diseases?

Two more. Not commonly, we see a small boil, usually near the outer end of the ear canal. This can be extremely painful and the child may cry and scream if you even touch it. Because of the looks and the pain, the doctor often has to see it. If the boil is ripe and there is enough pus in it, the doctor may open it, drain the pus, take a culture, and thereby relieve the pain.

Cauliflower ear is something rare in children but worth mentioning. It follows a blow on the ear and is common in boxers. Bleeding will take place under the layers of the painfully red and tender skin. The swelling should be relieved right away by the doctor or surgeon. If this is not done, an irregular deformity of the outer ear will be the result, more or less in the shape of a cauliflower!

When a child receives a blow on the ear, and when he or she screams with pain and shows a mean red swelling of that ear, you better call the doctor right away rather than just apply cold compresses and wait. The blood supply to the cartilage will be cut off by the swelling, thus leading to the cauliflower ear. If the hematoma (collected blood under the skin) is relieved, however, the chances will be good enough for a normal ear.

These are some of the common disease of the outer ear; there are others but fortunately they are rare. Most such diseases will make it necessary to see the doctor, and in some, the earlier you go the better.

THE INFLAMED EAR CANAL OR "THE SWIMMER'S EAR"
OTITIS EXTERNA

The child complains of pain in the ear, but doesn't cry and you are apt to ignore it. But subsequent constant complaining cannot be ignored for long.

The ear looks O.K. to your eyes. However, when you press at the hole that leads to the ear canal, the child may jump with pain, or give you a good "ouch" and move his or her head away from you. When you press your fingers at the back of the ear, pushing it forward, the child will say it hurts, but will not cry.

Do I have to see the doctor?

Yes. Infection of the external canal of the ear can be of various degrees, and occasionally it can be to such an extent that the canal is practically closed. Some oozing (discharge) from the canal may show up at the outside too. Luckily the majority of cases are mild or moderate infections.

When such infections take place during summertime, they are nicknamed "the swimmer's ears" because they are frequently seen in children who swim.

The doctor has to see the child to assess the degree of severity of the infection and to see if there is also an associated middle ear infection. The treatment will of course depend on the evaluation of the condition and its severity.

What causes such an infection?

In most cases it is a result of water in the ear canal. The water will soften the wax in the ear canal, and this becomes a good medium to grow many kinds of bacteria. When this happens, it will lead to the infection.

During summertime, swimming is the obvious means to lead to this infection in most children. However, this infection can show up quite often in those who don't swim. In such children (and in others during the non-swimming season), the water enters the ear during bathing or taking a shower.

What will the doctor do?

Other than diagnosing and evaluating the condition, the doctor may take a culture of the ear canal, especially if there is some discharge. In some cases, it may also be necessary to wash out the pus and wax in the ear; this will clean the canal so that the eardrops will have a better access to the inflamed area.

For most cases of ear-canal inflammation, eardrops used as directed by the doctor will be sufficient. However, if there is an associated middle-ear infection, a ten-day course of an antibiotic will have to be used in addition.

Can I prevent swimmer's ear?

Yes, you can prevent a good many of these infections. Since swimmer's ear is usually caused by water entering the ear canal, special care must be directed towards preventing the water from entering. This can easily be done by an earplug. However, a well-fitting plug for the child may not be easy to find, and the child may dislike it, rebel against it, or simply forget to use it every time. Gator ear plugs (nonprescription) may be used.

Removing the earwax is an important step in preventing swimmer's ear. If it is soft wax in small amounts, you may be able to remove it by using Debrox or Murine eardrops (nonprescription). If the wax is plentiful or seems to be too hard, the doctor will have to remove it in the office by washing it out.

If the child doesn't like the earplugs, you may put three to four drops of VoSol eardrops (prescription) in each ear after swimming. If you don't have that, you may mix one teaspoon of vinegar in one cup of water and use three to four drops in each ear.

Keep the rest in a small jar to be used in the days ahead.

You may keep doing that during the whole swimming season.

Hydrogen peroxide may also be of some help, and it can be used in the same manner as the VoSol drops or the diluted vinegar solution.

Rubbing alcohol (which some people like to use) is not worth trying, since it doesn't work in most cases and it may irritate. Remember please, not all children are susceptible to swimmer's ear, and you may not have to go through the above steps if your child gets swimmer's ear only once in a while. The above steps apply mainly to children who get this infection often, in summer or winter.

Usually keeping the ear canal clean of wax and dry enough, goes a long way in preventing this nuisance of a disease.

EARDROPS

Eardrops come in various forms and combinations. They are designed for specific conditions. Many parents use them mistakingly in the hope that they stop earaches.

It is true that certain eardrops will relieve the earache to some extent, but you have to know what disease is causing the earache before you use them.

Why is that?

As mentioned before, the commonest cause of earache is infection of the middle ear. It is usually the most intense pain of earache. Such pain, however, responds only partially to the use of eardrops. It is perhaps advisable not to blindly use these eardrops (such as Auralgan). The reason is that the drops may mix with the wax of the ear and make the wax swell, and when the doctor wants to check the ear, the ear canal may be so full of "soggy" wax that he or she will not be able to see the eardrum at all.

Eardrops that "numb" the eardrum may give a feeling of false security by taking the pain away. When this happens, a parent is less tempted to take the child to the doctor. If a middle-ear infection is left untreated with an antibiotic, it is likely to lead to a ruptured eardrum, or form fluid leading to the gluey ear (see page 213).

When shall I use eardrops?

Eardrops are most useful in infections of the outer ear canal. Eardrops containing antibiotic and cortisone are most frequently used. Others consist of special combinations of acetic acid and cortisone, and they are useful too. But again, the use of such medication depends on the advice of your doctor, usually after seeing and checking the child.

Aside from that, certain eardrops can be used for special purposes.

What kind of eardrops?

Debrox or Murine eardrops (nonprescription) are quite useful in softening and getting rid of the wax of the ear. They succeed not in all cases, but in a good many. They are quite safe. Follow the instructions on the bottle

To help prevent swimmer's ear in those susceptible, VoSol or Domeboro eardrops may prove to be quite effective. Even vinegar and water (one teaspoon vinegar to a cup of water) may prove effective. You may put four to five drops in each ear, after coming back from swimming. The drops will acidify the ear canal and make it less inviting to bacteria.

VoSol and Domeboro eardrops are special forms of acetic acid and they do a better job than vinegar/water. However, you need a prescription before you can get them.

What is the best way to use eardrops?

Most parents put three to four drops in the ear, plug the ear with a piece of cotton and call it quits. This is O.K. for many. However, a better way is as follows: let the child lie down on his or her side with the diseased ear up. Put in the number of eardrops prescribed, hold the external ear and move it in a gentle circular movement. Let the child open and close the mouth to "massage" the external ear canal from inside. You will see that the drops will slowly and gradually go down, and you may even see air bubbles coming through the drops. This procedure is especially useful if the ear canal is quite swollen or full of wax.

When you put in the cotton to plug the ear, use a fairly big "ball." I have seen some children who have had a piece of cotton lost deep in the canal near the eardrum!

Some doctors suggest putting a wick in the ear canal, but it is doubtful if this is necessary for general use. When you put the cotton in, make sure to roll it to a point and let the pointed end go first. This will absorb part of the eardrops and make it come in contact with the wall of the ear canal. Also make sure to leave the cotton in place for about half an hour or so.

If there is swimmer's ear, can I use the drops?

If you are sure the child has swimmer's ear and you already have eardrops for that (e.g. from previous use), feel free to use them. You can have a good measure of success. But be careful, since there may be a combination of middle-ear infection along with swimmer's ear. If this happens to be the case, you will miss treating the middle ear! It is truly a tricky situation. If the earache is bad enough, have the child looked at, because without taking a look with the otoscope, it is almost impossible to give an accurate picture.

Therefore eardrops for earache are no good?

Eardrops for earache caused by middle-ear infection are O.K. if the case is already diagnosed. They are of limited value even then. Using them blindly is not advisable. When a child is screaming with earache, and it is evening or midnight, call the doctor for advice. Use a heating pad on the ear and give the child aspirin or Tylenol for the pain. If the pain is mild, the child will feel good in an hour or two. If it is severe, then calling the doctor is not only assuring but necessary.

FOREIGN BODY IN THE EAR

As strange as it sounds, it is not uncommon for a child to put a small object in his or her ear. In fact, a child is likely to put something in the nose, ear, vagina, or any cavity, thus giving the child, the parents, and the doctor a good deal of worry until the object is removed.

It is also common for a small foreign body to find its way into the ear canal without the child knowing it or even seemingly suffering from it.

How is that?

We have come across strange cases in this regard. Once we discovered a blue object in the ear canal. When it was removed, it proved to be a facial tissue, folded up tightly like a ball! Another time, a pretty glistening object showed itself during routine examination. It was difficult to remove. When it finally came out, it proved to be a small pearl! When the other ear of the same child was cleaned, to the surprise of the already shocked mother, another pearl was found! Fortunately many such foreign bodies do not hurt the ear canal or the eardrum and they can be removed easily.

What else can you find in the ear canal?

Some children become the victim of intrusion of insects. An insect can produce a good deal of pain in the ear. The insect not only becomes trapped in the canal, but also has to fight off the wax in the ear canal, which is poisonous to it. Therefore, the insect fighting for its life, may either sting or fly furiously, thus producing the pain and discomfort.

An ant behaves differently. Quite often it walks on the eardrum or bites it, and this can produce a lot of discomfort and even excruciating pain.

A gnat may fly inside the canal, bite, and hurt. This is fairly common in children. As a matter of fact, some children seem to be a special target for gnats, more so on hot sweaty days during summertime. Once I saw a patient with a yellow jacket inside the ear canal! Fortunately the wax of the ear canal was too poisonous for the yellow jacket, killing the insect before it could sting and cause excruciating pain. The yellow jacket was lying prostrate deep in the ear canal, dead.

Another patient had a cockroach in her ear. The roach was small but it caused a great deal of discomfort and noise because of the movement of its tentacles, and it was still alive when removed from the ear!

How do you remove such "beasts?"

In most cases the insect comes out along with the wax when the ear canal is flushed. Of course the doctor will have to do that for the patient.

At other times, the insect can be pulled out with some instruments. If a gnat happens to be there, you may try a nifty trick: take the child to a dark place such as a closet, let him or her stand with the affected ear toward you. Turn on the light in the room, or use a flashlight aimed at the ear. If the gnat is still alive, it may try to fly out of the darkness of the ear canal towards the bright light. If it succeeds, then you will have remedied the situation. If not, you will of course visit the doctor.

What other foreign body should you be careful about?

If a bean goes into the ear canal, you should be particularly careful, and so should the doctor. The child should be handled by the ear, nose, and throat specialist as soon as possible. The reason is that a bean is a vegetable matter and it will absorb moisture. By so doing, the bean will swell and may even press at the ear canal in a tight fit. The ear canal will often react to this, sometimes severely, by becoming swollen, painful, and even inflamed. The condition can become much worse if left unrelieved.

Other than beans, metal foreign bodies in the ear canal are not that rare either. They are likely to cut the ear canal, produce a feeling of fullness in the ear and pain. Bleeding from the ear canal can easily be seen by the parent and felt by the child. Naturally in such cases you better get in touch with your doctor or an ear, nose and throat specialist as soon as possible.

What are the aftereffects of a foreign body in the ear?

This all depends on the kind of foreign body, how long it stays in the canal, and the degree of injury it produces. A live insect will produce too much noise (by irritating or being near the ear drum) to be tolerated. Pain is noticeable too. But once the insect is removed, the trouble will be relieved, and the ear canal will be O.K. Twice we have seen spots of blood on eardrums from the bites of insects trapped in the ear. If a foreign body has cut the ear canal, the cut will heal quickly once the foreign body is removed, a local antibiotic such as Neosporin or Mycitracin (nonprescription) may have to be used. If a bean is there and it has swelled to a good extent, even after the bean has been removed the inflammatory reaction of the ear canal will take a number of days before it goes away. This may be the case despite the use of medication.

EARWAX

All of us have it, to a greater or lesser degree. It is there for a good reason, but at times it is produced excessively, thus leading to certain problems.

There are two kinds of glands in the ear canal; one kind produces wax and the other produces sweat. If the wax is runny, it will mean that the ear canal is producing too much sweat. On the other hand, if the wax is hard or brittle then there is not enough sweat to mix with the wax.

How shall I clean the wax out?

If the wax is soft and seems to seep out of the ear canal, you may take a Q-tip and clean the wax out of the opening of the ear canal. Please don't dig deeply into the ear canal or you may push the wax in too far; this will make it difficult for others to clean it out and it may compact the wax against the eardrum. If you dig into the ear canal, you may also manage to produce abrasions, resulting in some bleeding, and open an avenue for infection.

How will the doctor remove the wax?

Each doctor does it differently. A popular method is to use certain eardrops ahead of time to soften the wax. Then the area under the ear is covered with paper towel, the parent holds a deep basin under the ear, and the doctor flushes the ear out with a special fat syringe filled with water. The process of flushing might have to be repeated a good many times before all the chips of wax are out. The child's patience is essential for our success, and he or she may get somewhat wet in the process.

How often do you have to remove the wax?

In most cases, once a year or so. Occasionally you may have to do it less often.

In active wax secretors however, we may have to do this kind of cleanup job more often, perhaps twice a year or so. It all depends on the child's capacity to produce and accumulate the wax in the outer ear.

Can you wash out the wax in a baby?

Yes we can, but with more difficulty. Children up to the age of four years are more apt to be scared of this procedure. Thus they will deny us their cooperation, if not fight us mercilessly. That is why we usually postpone this procedure up to this age, unless it becomes essential to remove the wax.

What will the wax do if you leave it alone?

One of the most irksome things is that the wax may accumulate to such an extent that it fills the ear canal completely. If a child has an earache, the eardrum must be checked, but excess earwax will block the doctor's view of the eardrum. Therefore, the doctor will not be able to diagnose the problem properly, especially at a time when such a diagnosis is essential before proper treatment can be given.

Another problem arises when the wax becomes soggy due to water having entered the ear canal. The soggy wax can act as a focus of infection, and it will produce an acute inflammation of the ear canal.

Because of the itching wax can produce, a child may put a fingertip (or a sharp object such as a pencil) in the ear to remove some of the wax and to relieve the itching. This action may break the skin inside, thus opening an avenue that can lead to infection such as a boil.

Can I help get rid of the wax myself?

If the wax is not very hard and it is not excessive, then you can put three to four drops of Debrox or Murine ear drops (nonprescription) in the ear, then insert a piece of cotton big enough to block the ear canal. Do that once a day before going to bed, for about two weeks. Another way of using these drops is described in the instructions on the bottle.

In many cases the wax will dissolve away and come out by itself, if not you may try to flush it out with a bulb syringe. The latter has to be filled with water and squirted into the ear canal, while bending the head over a basin. Repeat this procedure several times for each ear until the wax is out.

CHAPTER EIGHT

THE MOUTH AND THROAT

mouth-breathing
geographic tongue
stomatitis (trench mouth)
aphtha (canker sore)
the permanent teeth
tooth abscess and gum boil
accidents to the mouth
the throat
lozenges, gargles, and mouth sprays
sore throats
herpangina
acute tonsillitis
T & A (removing the tonsils and adenoids)
hand, foot, and mouth disease

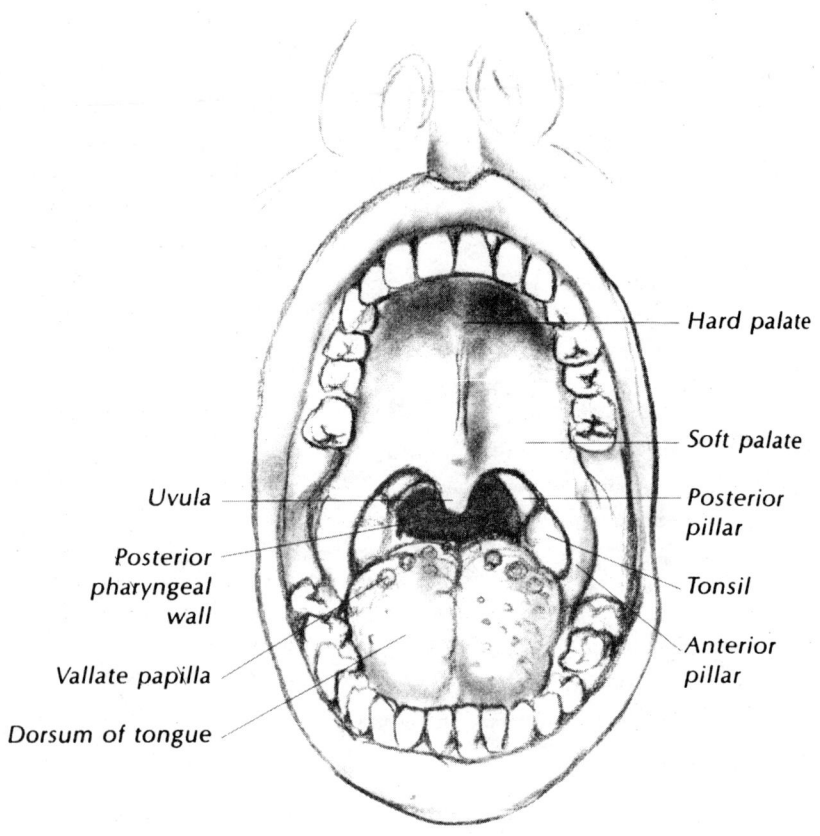

Courtesy Barbara Bates, M.D.
from a Guide to Physical Examination, p 62
Written permission from the publisher, J. B. Lippincott Co.

MOUTH-BREATHING

Some children's mouths seem always open; they seem to breathe through it all the time. When they sleep, they continue to noisily breathe through the mouth, and this seems to the parents to have been going on for too long. Their noses are not that stuffy, but somehow the children cannot easily breathe through them. This mouth-breathing becomes exceedingly bothersome to parents of these children, and to others.

What causes it?

There are two major causes: an enlarged adenoid or an allergy of the nose. Other causes are rare.

When the adenoids are enlarged, they will partially obstruct the passageway of the air that the child breathes through the nose. This area is called nasopharynx, and it is above the soft palate, at the back of the base of the nose. Generally speaking, the adenoids, along with the tonsils, enlarge naturally when the child is three or four years of age. This enlargement is not enough to obstruct the nasopharynx. Even when enlarged by infection, the adenoids will produce either no obstruction or at most only a temporary obstruction. Therefore, infected adenoids, though enlarged, will not be our problem.

In a small percentage of children the adenoids enlarge more than usual, to such a degree as to obstruct the nasopharynx. The child will then resort to mouth-breathing, since he or she cannot breathe through the nose. Early cases are usually not discovered. Usually a year or so passes by before parents start observing the mouth-breathing phenomenon and become concerned.

Should we really be concerned about it?

Yes, mouth-breathing is a condition to be concerned about before some permanent changes take place. If you leave it go, the structure of the face will slowly but progressively adjust to the new situation. It will lead to what is called adenoid facies.

With adenoid facies, the child will have an open mouth, droopy eyes, and a "blocked" nasal quality to the voice, and when asleep, he or she will exhibit noisy breathing. The bridge of the nose may also become thickened, and the palate in some cases highly arched. The profile and frontal facial features may change substantially. Even dental malocculsion can result in some cases.

Not all cases are like the above. In early stages, mouth-breathing, snoring, and a nasal quality to the voice may be all the symptoms you can detect. It is at this early stage that corrective measures have to be taken. If you wait for a few years and the changes in the features of the face take place, it is too late for the corrective measures to be successful.

What can be done about it?

If the obstructing adenoids are the cause, removal of the enlarged adenoids will cure this condition. But this is said with reservation. The timing factor for the correction is most important, since only early obstruction will not have caused any changes in the bones of the face. At this stage, removing the adenoids gives the best results. When the obstruction is removed, the nasal passages will open once again, and breathing will be back to normal.

If mouth-breathing has continued for many years, and the facial bone-structure has changed its configuration, removing the adenoids will hardly help. The bones will usually remain as is, in spite of adenoidectomy. In addition, the child may continue to breathe through the mouth, because it has become a habit!

Will removing the adenoids help the child in other ways?

In a number of cases, the adenoids may press on the eustachian tube, and indirectly lead to various degrees of serous otitis media (gluey ear). Naturally when this uncommon condition is discovered, the removal of the adenoids, if they are related, will be mandatory, and it will relieve the condition.

In others, the large obstructing adenoids will cause pooling of the secretions of the nose, as the secretions drain backwards. Infection will often set in, and not rarely sinusitis may occur, along with postnasal drip. Upon removing the adenoids, the drainage will be established, and the infections and sinusitis will clear up promptly.

How about mouth-breathing caused by nasal allergy?

Mouth-breathing caused by allergy of the nose is fairly common and it behaves in a different manner. Usually the child has some allergic manifestations such as runny nose, sneezing, shiners under the eyes, postnasal drip, etc.

In some children however, the allergic rhinitis (see page 278) is not as bad as mentioned above, but the nasal mucous membrane seems to continue to be boggy and engorged. This will obstruct the airway within the nose, and the child will have no choice but to breathe through the mouth.

Usually if the nasal allergy is severe enough to cause mouth-breathing, it may be severe enough to initiate allergy control, such as the use of nasal decongestants and antihistamines of different forms (see page 305), humidifiers (see page 290), and even electronic air filters (see page 292). In a number of cases, the nasal allergy becomes reasonably controlled, and gradually the nasal passages open. In other cases, the nasal allergy is too advanced to respond to the above treatment. Allergy tests and allergy shots will have to be instituted, and will usually be followed by some degree of improvement in a few months. The improvement will be slow and gradual; not only will the allergy disappear, but so will the mouth-breathing.

It is safe to say that more mouth-breathing is related to nasal allergy than to enlarged adenoids. Other causes, as stated before, are not that common.

GEOGRAPHIC TONGUE

The name must arouse your curiosity. The name stems from a condition wherein the tongue's surface takes on a "maplike" appearance. Instead of even coloring, the tongue will have a patch with edges that are irregularly wavy and clearly defined. Usually only a part of the tongue is affected this way; the rest of the surface will look beefy red or bright red, but without tenderness or pain. Therefore, the patch will stand out in sharp contrast to the rest of the tongue. Yet, there will be no pain or complaints. To your surprise, however, a few days later you may notice that the patch will have changed its shape. This is to be expected.

Is this a dangerous thing?
Geographic tongue is a fairly common thing, and there are many theories about its causes. Although it may scare you when you discover it, soon you will find out that this is a benign condition and there is no cause for alarm. It will come and go, and it is better to ignore it.

It does not deserve any kind of treatment, nor any special precautions, and the child can eat and drink as usual, without any restrictions.

How does the disease progress?
Geographic tongue is a curiosity disease and is harmless enough to be merely a conversation piece. You cannot prevent it and you do not have to, since it is such a benign condition. It often shows up for several months if not several years, usually changing shape from week to week, before it finally goes away.

How about using gargles or mouthwashes?
Since the condition is benign, and since it may go on and on for several years, it makes no sense to use anything in an attempt to help the situation. Besides, lozenges, gargles, or mouthwashes are completely ineffective. On the contrary, they may even irritate the tongue and cause problems. Therefore, it is best to ignore geographic tongue, once you learn about its nature.

STOMATITIS (TRENCH MOUTH)

Don't dread it, stomatitis is not as serious as you may think. It is not uncommon, and many a baby or a young child will become afflicted with it every so often. The term trench mouth is a popular, colorful misnomer used by many doctors for the condition known as stomatitis. Stomatitis is an inflammation of the mucous membrane of the mouth. It is usually mild, but can be severe at times.

What does stomatitis look like?

The child's mouth looks and feels very sore. The gums may be swollen, and congested at the edge. In some cases they become ulcerated and may even bleed. The tongue may also be red and sore, making it difficult for the child to eat. The sides of the mouth and the palate may show a few shallow ulcers. The poor little one will be drooling a lot, since the mouth is too sore to even swallow the saliva. The child's breath may have a faint odor too.

The temperature is often normal or slightly high, though it can reach 103 to 104 degrees F in severe cases. The child is hungry and thirsty, since it is too painful to chew on food. These conditions often lead to extreme fussiness and irritability.

How long will this last?

In mild cases it may take five to seven days before going away, with a fairly severe period of only two or three days. In severe cases, however, it may take ten to fourteen days before going away, and will be fairly bad for four to five days. Fortunately the majority are mild cases.

What causes stomatitis?

Very possibly it is caused by a virus, though many claim otherwise. Upon having the infection, the child will build a resistance to it, and future reinfections are rare or not that severe. Younger children and babies also don't have a natural resistance to stomatitis until they come down with it but they will develop various degrees of immunity to it once they have the disease.

What can we do for it?

You may be able to treat mild cases at home since such cases are self limited. Most cases of stomatitis must be diagnosed and evaluated by the doctor, since some medication is needed to take away the soreness. As mentioned before, the soreness of the mouth is the main reason the poor child cannot eat, and not eating for too long will alarm the parents.

Therefore, bland nourishing foods have to be given, and sour, hot, or rough foods have to be avoided. Feed the child cold milk, milkshake, ice cream, slightly warm soups, baby foods, jello, pudding, applesauce, soft-boiled egg, egg nog and the like. These are used as a temporary measure until the condition goes away and the stomatitis becomes history. Don't worry about starvation.

Avoid hot foods, including hot soups, since they will hurt the already sore mouth. The same applies to spicy foods, or foods that need chewing, including peanut butter sandwiches -sore gums become very painful upon chewing. Juices such as orange juice or carbonated beverages in all their forms often burn the sore mouth, and they ought to be avoided, too, until the stomatitis is gone.

Once the condition clears, children often attack the food with vengeance, and their hamburgers, and peanut butter sandwiches may seem as if sent from heaven.

Does it come from dirt?

Although putting dirt in the mouth is indeed unhealthy, it has nothing to do with such a disease. Stomatitis affects children who are clean or dirty, rich or poor. It has to affect them for them to build a future resistance to it. There are even some cases so mild as to skip your attention, but in the meantime the child will develop an immunity.

What will the doctor do?

Other than checking and evaluating the child, the doctor may suggest a medicine to take the soreness away. Chloraseptic gel (nonprescription) but not other forms of chloraseptic, is pretty good, and may be used on the gums and sides of the mouth before and after eating. Other medicines, such as Xylocaine Viscous Solution (prescription) or Orajel (nonprescription) may be used too.

In very rare circumstances a baby with stomatitis may completely refuse to take any food or drink. If this continues for too long, it may justifiably alarm every one: hospitalization and intravenous feeding may even be necessary. These are drastic measures, but fortunately it is very rare that a baby will need them.

How contagious is it?

It is somewhat contagious but usually only among the young children who haven't already developed immunity to it from previous infections. The contagiousness, however, doesn't amount to too much, even among children; it is rare to find that two members in a family have developed the stomatitis.

Most cases of stomatitis seem to come out of nowhere. Therefore prevention can be next to impossible. If your infant or young child is to be in a day-care nursery or another place that has children, and if you know that one of these children has stomatitis, it will be wise to keep your child away.

Is there a real "trench mouth"?
The real trench mouth is a special infection by itself, claimed to be caused by certain bacteria. It affects adults and children, and usually has a different appearance in the mouth than stomatitis. It may even be difficult for some doctors to differentiate trench mouth from stomatitis. Most people, however, use the term trench mouth loosely, to mean stomatitis, and the treatment of, and approach to the two diseases are indeed similar to each other to some extent.

APHTHA
CANKER SORE

They are commonly called canker sores. They are fairly common, and they may affect children as well as adults. In some people these aphtha ulcers show up repeatedly for a good many years, though they are more likely to show up only every once in a while in a child.

What is aphtha?
Aphtha is a small shallow lesion, in the form of an ulcer. It affects the mucous membrane of the mouth, mainly the sides of the mouth, the gums, and the trough between the gums and the lining of the cheek.

It shows up as a sore, painful red spot that soon becomes a shallow ulcer, usually oval in shape, with a fairly sharp margin. The base of the ulcer may be yellow, but the edges and the area around are often red in color.

Sometimes there may be a double ulcer (kissing ulcer) whereby there is one such ulcer on the gum, and the other ulcer on the lining of the cheek that touches the ulcer. It is also more common to have several ulcers in the same vicinity or on the other side of the mouth.

What causes it?

The cause of these ulcers is unknown for sure. They seem to appear whenever the resistance of the body seems to suffer. Therefore aphtha can show before or along with other diseases, be they of the mouth or other parts of the body. Aphtha can also show up when the person is under stress, e.g. taking exams, working exceptionally hard, or having constipation among other things.

How long do these ulcers take?

They take a few days before reaching maturity. Gradually, the ulcer will become less painful and the healing process will become obvious. In about seven to ten days the ulcer will be almost gone.

During the first few days of its life, the aphtha is quite painful and the child will often complain of the soreness. Yet, the soreness is not bad enough to prevent eating or cause drooling.

It is not unusual to see one ulcer having taken its course and ready to disappear before another one shows up, or two to three others to show up at the same time. Thus, the soreness caused by the ulcers can be prolonged to a troublesome extent.

What can we do about them?

If they are limited to themselves, you don't have to go to the doctor.

The local treatment is quite simple. You may want to use Gly-Oxide (nonprescription); make sure to follow carefully the directions on the bottle. Or you may dip a Q-tip in pure undiluted Cepacol (nonprescription), then touch the aphtha ulcer with the moistened Q-tip . Do this regularly a few minutes before meals. Keep doing it as long as the ulcer is sore and painful. Another way of using Cepacol is to dilute it with water and use it as a gargle. Many children however, don't like either the action of gargling or the taste of gargle. If the pain is fairly severe, you may want to use Chloraseptic gel (nonprescription). It is a fairly good local anesthetic. Apply it to the ulcer four times a day for a few days.

How dangerous is aphtha?

It is more of a nuisance than a disease of any significance. Some persons are more susceptible to it than others, and there seem to be some who may continue to get it on and off for a good many years. I hope you and your child won't have that problem, but even so, you will learn to adjust to it and treat it accordingly.

How about preventing these ulcers?

Unfortunately there is not much in the way of prevention. Good oral hygiene is of little help, and it seems that these ulcers are as common with smokers as they are with nonsmokers.

Taking extra vitamins, being careful about spicy or greasy foods, or taking any other extra measures seem to be of practically no help in preventing these ulcers.

Usually the resistance of the body will play its part and all of a sudden you may see that these ulcers will have stopped appearing so frequently.

THE PERMANENT TEETH

After having had a loose front tooth for so long, it is a happy time when your six- or seven-year old child loses his or her front tooth, and sleeps with the expectation for the tooth fairy. The incisors will then slowly and gradually come to replace the baby teeth.

There are thirty-two permanent teeth. The period of dentition is a prolonged one, almost up to the age of eighteen to twenty years, when the wisdom teeth finalize their appearance. By this time the slow growth of the jaws is completing, thus giving space for the teeth. The teeth may appear crooked or crowded, especially the front teeth. Many such cases will correct themselves given a number of years for the growth of the jawbones. However, a certain percentage of such teeth will need the help of the orthodontist.

When the incisors have completely erupted, they are followed by the front jaw teeth. The latter two will replace their corresponding baby jaw teeth. By now the child is almost ten to twelve years old, and the canines finally erupt, making the row of teeth look even. The third set of back jaw teeth will appear gradually, and this is followed by the emergence of the wisdom teeth, as space in the jaw bones becomes available for them.

TOOTH ABSCESS AND GUM BOIL

The child's tooth has been hurting a lot, then somehow the pain subsides. You have thought of going to the dentist but the idea by now seems to have evaporated. But soon you see swelling of the cheek and/or the gum, or even of the area of the base of the lip. The swelling seems to progress steadily, and you become more scared and concerned. The swollen area is tender, slightly pink, tense, and accompanies a rise in temperature.

The child will usually point to some discomfort in the gum area adjacent to the swelling. You take a good look out of curiosity and see swelling of the gums, coming to a head somehow, and when you touch it, it will feel quite sore.

And your doctor will say bring him in:

The doctor will check the area and tell you that it is a tooth abscess, or a gum boil. Usually the tooth nearby either has a cavity, has died, or has been broken or chipped because of an accident before.

How can a nearby tooth cause an abscess?

Because the mouth is loaded with a variety of germs; when a tooth is diseased, the germs find a haven in which to multiply and cause trouble. The decayed area will act as a focus - the infection will burrow itself, making a tunnel through the bone. This tunnel starts at the base of the tooth, becomes loaded with pus and infection, and reaches outside to the gums and the tissues around, i.e. going through the jawbone! If it points mainly to the gums, the gums will be red, inflamed, sore, and may even ooze some of the pus, leaving a bad taste and smell in the mouth. The infection may also go to the soft tissues of the cheeks making them swollen and painful. There may be quite dangerous consequences if the infection spreads to certain other areas.

Where does the infection spread?

If the swollen area is the upper lip and the base of the nose, it can be potentially dangerous. This indicates that the tooth abscess comes from diseased front teeth, a broken or chipped upper incisor tooth. It is dangerous because there is a network of veins in that vicinity that can pick up the infection and transfer it to certain areas in the brain leading to grave consequences. It is scary to think of, so we must beware.

What would the doctor do for the tooth abscess?

An antibiotic, usually penicillin or its equivalent, will suffice, if used for ten days or so in the proper dose. It can be given either in the form of one shot or a course of oral medication. The infection will gradually subside, the swelling will be under control and the temperature will drop down to normal. Occasionally, the abscess has to be opened from inside, to drain the pus.

Will the abscessed tooth have to come out?

In the majority of cases, yes. Your dentist will be of help in this decision. Occasionally the tooth can be fixed in such a way as to prevent the recurrence.

Is tooth abscess preventable?

Yes, if you have taken good care of the teeth. If a dentist has taken care of any cavities or the chipped tooth, the likelihood of a tooth abscess will be extremely remote, and you and your child will feel quite safe.

ACCIDENTS TO THE MOUTH

Accidents in general are common, especially those that involve the mouths of children. This is true in children who are a few years old and younger. There are certain aspects worth learning about in regard to accidents of this nature.

Accidents to the mouth can be divided into three groups:

1. those caused by physical force, e.g. from a fall or enduring cuts inside.
2. those caused by foreign bodies (not common).
3. those caused by drinking some chemical or hot liquid.

Each group of the above can lead to a different difficulty.

How is that?

In the first group, it is fairly common for the tooth to go through the soft tissue of the lip, cutting deeply, and even emerge through it to the skin. It is not unusual either for the upper frenulum (the ridge that connects the upper lip to the gum area) or the tongue to be cut. A cut on the tongue is usually small, but every once in a while the laceration is through the tongue, and it may be quite big.

There is also another form of accidents caused by physical force. This happens when a child has a stick in his or her mouth, and falls on it; the stick will cut the palate, often in a gruesome way.

All these lead to a lot of bleeding and crying from the scared, bloody child.

What will you do?

Most such accidents are minor and insignificant. If the cut is small, be it in the lip, frenulum, or tongue, it will heal without stitches. Bigger cuts should be cheked by the doctor, but rarely will stitches be needed, because stitches don't stay well enough in these areas.

The cut will look pussy for a few days, and of course there will be pain. If the cut interferes with eating, feed the child bland cold liquids or a soft diet, e.g. milkshakes, milk, ice cream, jello, applesauce, etc. Using ointments on the mucous membrane will be of little value since it will be washed away with saliva. Antibiotics are not needed in most cases, because the blood supply here is very rich and healing will often take place in a few days. But check with the doctor to see if the child needs a tetanus shot.

How about mouth accidents caused by a foreign body?

These are not common. We have seen some metal portions of toys being the cause of such accidents. This usually leads to lacerations in the palate.

The laceration of the palate may prove to be large and the bleeding may be severe. Some patients we have seen had almost cut one tonsil in half! And some were so bad that they even damaged the bone of the palate. If such accidents involve the two big arteries of the palate, the bleeding will be ferocious.

And what of the mouth accidents caused by chemicals?

Of course such accidents depend on the nature of the chemical. A child loves to put things in the mouth, and loves to explore and experiment.

If the child happens to experiment with a caustic material (lye), acid, or with other numerous available chemicals, he or she will develop a chemical burn (drinking hot liquids will lead to thermal burn).

The tongue may be the victim, especially its tip, developing chemical glossitis. The lips, the palate, and the pharynx often get burned too. Parents, please let the doctor see such cases and treat them accordingly or go to the poison control center of the nearest hospital.

Parents must try to do preventive work such as keeping hot liquids and chemicals away from the child, and keeping a cautious eye out.

How about the teeth?

Often enough, the teeth do become involved in mouth accidents, and it is usually the upper front teeth that are most affected. They can be chipped or cracked, or they may die and become discolored. In some severe accidents, the bone that holds the tooth may even break or chip, leading to other complications.

Whenever there is suspicion that the teeth have been involved in the accident, the dentist ought to be consulted as soon as possible. Not only will he or she help assure you about the teeth, but also may remedy the problem in its earliest stages thus giving it the best chance for success.

THE THROAT

See your throat in a mirror, or take a look at the throat of your child. When the mouth is wide open and the tongue is not in the way, you will see the soft palate which arches nicely, having the uvula dangling from the middle of its edge. The uvula looks like a tiny "tongue," extending down, sometimes even to the base of the tongue.

The back wall of the mouth forms part of the pharynx. The wall of the pharynx has tiny protrusions, which are lymphoid follicles. At the sides of the pharynx, the tonsils sit like lumps, the size of small walnuts or smaller. Sometimes they are so small as to be hardly noticeable. Often the wall of the tonsils is not smooth, but seems to have pits or irregular shallow convolutions. The tonsils are hugged by two ridges, one in front and one behind each tonsil. They stand like pillars or folds of adjacent tissue. These are called pillars of the tonsils.

Why do the tonsils vary in size?

Variation in the size of the tonsils is quite natural and normal. Also the tonsils undergo changes in size in the same person at different ages, which are also normal.

When a baby becomes one or two years old, the tonsils become bigger. This is part of the increase in the size of lymphoid follicles in the area. The tonsils become fairly big at the age of three to four years, and continue to be large for a few years. When the child reaches the age of eight to nine years, the tonsils gradually start to shrink. Upon entering adolescence, the child's tonsils become small, and sometimes they shrivel to such an extent that they will hardly be visible.

One word of caution: depending on how far the child can open his or her mouth and how far the tongue can protrude, you may get a false impression that his or her tonsils are huge. A better way of assessing the size of the tonsils is to depress the base of the child's tongue with the handle of a spoon, then take a quick look at them.

Can we see the adenoids?

The adenoids hide above the level of the palate, therefore they are not directly visible. They consist of a lump in the back of the throat, high up near the opening of the eustachian tubes (one on each side). You may be able to feel the adenoids, but in the process the child will either gag or bite your finger. Good luck!

Usually the adenoids become larger in size at the same time the tonsils do, and they undergo shrinkage too as the child becomes older. When they become large, however, they are apt to partially obstruct the eustachian tubes and may indirectly cause trouble for the ears. When there are frequent ear infections or the "gluey" ear, an ear, nose, and throat specialist may deem it necessary to remove the adenoids. When the adenoids become very big, they may partially obstuct the throat (nasopharynx). When this happens, the child will become a mouth-breather, and may even develop what is called adenoid facies or "adenoid looks" (see page 231). If this is the case, the adenoids have to be removed early enough so that the child can have an easier time breathing.

How come the throat becomes infected so often?

The throat is a gateway, joining the nasal passages with the respiratory tree and esophagus, and at the same time it joins the mouth with the esophagus and larynx. Therefore the pharynx, tonsils, and adenoids are the victims of a good many viruses and bacteria. They have to put up an almost constant struggle against these viruses and bacteria.

Not only that, but things like postnasal drip, nasal discharge, offending agents from the mouth, etc., must be stopped. This should be coupled with the fact that the child's resistance is building up during the very first few years of life, thus making him or her vulnerable to frequent infections of the throat. It is said that an average American child will get about six attacks of such infections in a year's time.

What kind of infections are they?

Sore throats are about the most common infection in childhood. Viruses are the cause of most such infections, but some bacteria are also responsible, and of those, strep is the most troublesome. The latter may lead to pharyngitis, acute tonsillitis, and other local infections, and it is the main reason doctors take cultures so often.

Herpangina (see page 250) is also a fairly frequent disease of the throat, especially during summertime. It is caused by coxsackievirus, and shows like small shallow ulcers on the pillars of the tonsils and on the soft palate.

Can you see postnasal drip in the pharynx?

Not in all cases. When you see it, it will be a clear or pussy discharge in the form of a sheet on one side of the pharynx or lining the whole pharynx. Occasionally it smells but in general it does not. The pharynx usually does not show congestion though the child complains of a sore throat.

Pus on the tonsils (exudate) is fairly common. Usually if the tonsils are acutely infected, pus is a fairly good indication of strep infection. If the tonsils seem to have almost no inflammation, the white material on their surface is debris, i.e. food mixed with bacteria and dead cells, dried up and imprisoned in one of the crypts of the tonsils.

Pus on the tonsils may indicate infectious mononucleosis, whereby the exudate is usually white with a yellowish tinge, fairly stuck to the tonsils, almost like a membrane. The nodes at the angle of the jaw bone enlarge and so will the spleen in many such cases.

The throat can thus be a mirror of many conditions in the body. Not every sore throat is simply a virus infection to be ignored.

LOZENGES, GARGLES, AND MOUTH SPRAYS

Many times questions are asked: How about using lozenges, gargles, or mouth sprays? How useful are they? When are they to be used?

There are many over-the-counter preparations for the purpose, many with claims that are hard to believe and may even be misleading. To understand how and when to use such preparations, a person must have an idea about their purpose and the mechanism involved.

How is that?

It is worth mentioning that in each cubic centimeter of saliva there are about 125 million bacteria. Most of these bacteria are not harmful. They are there because the mouth is a good incubator, i.e. the conditions for the growth of all these bacteria and viruses are quite favorable.

For a mild sore throat, some mouth ulcers, sore gums, or a bad taste in the mouth, a person may wonder about using such preparations. Upon asking the doctor, he or she may be surprised to see that the doctor is hardly in favor of using these preparations and may say: they are useless.

Are these preparations useless?

Most over-the-counter preparations are of limited value, and many are truly useless. Let us take some examples.

Sore throats are caused by viruses or some bacteria; and if it happens to be caused by bacteria, an antibiotic is mandatory. If the sore throat is caused by postnasal drip, however, lozenges will be of some help. In that case, they will act as a demulcent (lubricant to the throat), and they will soothe the area. This may be true of other minor sore conditions in the mouth too.

What about lozenges?

Cepacol lozenges and Chloraseptic lozenges are tolerably goodtasting. They have very mild medications and they may leave a medicinal-tasting but slightly refreshed mouth.

Lozenges are to be sucked and not chewed. If they are used on a trial basis, use them for mild conditions in the mouth or throat, but no longer than two or three days. In other words, don't be lulled into wishful thinking or false security. If the condition is checked by a doctor who suggests using such lozenges, go ahead and use them for many days until the throat or mouth feels better.

How about gargles?

Gargles used to be in vogue many years back. Doctors rarely recommend them nowadays, because they simply wash the surface of the mucous membrane of the mouth and throat, and not even effectively at that. Most children cannot gargle easily. The diseased throat or mucous membrane of the mouth does not improve much with a gargle because the disease-changes in the tissues are deeper than the surface.

On the other hand, a gargle gives a clean feeling to the mouth. If it is to be used, a gargle consisting of one glass of water and one-fourth of a teaspoon of salt will suffice. It can be used as often as a person wants. Another worthwhile gargle consists of a glass of water and one teaspoon of Cepacol mouthwash. This will have a medicinal but refreshing taste in the mouth. These gargles may help wash some of the debris off the surface of the mucous membrane of the mouth.

How about mouth sprays?

The same rule applies to both mouth sprays and mouthwashes. Some have a strong and nasty taste. Often the user sprays the tongue, the palate, and the throat, and ends up with a strong funny taste that makes the eyes water. Chloraseptic and other sprays may be used at times.

The value of such medications is very limited indeed, but may make you feel better.

In short, lozenges, gargles, mouthwashes, and mouth sprays are often not suitable for children's use, are of very limited value, may be refreshing; and that if they are used for two to three days without an improvement in the child's condition, it will be wise to look into the cause of the sore throat.

SORE THROAT

This is the most common complaint in a pediatric practice. The child's throat may feel raw, it may hurt to swallow, and he or she may shoot up to 104 or 105 F and scare the devil out of you. Your child will look flushed, pale around the mouth and may even have foul-smelling breath. You use antipyretics such as aspirin or Tylenol regularly every four hours (see page 131), but the child's temperature may or may not come down to normal in a day or two.

At times the sore throat is the only symptom, and it seems to last forever. At other times, headache, stomachache, nausea, and even vomiting once or twice may occur, and occasionally there may be a hacking raspy cough.

What causes these sore throats?

Sore throat is only a symptom. Most sore throats are a symptom of inflamed throat or tonsils, the causes are usually viral or bacterial.

The sore throat can be caused by postnasal drip and it can also be one of the symptoms of upper respiratory infections, some generalized disease, or it can be caused by local diseases in the area of the throat.

When can I ignore a sore throat?

Most sore throats should not be ignored, especially if they are accompanied by other symptoms. If the child is also feverish, or has a headache, stomachache or other symptoms, and if these symptoms persist for a day or two, then it would be wise to see the doctor. If it is a sore throat with no other problems, and if it doesn't take long before it goes away, then you can subsequently ignore it.

Is sore throat contagious?

Most cases of sore throat are contagious, and you ought to be careful about being in close contact whether the child has bacterial or a viral infection.

What would the doctor do for it?

Very much depends on the diagnosis. If it is mainly the tonsils or the throat being inflamed, then a culture ought to be taken first, and treatment will follow accordingly (see page 143). If it is a case of postnasal drip (see page 281), an upper respiratory infection (see page 307), croup (see page 313), laryngitis (see page 309), treatment will concentrate on the specific trouble.

In other words, treat what is leading to the feeling of sore throat and the child's well-being will improve. Just don't be disgusted or discouraged if your child gets these sore throats often; all parents pass through such experiences.

What happens if I don't treat sore throats?

If the sore throat is caused by a strep infection of the tonsils or the pharynx, you will be taking a chance with rheumatic fever or glomerulonephritis if you don't treat it. In addition, you will be taking a chance with a number of complications of the strep such as inflamed ears, inflamed lymph nodes (at the angle of the jaw), sinus infection in older children, etc.

In the not so "good" old days when medical facilities were not as advanced, children and adults used to suffer so much from such infections. There is no reason to take a step backward in our progress.

If other causes of sore throat are not treated, there may be a chance for complications to show up, some of which are harder to treat than the disease itself.

HERPANGINA

Suddenly the child's temperature is up, not unlikely to around 103 degrees F or even higher. The color of the skin appears "off," and the child complains of a sore throat and being tired. There may be nausea and some stomachache. More often, however, the little one complains of a headache that occasionally becomes severe.

The above symptoms may not show up in their entirety, yet, on the other hand, others may occur: swollen glands under the angle of the jaw, some vomiting, loss of appetite, and/or irritability. The doctor may diagnose herpangina.

What is herpangina anyway?

It is a fairly common disease, and it usually shows up in the form of a "small epidemic," affecting a good many children in a short period of time; in about two to three weeks the "epidemic" seems to go away.

It usually shows up when it is quite warm outside, often during July and August, when the swimming pool is used quite frequently.

Herpangina is caused by the Coxsackievirus.

What will the doctor do?

The doctor will check the child and see redness of the throat, often with small "bumps," on it; there may also be shallow tiny ulcers, especially on the pillars of the tonsils. Some children may have a few pinpoint spots of hemorrhage on the palate.

The doctor may also take a throat culture, because strep may complicate herpangina, or it may simply simulate it, not only in its course but also during the examination.

What shall we expect of this disease?

Since herpangina is caused by a virus, treatment with an antibiotic will not help at all. Therefore, this disease has to take its course. In mild cases, the temperature may come down to normal the next day.

In a good many others, however, it may take three to four days of feeling tired and achy, of having a headache and fever, until the condition is over. In more cases, a course of fever of up to seven to eight days is not unusual; when in addition to the above symptoms, the child will not eat, will complain, and will feel tired and out of sorts. When you call the doctor for help, he or she will still say an antibiotic should not be used, because of the viral nature of herpangina and the negative throat culture. You will feel helpless, of course, and so does the doctor, but your child will improve slowly with time.

Is this a contagious condition?

Yes, especially from child to child. Playing together, coughing in each others' face, and swimming together may be the main methods of spreading the virus. Kissing the parents may also spread the virus, although adults are far less likely to catch this disease.

Can I prevent herpangina?

A few steps may help prevent it. However, even if the child gets this disease, it is no more than a self-limited condition that often lasts for one to three days or so, and only on rare occasions is it severe.

If the "epidemic" is in, simply prevent your child from going to the swimming pool or mixing with crowds. Not only that, but once your doctor says your child has herpangina, separate the child from siblings and don't let the child kiss you until the symptoms have been cleared away for about twenty-four hours.

Can I help the child to be comfortable?

Yes, you can. If the child sucks on hard candy, Chloraseptic lozenges, or Cepacol lozenges, the throat will be soothed (but not healed). For the fever you will, of course, give the little one an antipyretic such as aspirin or Tylenol in the appropriate dosage, every four hours as needed. Bland liquids and soft diet will be more to his or her liking, and resting and watching TV or reading a book will help pass the time until the condition is back to normal.

ACUTE TONSILLITIS

Often children complain of a sore throat that may be severe; their temperatures may suddenly be up, even to 104 degrees F or higher, and their faces may look flushed but pale around the mouth. If they are old enough they may complain of a headache, feel queasy, be irritable, and may refuse to eat. Sometimes they feel nauseated or vomit once or twice. If the inflamed tonsils are swollen and big, they may talk as if they have a lump in the throat. Their breath may smell putrid, as if there is some degree of decay inside.

Not all cases of tonsillitis are like that, however.

How is that?

Mild cases of acute tonsillitis usually have the above symptoms to a lesser extent. Like any other disease, tonsillitis can be very mild, even to such an extent that it may escape your attention or you may ignore it; it can be moderately severe where the child has to see the doctor and receive medication, or it can be quite severe whereby a doctor's visit must be arranged as soon as possible.

What causes tonsillitis?

In most cases tonsillitis is caused by viruses although bacteria may be the cause too, especially the strep germ (in about ten to twenty per cent). It is said that the bacteria are opportunists, and may come on top of the viral infection, because the viruses make the tonsils receptive to the bacterial infection. This is also true of cases of pharyngitis and some other infections.

Why does the child keep getting these infections?

Sore throats, pharyngitis, tonsillitis, and respiratory infections are very common in the first few years of life. There are many reasons for that, and an advantage. The advantage is that with each infection the resistance of the child will be stimulated to a higher level, and by the age of five years or around the level of resistance will have gone to an excellent height.

If given time, the chances are very good that the frequency of these infections will become lower, and that healthier times are ahead. Perhaps most parents will think of having the tonsils and adenoids removed as soon as they hear that the child has tonsillitis, but most such cases ought to be treated with medications in a conservative intelligent manner, short of an actual T & A (see page 254).

What can be done about tonsillitis?

The child with acute tonsillitis should see the doctor for diagnosis, assessment of the condition, and a culture. A culture is a must since a number of these infections turn out to be the result of strep infection.

A course of penicillin or its substitutes will of course have to be given once we know that strep is the causative agent. A repeat culture after the course of treatment is also mandatory to determine if the strep has been eradicated. When treatment is initiated, the response is usually very good and within a day or two the child will bounce back to normal. However, if the tonsillitis is caused by a virus, it will have to take its course and it may take four to five days before the child is O.K.

Symptomatic treatment will have to be observed too, of course. An antipyretic such as aspirin or Tylenol for the fever and/or headache, liquids, soft diet, and rest are some important points to observe.

What about prevention?

As with any other disease, don't expose the child to someone sick, or allow close contact with others, or expose the child unnecessarily during inclement winter weather. If the case of tonsillitis is treated promptly, there will be less chance of it spreading to others in the family. In this day and age, tonsillitis is a nuisance disease that is easily treatable; gone are the days when the tonsils used to be removed for only a few episodes of acute inflammation. With culturing and the available present day medications, most episodes of tonsillitis can easily be cured.

What happens if we don't treat tonsillitis?

Cases of acute tonsillitis that have not received any treatment often subside gradually over a period of a week or so. In some cases it may take longer.

However (and this is a big however), chances for complications are much higher in such cases. If the acute tonsillitis has been caused by strep, not treating may lead to rheumatic fever, glomerulonephritis of the kidneys, or local complications such as infection of the "cervical " lymph nodes, among others.

The advantage of medicine now compared to yesteryear is that most if not all such complications can be prevented by having early diagnosis and treatment.

T & A (REMOVING THE TONSILS AND ADENOIDS)

The term T & A simply means the removal of the tonsils and adenoids. In the U.S.A., it is a half-billion-dollar industry a year, most of which is unnecessary.

T & A used to be done very frequently in the decades past, usually with the assumption that the tonsils and adenoids are useless and do get infected often. A doctor may have done fifty to seventy-five cases a year, if not more. Nowadays, a competent, conscientious doctor is likely to refer an average of about one child a year for T & A, if even that.

Why the change?

The tonsils and adenoids are there for a purpose, and as medicine has advanced, many unsuspected functions have been discovered, notable among them is an increase in the local resistance.

The throat and tonsils do get infected often, usually in the ages of one to five years. After that, sore throats may show up once a year or less often. Most such infections are viral and only ten to twenty percent prove to be caused by strep. Strep germ can be easily detected these days via throat cultures, and can also be easily treated and eradicated.

Even for the gluey ears (serous otitis media, see page 213) removing the adenoids is being discontinued more and more these days. It has been found out that only in a certain percentage of such children do the adenoids need to be removed.

And of course there is the possible danger of the operation and anesthesia.

How is that?

Though most cases of T & A -and the anesthesia for them- are without danger, every once in a while a child ends up with trouble. Severe bleeding after the operation is not unknown, and cardiac arrests have occurred in rare cases, and some children have lost their lives because of it.

Common sense dictates then, that if the operation is hardly needed, a chance should not be taken.

Then when will you remove the tonsils and adenoids?

There are some rare circumstances whereby T & A will have to be done. The following are the main examples:

1. If the tonsils and adenoids are so huge as to fill the throat and obstruct the nasopharynx. The child then becomes a mouth breather, and his or her sleep is quite restless. Perhaps once every few years a pediatrician will have a case like this.
2. If there are very frequent infections of the tonsils (and not simply sore throat), e.g. every six to eight weeks. This means five to eight infections a year. If this trend continues for two

consecutive years, then go for T & A.
3. In the uncommon case of gluey ear, whereby the adenoids are interfering with the function of the eustachian tube. The ear, nose and throat specialist will be able to tell about that.

What happens to the tonsils if they are not removed?

Tonsils and adenoids are part of the lymphoid tissue. They are supposed to become bigger naturally, and by the age of three to four years they are at their biggest. It is at this stage where some parents mistakenly consider the tonsils to have become too large, and ask to remove them.

But if you leave the tonsils where they are, they will start to shrink when the child is eight to ten years old. During adolescence the tonsils will have shrunk to insignificant pieces of tissue happily sitting in their cozy spots.

HAND, FOOT, AND MOUTH DISEASE

Yes it is a funny name, and it may put a smile on your face, but seriously speaking, such a diseae does exist. This oddly named disease comes more or less in epidemics, and usually during summer time. It may show up successively every summer for two or three years, then disappear for a few years just to reappear again.

Children, especially young ones, are more likely to get it. Usually most adults are immune to it since they will have built up an immunity to it during their childhood when they contracted the disease.

How does it show up?

It affects children to various degrees of severity. In an average case there will be an up-and-down temperature -may be even to 104 degrees F and more- and the fever may continue for two to three days or longer. The child may have a headache and/or stomachache, feel nauseated, and may vomit.

There will be complaints of a sore throat that can become severe enough to make it difficult for the child to even swallow saliva or be able to eat properly. His or her throat will be congested and may show many tiny red spots at the palate, or ulcers on the tonsils and the areas around.

The hands and feet will also show dark red, pinhead-sized spots that are concentrated on the palms and soles, especially near their junction with the rest of the skin. There may be half a dozen or more of these on each hand or foot. In some other cases, these spots might look like very small blisters, superficially situated under the skin; these are also the size of pinheads, more likely oval than circular in shape. Both hands and feet may be tender or even painful, and the child may therefore prefer to be barefoot.

Though a similar rash may show up here and there on the arms and legs or on the trunk, this is not common.

The characteristic three locations of the disease give it the straightforward name hand, foot, and mouth disease.

What causes it and is it contagious?

It is caused by a virus and is of a limited duration. Usually it takes five to seven days before it is gone. It is also contagious to a good extent, so that a number of family members will get it. It is more likely to spread in the crowds of swimming pools, churches, etc.

What can be done about hand, foot, and mouth disease?

The child may become sick enough to necessitate a trip to the doctor. The doctor will diagnose it, tell you what to expect, and may take a throat culture.

The usual treatment is to give an antipyretic such as aspirin or Tylenol for the fever (see page 131), and to keep the child off his or her feet if they are tender or painful. Because of the soreness of the throat, it is best to give a cold, bland diet for a while. Milkshakes, ice cream, milk, jello, applesauce, cottage cheese, and the like will be tolerated. Of course the child should avoid foods like coke, orange juice, pickles, and spicy or hot foods, because they will irritate the throat further and may drive the child crazy. Antibiotics are not needed if the case is not complicated.

If the throat is sore to a good extent, Cepacol lozenges, Chloraseptic lozenges, or hard candies may be tried. If sucking on them seems to soothe the throat, let the child keep using them.

By the way gargles are of little use if any, not only in this condition but many others like it.

Can I prevent it?

Yes and no. Hand, foot, and mouth disease is quite contagious and if your child has been exposed to it, you can do nothing but wait and see. However, if one of your children gets it, the fairest thing to do is to isolate the child from others, to narrow the base of the disease spread. It will protect some of the children from getting it, though they are still susceptible to transmission through crowds especially in swimming pools.

If this disease is in an epidemic proportion, it may be wise to keep your child from the swimming pool altogether until the epidemic is over. Of course this does not apply if you have your own pool and the child swims alone.

CHAPTER NINE

THE NECK

the neck
wry neck
he has a lump under the jaw

THE NECK

The Adam's apple (the larynx) is the bulge in the middle of the neck. The trachea (wind pipe) comes down from the larynx to behind the breast bone (the sternum) where it divides into bronchial tubes. A little below the larynx, the thyroid gland hugs the trachea snugly. If the thyroid gland is enlarged or if it has any lumps you may even be able to notice it and feel it, although those conditions signal certain important diseases. This is not common in children, but adolescents, especially females, may show some enlargement of this gland. It is called adolescent goiter, or is an indication of Hashimoto's disease. Usually there are no other symptoms, and the enlargement is best seen when the child looks up at the ceiling.

In some children, a node may appear above the larynx, also best seen when the child looks up.

What does a visible node mean?

If you see a node, the size of a tiny walnut, situated above the larynx, almost at its junction with the "double chin," see the doctor. It is usually situated in the middle line, is not tender, and does not seem to bother the child. Such a node often proves to be a cyst related to the thyroid, and it will have to be operated on before it ruptures to the outside. It is more likely to be seen in younger children.

If it opens up to the outside, the area will show a tiny hole that oozes thick sticky material. If this happens before you discover the lump, the operation will be a little more difficult. This is called "thyroglossal cyst."

Are there other nodes?

There are numerous lymph nodes in the neck, often no less than one hundred. Some of these nodes are situated along the muscle that connects the breast bone to the bottom of the skull. This muscle (sternomastoid) is readily seen standing out as a ridge on each side of the neck, especially when the child turns the head to one side.

The lymph nodes along this muscle fall in two lines, those which are situated between this muscle and the skin (superficial nodes) and those that are deep to the muscle. The superficial nodes are the ones that parents notice most often, especially when the nodes are slightly enlarged.

Should we worry about them?

Usually these nodes are so small that they skip your attention. Every once in a while, one or two of them become slightly enlarged. This is more true in a child who is a few years old and happens to be thin. When the child turns his or her head to one side, the lymph node will show up and may even stand out. The node is not tender and may move under your fingers.

Most such nodes prove to be normal, and the doctor will assure you accordingly. Every once in a while, however, they may indicate a special disease of the blood, lymph system, or otherwise.

Are there any other lymph nodes?

Yes. Other important ones are the tonsillar or upper cervical lymph nodes (the ones under the angle of the jaw). These lymph nodes drain the tonsils and pharyngeal area, and often become enlarged and inflamed when the throat becomes inflamed (see page 265).

You can easily discover such an enlargement when you ask the child to look at the ceiling. If this node (or nodes) is enlarged, it will stand out like a walnut on either side of the jaw. In some cases it may even be the size of a golf ball. Once you see this enlarged node, consult the doctor. Usually it proves to be an acute inflammation related to the throat, and an antibiotic will have to be given.

If left without treatment, the acute inflammation can keep progressing. When this happens, an abscess may form, necessitating an operation to drain the pus.

Are there other diseases causing this enlargement?

These tonsillar nodes can enlarge in cases of infectious mono (see page 168). The degree of their enlargement is variable, but it is not rare to see them reach a relatively enormous size. Naturally other manifestations of infectious mono will be present at the same time, and the diagnosis may be obvious.

There are various serious but rare diseases of the lymphatic system or blood system that can cause such an enlargement too.

By the way, enlargement of the "tonsillar node" is often mistaken by parents for mumps (see page 164). Mumps is a diffuse swelling of a salivary gland, situated at a slightly higher place, "hugging" the lobe of the ear. Mumps' swelling does not stand out when the child looks up at the ceiling.

WRY NECK (TORTICOLLIS)

Sometimes children suddenly feel as if the muscles of the neck are stiff, and they will have to hold their heads to one side, giving the impression of a twisted head. They will have a good deal of pain if they -or their parents- try to straighten their heads. This is called the acute wry neck or torticollis. It can also be intermittent, chronic, or even permanent.

You may be scared upon seeing your child with a sudden torticollis, and you may look for other symptoms, but in most cases there will be none.

What causes this problem?

It depends on the kind of wry neck. Fortunately, most of these are of the acute transient type that lasts for only a few days, after which the child will be perfectly all right. Upon questioning such a child, you may discover that before developing the wry neck, he or she was running excessively or riding a bicycle hard, thus sweating a good deal. When the sweaty area is exposed to a breeze of air, the muscles of the neck will go into spasm and will act as if there has been some degree of inflammation. This will cause the muscle to contract and cause pain upon being stretched or moved.

Occasionally an inflamed lymph node in the area will make the muscle nearby contract in a move to protect the inflamed area, but in the mean time lead to wry neck.

There are many other causes besides the above, but they are rare.

How about the permanent wry neck?

Many such cases arise from babyhood. This can happen if the baby had a sternomastoid mass (see page 82) that was not corrected, and/or the baby was allowed to sleep on his or her preferred side with the head turned most of the time in one particular direction. This will often lead to a face that is not symmetrical, which can become permanent if left uncorrected.

Occasionally a weak muscle in the eye may force the baby to rotate his head to look at a subject, and that can become a habit out of necessity. This may lead to the chronic wry neck, but fortunately this is rare.

What will the doctor do?

The doctor will try to ascertain the degree of severity of the wry neck, and will determine which group of wry neck muscles are in spasm. He or she will also check the child all over, paying special attention to the throat, tonsils, and the lymph nodes of the neck, and may take a throat culture if some degree of inflammation is suspected.

In a baby or a young child, the chronic type of wry neck may be obvious, and it is this type that can become permanent if not treated energetically and persistently.

What kind of treatment will the doctor choose?

For the acute wry neck, if the throat or the lymph node of the neck is inflamed, the doctor may put the child on a course of an antibiotic. For the wry neck caused by spasm of the muscles of the neck and back treatment will consist of the following:

1. Applying heat to the sore muscle, be it wet heat or using a heating pad or hot-water bottle, for about ten minutes at a time, three times a day.
2. Applying Myoflex cream or Ben Gay ointment (nonprescription) to the sore area, and massaging it consistently and hard for about five to ten minutes, three times a day. Your doctor will show you the area to be massaged.
3. Giving the child aspirin internally in the appropriate dose, every time you do the above procedures.

In many cases the neck will slowly improve, and in a few days it will look normal and suffer no pain or spasm at all.

How about the chronic wry neck?

In chronic wry necks treatment is completely different, depending on the cause. If a baby has a bad posture of his or her head during sleep, you have to take countermeasures early to correct the defect before it becomes permanent. You will move the head to the opposite direction to help stretch the tight muscle of the neck, as well as forcing the baby to sleep on the protuberant side of the lopsided head (see page 82).

If the wry neck is related to the eyes, proper treatment by the eye doctor will help eliminate it.

Fortunately wry neck is not that common, and in most cases it is of the acute transient type. But when it is chronic or if it becomes permanent, it can affect the child psychologically in later years, as it becomes necessary to always hold his or her head in a slightly rotated manner.

A LUMP UNDER THE JAW

The child is fussy, pale, out of sorts, and may have circles under the eyes (shiners). The temperature may or may not be up, the appetite is not so good, and the throat is sore. As the child looks at the ceiling, you will see a lump below the angle of the jaw, sometimes walnut-sized or bigger, on one side or both. You take the little one to the doctor, who tells you :

It is upper cervical lymphadenitis:

Lymphadenitis is an infection of the lymph nodes that drain the tonsils and the throat. The nodes "catch" the infection from the throat and help prevent it from going deeper to the system, before it causes more damage. By so doing, these nodes get infected, enlarged and tender. The germ may be staph, or strep, but rarely it can be others.

How bad can it be?

If you wait too long, the inflamed gland can become larger, more tender, and painful. Sometimes it can become the size of a golf ball!

At certain stage it can become abscessed, thus needing surgery.

If you let it go without treatment, and if the "bug" happens to be strep, you will also be taking chances with consequences coming after this germ (see page 145).

And what if I am prompt?

Proper and early treatment is essential to such preventable consequences. Enlargement of these lymph nodes can be part of other symptoms that drive you to the doctor right away. But sometimes the symptoms are not too bad, or hardly apparent. In such cases a person may postpone going to the doctor and end up with trouble.

Does it look like Mumps?

The trained eye of your doctor and his examination will determine whether the child is mumpy or lumpy. If you are absolutely sure that the child has mumps (see page 164), you don't have to see the doctor. The smooth, diffuse swelling of mumps starts from the area in front of the ear lobe and sweeps around to below and slightly behind the ear, and it won't bulge when the child looks up at the ceiling.

Are all lumps in the neck important?

Yes; lumps in the neck or in other places of the body can be caused by many diseases. Some of these diseases can be serious, and extensive investigation may be required. The investigation may concentrate on the blood, endocrine glands, tuberculosis tests, etc. In some cases the doctor may even ask you about cats.

Why cats?

Believe it or not, there is a disease called cat-scratch fever. The cat scratches the child, and the child reacts by developing a lump in the neck, armpit, or groin, depending on the location of the scratch.

The lump can become fairly big over a period of a few weeks. Many tests are needed to verify the diagnosis, and to differentiate it from other diseases. Since there are so many diseases that can cause enlarged lymph nodes or other lumps, and since some of these diseases are serious, it is prudent to consult the doctor for an opinion and medical expertise.

Are the lymph nodes all over us?

No, they are not. A good many lymph nodes are concentrated in three special regions of the body:

1. The neck, in several groups, arranged in two ring forms,
2. The arm pits, arranged in a few groups,
3. The groin, arranged in a few groups.

Lymph nodes have special important functions, one of which is to halt creeping infection from going deep into the system. As we have described, the poor nodes themselves become infected in the process, and such infected nodes should be treated without delay.

CHAPTER TEN

THE NOSE

    the nose
    colds
    the stuffed-up nose
    nasal allergy (allergic rhinitis)
    nasal discharge
    postnasal drip
    nose bleeds
    fractures of the nose and deviated septum

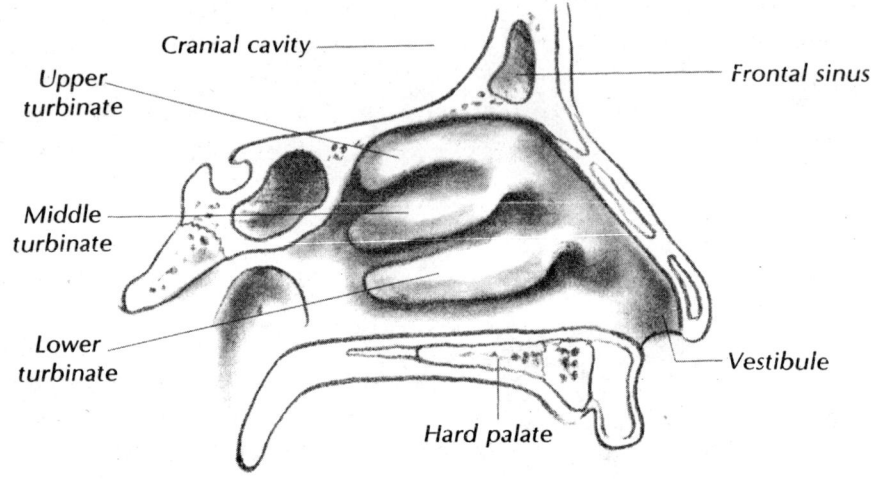

LATERAL WALL — LEFT NASAL CAVITY

Courtesy Barbara Bates, M.D.
from a Guide to Physical Examination, p 60
Written permission from the publisher, J. B. Lippincott Co.

THE NOSE

Press at the tip of the nose and take a look. You will see a septum in the middle separating the left from the right nostril. At each side of the nasal cavity, you will see slight bulges. These are called the turbinates, and there are three on each side. You are likely to see only the lower turbinate. The others can be seen to some extent if you use a flashlight. They constitute ridges, one overriding the other.

What are the turbinates for?
The bulging ridges stretch from the front to the back of the side of the nose. The smallest is high up and it can hardly be seen by you, if at all. These ridges are covered with the mucous membrane as is the rest of the nose. They help increase the surface area of the nasal cavity, thereby increasing the exposure of the inhaled air to the influence of the mucous membrane. This is essential to effectively modify the character of the air going to the lungs, temperature, moisture, and contamination-wise.

What do you mean?
The air we breathe may be at various degrees of temperature, depending on the season or the climate. The air may also have pollutants or carry pollen particles and similar material. The mucous membrane affects the air to suit the lungs in a better manner. The air will become moistened as it passes through on its way to the respiratory tree, thus it will become less irritating to the lungs. Its temperature will be adjusted to fit the respiratory tree in a better way. A good deal of filtering of the air will also take place. This is accomplished first by the hairs at the entrance of the nose, but more importantly, the particles in the air will be trapped by the moist, sticky mucous membrane of the whole nasal cavity (the turbinates facilitate this by creating a bigger surface area), and prevented from going down to the lungs to a great extent.

Will the air quality affect the turbinates?

Yes it will. By doing their duty, the turbinates will react in varying degrees; they and other parts of the nose may become swollen or slightly congested in response to the kind of air passing through. When the turbinates swell, the nasal cavity will consequently become narrower.

Secretion of the quantity and quality of mucus will also vary depending on the quality of air. The mucus may become dried up forming crusts. Both the mucus and the crusts may lead to a certain degree of nasal obstruction, just as swelling and congestion of the mucous membrane do.

Is that the reason for the postnasal drip?

It is indeed one of the reasons. Infection and allergy of the nasal cavity, as well as various degrees of sinusitis in grown-ups are other reasons.

The secreted mucus, infected or not, must drain. The drainage is mainly to the back of the nose, down to the throat, leading to cough. The cough may persist for some time until the postnasal drip is controlled.

How do the sinuses open into the nose?

The sinuses are simply small cavities adjacent to the nose, and each of them opens into the nose by a small hole or inlet. There is one maxillary sinus on each side of the nose, three ethmoidal sinuses (lying high up) on each side of the nose too. In addition, there are two frontal sinuses, each situated above the bridge of the nose, one on the right and one on the left.

What are the sinuses for?

The sinuses help in resonating the sound as we talk, and their presence helps give shape and configuration to the face. They are somewhat vulnerable, though. The mucous membrane of the nose will extend into the sinuses, thus lining them. The sinuses become involved to some extent in the infections and allergies affecting the nose. Infection of the sinuses (sinusitis) is well known in adults and a small percentage of older children.

Sinusitis in younger children is rare, since the sinuses do not develop completely until the child is several years old, up to age six or seven years. In young children the sinus cavities simply become involved when the usual afflictions of the nose take place.

COLDS

The nose keeps running, its tip may look red, and the child sneezes and develops an occasional dry hacking cough. The child's temperature may go up for two or three days and he or she may feel tired and look slightly pale; if the cold is mild and self-limited, it will go away in a few days. Some, however, will develop complications. Not only that, but there are other conditions that mimic colds and fool the parents.

What causes colds?

Colds are caused by a variety of viruses, perhaps as many as seventy types! Colds, of course, are more common during wintertime since the cold weather seems to favor the spread of these viruses, which in turn affect many schoolchildren. The integrity of the mucous membrane of the nose is very important too; the cold air irritates the nose to a good degree, thus making it less able to fight off these viruses. Many other factors, known and unknown, are involved, making the mechanism of understanding colds complex.

What complications are likely to show up?

A good percentage of colds come and go without complications. Some, however, can lead to sore throat, tonsillitis, and ear infections. The latter may be suspected when the baby seems to cry and cry, or when the older child complains of earache.

Upper respiratory infection, postnasal drip, bronchitis, and even pneumonia may also prove to be complications of colds. The symptoms of these complications will tip you off, or the fact that the cold seems to persist for more than a few days.

If you can't prevent colds, can you treat them?

Colds cannot be prevented easily, and antibiotics are reserved only for their complications. A viral cold will run its course and go away. Its treatment is symptomatic; in other words, we treat the symptoms and let the natural resistance of the child take care of the virus.

When the nose shows thin liquid discharge, nosedrops are not needed. Nasal decongestants may be of some value (see page 305). Sudafed or Novafed may be used. Antihistamines such as Novahistine or Triaminic may also be used.

Later on, the nose may become full of thick sticky mucus, and it may be hard for the child to breathe. When this happens, nosedrops may be used. Neosynephrine or Alconefrin (1/4 percent for a two-year-old child or older, and 1/8 percent for a six-month- to two-year-old) may be used for two to three days. Remember, using these drops for longer than three days often leads to "rebound phenomenon" i.e. the drops will give the opposite effect and make the nose stuffy instead! For a baby up to the age of six months, use saltwater nosedrops, four to five drops every three hours, of a mixture of 1/4 teaspoon of salt in one cup of water.

Vaporizers or humidifiers are worth using for a few days (see page 290). Don't overuse these, however, because condensation on the windows can encourage the growth of fungus. Usually you need to use them at night only.

For fever, an antipyretic such as aspirin or Tylenol can be used (see page 131). They do not cure a cold, as so many parents believe. They simply reduce the temperature if it is high enough (102 to 104 degrees F), and are not worth using for low temperature (99 to 101 degree F). If the child feels achy and tired, aspirin may help.

If I have a central humidifier, do I have to
use a regular humidifier for a cold?

Yes, you better use the regular (portable) humidifier (or vaporizer), even though you are using a central humidifier. The regular humidifier is needed for only a few days, and mainly while the child's cold and respiratory infection are acute. Central humidifiers help prevent nasal and respiratory tract irritation, thus the child is less likely to develop trouble in those organs. But if he or she has already started with such problems, then extra humidity supplied by the humidifier or the vaporizer will be needed. They should be used for a few days until the child's nose and respiratory tract have improved to a reasonable extent.

How about high doses of vitamin C?

Numerous well-controlled studies have been published, indicating that high doses of vitamin C do not help colds, nor prevent them. The vitamin C enthusiasts will of course continue to consume large amounts of vitamin C, convinced that they are preventing and/or treating colds. While this consumption is usually harmless, recent reports of some trouble resulting from very high daily doses of vitamin C have appeared in the medical literature.

What can I do about the complications?

See the doctor if:

1. The child develops an upper respiratory infection following a cold, and if his or her cough becomes frequent, tight and hacking, and if your treatment with cough medicines and other medications fails;
2. The temperature is too high (103 to 104) or goes on for many days even though it is low-grade;
3. The mucus discharge in the nose becomes yellow or yellowish-green in color;
4. The child complains of an earache;
5. In case of a baby, he or she cries excessively;
6. There is a sore throat.

Many a cold leads to a croupy respiratory infection, or in an allergic child, to a bout of asthmatic bronchitis, with its troublesome wheezing, and occasionally to pneumonia. Be on the alert.

Do allergies look like colds?

Yes, they do in many cases, and colds may be superimposed on an allergy. If a cold continues beyond five to seven days, it is very possible that it is not a cold, but an allergy or a cold with complications. A child with allergy is more susceptible to colds than other children, thus complicating the matter.

THE STUFFED-UP NOSE

Stuffed-up nose is one of the commonest complaints. The child's nose becomes stuffed up, making it somewhat difficult to breathe, and the trouble can be quite annoying at times. It may start all of a sudden, as a symptom of a cold, and it may continue for only a few days, in conjunction with a runny nose, occasional cough, and sometimes a rise in temperature for a day or two.

Can it be caused by anything else?

Yes; let us give some examples:

1. A stuffy nose can be a symptom of allergy, and this is particularly true during the "allergy seasons." In such cases there will be a good deal of sneezing, running, and itching of the nose, and perhaps some itching of the eyes. The symptoms may go on for weeks.
2. A stuffy nose can be a symptom of sinus infection, and in such cases there may be a boring dull frontal headache, a nasty cough, and occasionally a prolonged low-grade temperature.
3. A stuffy nose can be prolonged, resulting from a cold complicated by some bacterial infection in the nasal passages. In such cases the mucus that drains will look thick yellow or yellowish-green in color.
4. Occasionally, a prolonged stuffy nose may be associated with a "rotten" odor to the breath. Often this proves to be the case of a foreign body lodged in the nose by the child. We have seen band-aids, lollipop sticks, crayons, sponges, etc. lodged in the nose by children!
5. Very large adenoids can obstruct the nose from behind.
6. Of course, there are also rare diseases that can cause obstruction in the nose, some are of a serious nature.

What are the main problems an obstructed nose can cause?

At the very least it is a nuisance to be forced to breathe by mouth.

A stuffy nose is more likely to get infected, or lead to infection of the sinuses; it can easily lead to postnasal drip. A stuffy nose with a penetrating foul smell that cuts your breath ought to be seen by the doctor right away since it may indicate a foreign body.

For a baby a stuffy nose is a big problem, since he or she cannot breathe through the mouth easily (see page 77).

If the nose is obstructed for very long (years), it will lead to adenoid facies (see page 231).

What can I do about it?

If it is because of a cold or a mild allergy, nosedrops (see page 274), and or a decongestant (see page 305) may be used. A humidifier by the bed will also help (see page 290).

If the obstruction of the nose persists for more than a few days and especially if there is also a cough, low-grade temperature, and a persistent headache, then consult the doctor. It may mean a superadded bacterial infection. The same applies if there is a nasty smell to the child's breath, or a yellowish-green discharge from the nose.

PLEASE NOTE: Some cases of persistent runny noses will develop nasty-looking red skin at and around the nostrils. This may lead to impetigo of that area. The child may even wipe the nose then rub the eyes, transferring the infection there, and resulting in "pink eye."

What about the shiners?

Shiners are dark circles under the eyes, usually giving the child a sickly appearance. They often appear when there is some nasal obstruction of any sort. If this obstruction happens to be caused by a cold, allergy, or infection, the shiners may show up and make you concerned. Shiners occur when a nasal obstruction interferes with the venous drainage of the area. So, when the nasal obstruction is treated and relieved, those shiners will disappear, and parents will be happy again.

If I have a central humidifier, do I have to use a regular humidifier for a cold?

Yes, you better use the regular (portable) humidifier (or vaporizer), even though you are using a central humidifier. The regular humidifier is needed for only a few days, and mainly while the child's cold and respiratory infection are acute. Central humidifiers help prevent nasal and respiratory tract irritation, thus the child is less likely to develop trouble in those organs. But if he or she has already started with such problems, then extra humidity supplied by the humidifier or the vaporizer will be needed. They should be used for a few days until the child's nose and respiratory tract have improved to a reasonable extent.

NASAL ALLERGY
Allergic Rhinitis

The child is annoyed, uncomfortable, and may keep sniffing the nose. There may be bouts of sneezing to be followed by an outpour of thin clear liquid from the nose, causing the child to have to blow his or her nose. At other times, he or she may feel as if the nose is blocked, making it cumbersome to breathe freely and comfortably.

You may see that the child will wipe the nose with a hand, or a sleeve, or may even move the tip of the nose in a rotating manner in an effort to clear it. Even the eyes may become watery and look boggy, and there may be circles (or shiners) underneath them.

You mean all this is caused by allergy?

Yes, this is the general picture of nasal allergy, or what is called allergic rhinitis. It is a very common thing, and a good many of the so-called cases of "sinuses" are truly cases of nasal allergy.

Nasal allergy is often mistaken for a cold, yet it is quite different from a cold in many ways.

How does allergy differ from a cold?

Nasal allergy tends to go on and on, while a cold will take its course and go away in a few days, unless it is followed by complicatons. Nasal allergy is likely to go through exacerbations (flare ups) too, and when that happens, the poor nose will suffer acutely, and the child will feel quite uncomfortable. This is more true during the "allergy seasons" (see page 294).

Nasal allergy also differs from a common cold in that the mucous membrane of the nose will often look pale, boggy, and swollen. Not only that, but the mucus tends to be clear, and it often drips down the throat producing the postnasal drip (see page 281).

What causes it?

Nasal allergy is an inheritted tendency, and a high percentage of people do suffer from it. It comes in two forms, the seasonal and the perennial. In most parts of the United States, the seasonal allergy (see page 294) shows up during springtime, mid-summer and late fall. Some persons prove to be allergic in one season, others in two seasons, yet there are those who may prove to be allergic in every season.

In the perennial nasal allergy, the nose seems to be stuffy and partially full of mucus during much of the year, but especially during winter months. This often proves to be allergy to dust indoors, to some pets (cats, dogs, birds), or to mildew in damp areas such as basements.

By the way, food and other factors may play a part too, but this part is very small indeed compared to the above.

How contagious is it?

Nasal allergy is not contagious, although the common cold is quite contagious. On the other hand, you may find a number of family members suffering from the same problem at the same time, because of the inheritance factor, and because of their exposure to whatever is allergenic.

What can we do about nasal allergy?

It all depends on the severity of the nasal allergy, and on the previous experience of the person with it.

It is worth using an antihistamine, with or without a decongestant (see page 305). Good examples are Triaminic, Novahistine, Actifed, Demazine, Sudafed, Novafed (nonprescriptions), or Fedahist, Naldecon, etc. (prescription). These medications can be used four times a day or less often, usually in the amount of 1/2 teaspoon for a small child, but proportionately more for a bigger and an older child. The main drawback to these medicines is the drowsiness, sleepiness, and grouchiness they can lead to.

In addition to the above, nosedrops may be of help occasionally.

In case the nasal allergy is more persistent and more severe, and if it seems to come back every year, allergy tests and allergy shots may have to be done.

There are a few practical steps you may take for prevention:

1. During the pollen season, make sure the child comes home before early evening, because at that time a change in atmospheric temperature and humidity will take place, bringing the pollen to a lower atmospheric level and a higher concentration- i.e. the outside will be more allergenic.
2. Keep the child away from areas of high concentration of pollen, e.g. where grass is being cut in April and May, or piles of fallen decayed leaves.
3. Consider putting an electronic air filter on the furnace (see page 292). This can filter better than ninety percent of the pollen, dust, and other troublesome factors of allergy, making the air indoors more wholesome and healthy.
4. Since smoking is very irritating to an allergy sufferer, every effort must be taken to keep the smoke away from the allergic person. Better still cut out smoking altogether. This also applies to other irritants, such as fresh paint, perfume, etc.
5. Allergy tests and shots may have to be given.

POSTNASAL DRIP

The child's cough is annoying, hacky, dry, and fairly frequent; it occurs mainly at night, and it may not be associated with any other symptoms. The child may even act and look normal during daytime, but starts coughing at sleeptime. This cough may be mild, may occur every once in a while during sleep, and may not bother the child much. However, in severe cases, the cough may be bad enough to wake the child up a few times, disturbing everyone's rest and sleep. Other symptoms of postnasal drip are bad breath and sniffles.

Postnasal drip may be part of other respiratory problems the child has. If so, other symptoms may be present too, such as fever, headache, poor appetite, pallor, stomachache, etc.

What causes postnasal drip?

Children with a tendency for respiratory allergies are more likely than others to develop postnasal drip. It can also be chronic, but more frequently it shows up for a short period of time following a cold or an upper respiratory infection. In such cases, there will be excess mucus production, which may become milky or yellowish in color and fairly thick in consistency. This may indicate bacterial infection, making it necessary to use a course of an antibiotic.

Why does it make my child cough?

Upon going to bed, the mucus in the nose will accumulate, then slowly drain down the throat to near the larynx. It will "tickle" the throat and set up a reflex cough. This cough may also accur during daytime, but it is more common at night. It may also be caused by certain mechanisms other than the above.

Is postnasal drip dangerous?

It is more of a nuisance than a danger. In an acute but mild case, the postnasal drip may dry up in a few days by itself, either with or without a decongestant. If there is heavy bacterial infection, the postnasal drip will take some time to clear up, however, and that will usually be after having a culture taken and using a proper antibiotic. If the postnasal drip is chronic, it will require prolonged therapy.

How contagious is it?

In most cases, it is not contagious, and it is safe for the child to be with others. However, if postnasal drip is complicated by bacterial infection, and especially if this happens to be strep, then the child will be contagious for sure. Luckily, this strep complication is not common.

What can I do for the postnasal drip?

For mild cases, use a cool-mist humidifier or a vaporizer (see page 290); for "hard" episodes of coughing spells, sit the child in a bathroom while the hot shower is turned on until the room is well steamed, and keep him or her there for about an hour or so.

Nosedrops before going to bed may also be needed. Neosynephrine or Alconephrine 1/4 percent, four to five drops in each nostril, can be used. After you administer the drops turn the child over onto the stomach while on the bed, with his or her head dangling over the side, and let the child sniff up several times, over a period of one minute. This method will help disperse the nosedrops on the mucous membrane of the nose equally, thus shrinking the membrane.

Decongestants given by mouth may prove to be helpful too (see page 305). Sudafed or Novafed (nonprescription) are good examples. Antihistamines such as Triaminic and Novahistine (nonprescription) can also be used.

If the above measures don't help after two or three days, see your doctor. Your child may have a bacterial infection complicating the postnasal drip, or something else that you had not suspected; stronger measures have to be used to help in this matter.

Your chance for success with the home treatment is better than fifty percent, an encouraging statistic.

NOSEBLEEDS

Nosebleeds are fairly common in children, and tend to recur in some. The child may act scared but more often will cooperate with the parent in trying to stop it. Nosebleeds come in various degrees of severity, and the severe ones can be alarming. Fortunately most nosebleeds are short-lived, mild, and easily controllable.

What causes them?

The middle wall of the nose is called the nasal septum. It divides the nasal cavity into left and right sides. At the lower part of the septum, near the nostrils, there is a rich network of tiny veins and capillaries. When these break, the nose will bleed.

What makes them break? The answer is that many children will pick at the dry crusty material inside their noses; the material may be attached to the area containing the network of delicate veins, which easily break.

Bumping the nose can lead to nosebleeds, yet sometimes the nosebleed seems to come from nowhere. In such cases, the doctor will look for evidence of allergy. Allergy leads to a good many cases of repeated nosebleeds because the mucous membrane of the nose becomes boggy, swollen, and more fragile than usual.

In rare cases the nosebleeds can be a sign of some blood diseases, some of them quite serious.

What can we do about nosebleeds?

If they are not that frequent, i.e. three to four times a year, keeping an eye on them is sufficient.

If they show up too often (two to three times a month or so) the doctor may have to cauterize the area. It is done in the office, and it is a relatively painless procedure. With cautery, the nosebleeds will usually stop for nine to twelve months. If they become frequent again, the nose may have to be cauterized once more.

If there is nasal allergy, an antihistamine may have to be used (see page 305).

Can we prevent nosebleeds?

Yes, you can do a good job. Since the majority of nosebleeds are related to children picking dried-up mucus (boogers), using a central humidifier on the furnace will help prevent the drying effect of the air, and help the mucus to be more moist and thinner.

For children with nasal allergies, an antihistamine used on and off will be of preventive help too.

The blood is pouring from my child's nose now, what shall I do?

Be calm first, and set to work. Don't shake nervously if you can help it.

1. Stand the child straight up.
2. Pinch the lower part of the bleeding nose (the soft part) with your thumb and index finger well, and keep holding it that way.
3. Keep holding (pinching) the nose for ten minutes.
4. Let the child breathe through his or her mouth and you be reassuring.

Don't:

1. let the child stoop over or lie down while you are pinching the nose (it will increase the pressure in the veins, making the bleeding worse);
2. pinch on the bony part of the nose (it is useless);
3. put ice on the back of the child's neck or forehead (it is ineffective and bothersome);
4. let the child blow his or her nose hard (it may start the bleeding again).

In some children, aspirin may increase their tendency to nosebleeds. If this is the case with yours, please avoid the use of aspirin; instead use Tylenol.

FRACTURES OF THE NOSE
AND DEVIATED SEPTUM

Occasionally, when a child falls on his or her face, the nose gets involved directly or indirectly, and you will wonder if the child has fractured a bone in the nose.

What are the bones in the nose like?

There are two small nasal bones that form the upper half of the nose, and part of the bridge of the nose too. The lower part of the nose consists of pieces of cartilage, which are attached to each other and to the nasal bones by special tissue.

From the inside, the septum forms an approximate midline partition from the top down to the floor of the cavity.

What happens when there is a fall?

If the child falls on his or her nose, and if the fall is severe enough, there will be a soft-tissue injury, often a nosebleed of variable severity, and swelling of the injured area of the nose.

A more severe fall, blow, or hit, may dislocate the septum of the nose, and/or fracture the nasal bones. In such cases treatment will be almost nil. In some cases, however, the fracture will be depressed or complicated, making it necessary for energetic and prompt treatment. The septum is the main point of concern in all nasal injuries. If the injury is severe enough, the septum may dislocate to the right or left side, blocking one side of the nose. This may lead to other problems.

How will I know there are problems?

When the child falls or gets hit or bumped on the nose, there often is bleeding. Once you stop the bleeding, evaluate the degree of swelling at and around the nose. Touch the nose gently to see if it hurts a lot. Look at the nostrils with a flashlight and see if the septum is in the middle line, and if both nostrils seem to look similar and be of equal size.

If all the above conditions seem to check out positively, you probably have nothing to worry about. If not, call the doctor.

What will the doctor do?

He will evaluate the child's nose and may decide that X-rays should be taken. If the X-ray shows some fractures, you will be referred to an ear, nose, and throat (ENT) specialist.

If the septum is not deviated at the time but the deviation shows up later on, you will also be referred to an ENT doctor. Many ENT doctors won't work on the child until growth of the nose has been completed, when the child becomes eighteen years old. But if the deviation of the septum is severe, do not hesitate to consult with the ENT doctor anyway.

Remember that sometimes deviation of the nasal septum still takes place because of minor hits that will skip your attention and the child's.

Suppose we leave the deviated septum alone?
A deviated septum of the nose, if left uncorrected, may lead to some complications. It causes obvious cosmetic problems, but in addition, it may block one side of the nose almost completely, or give rise to sinusitis or other problems. This happens only in a certain percentage of uncorrected cases. So weigh your decision carefully.

Do nasal fractures have to be treated right away?
A nasal fracture is usually accompanied by a profuse nosebleed and swelling of the surrounding soft tissue. The severity of the nasal bleeding may be a rough guide for you to suspect trouble. It is best to treat the nasal fracture right away (within three days from the time of injury). The treatment depends on the extent and nature of the fracture and its complications. Such early treatment can help prevent later consequences.

After a lapse of three days from the date of injury, it is probably too late to be able to do anything.

CHAPTER ELEVEN

THE RESPIRATORY TRACT

the respiratory tract
cool-mist humidifiers, and vaporizers
electronic air filters
allergies of the respiratory tract
allergy shots
cough
cough medicines
upper respiratory infections (chest colds)
laryngitis
congenital laryngial stridor
croup
tracheobronchitis
asthmatic bronchitis
foreign body in the lung
TB (tuberculosis) and its tests
pneumonia
pleurisy

The Lungs

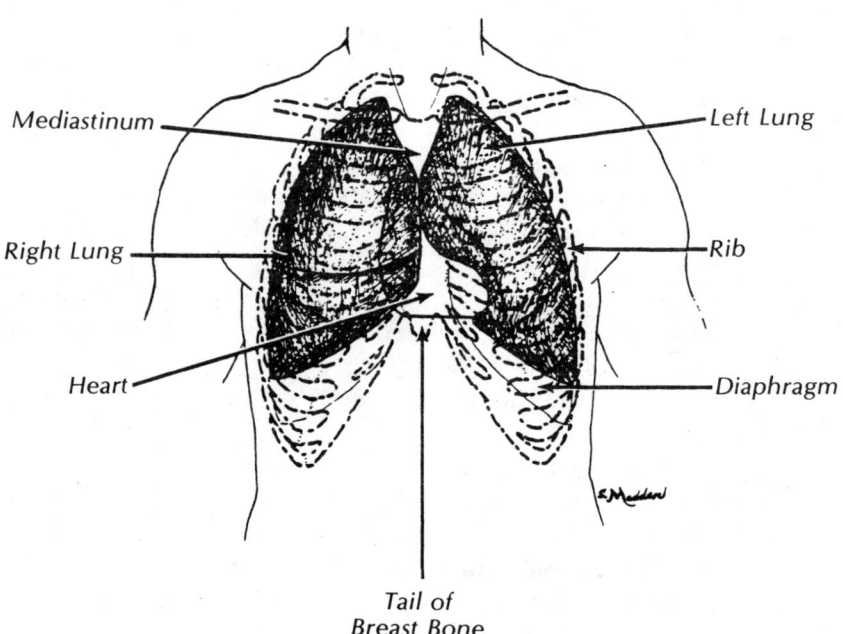

THE RESPIRATORY TRACT

The respiratory tract is the complex system where the air goes through us as we breath; it looks very much like a tree turned upside down. That is to say, the roots of the tree may constitute the grooved nasal passages and the sinuses, and the trunk consists of the pharynx (throat), the larynx (voice box), the trachea (wind pipe), and the big bronchial tubes. These are what we call the upper respiratory tract. The branches of the tree consist of the bronchial tubes and the air sacs; this is the lower respiratory tract.

<u>Tell us about the upper respiratory tract:</u>
The air goes through the nose to become:

1. warmed up,
2. moistened,
3. filtered from polutants (they are trapped by the mucous membrane).

The sinuses are pockets opening into the nasal cavity. They usually resonate the sounds we make.

As the air goes further down, it passes through the nasopharynx for further humidification. Then it will go through the larynx, which produces vocalizations (voice sounds) through a complex mechanism.

The air has smooth sailing after that, since it goes through the straight trachea, which branches into two big bronchial tubes. That is why so many diseases affect the upper respiratory tract. The air can carry pollutants and pollen, can be dry, cold, etc., and the upper passages have the bothersome and thankless job of having to modify the air to make it warm, moist, purified and less toublesome to the bronchial tubes and lungs.

By doing so, the many components of the upper respiratory tract may suffer and become diseased. Viruses, bacteria, pollen, and environmental factors are particularly responsible. In children, this is even more true, since their defenses are not as well-developed as an adult's.

What about the lower respiratory tract?
The bronchial tubes will divide and subdivide into smaller and smaller branches. Finally, the tiny branches of the bronchial tubes end up in air sacs for the exchange of oxygen and other gases within the system. The complex system of air sacs and bronchial tubes constitute what we call the lungs. The lungs are also covered with a smooth sac called the pleura.

What can go wrong with the lower respiratory tract?
It can get infected, leading to bronchitis or pneumonia. The bronchial tubes can go into spasm and lead to asthma. A bronchial tube can become blocked, leading to collapse of the part of the lung it leads to. As you suspect by now, there are numerous other diseases that can affect this tract. Also, the pleura can become troubled with pleurisy and other diseases.

Diseases of the upper respiratory tract are not as serious as those of the lower respiratory tract; however, they are far more frequent, and quite troublesome at times.

COOL-MIST HUMIDIFIERS, AND VAPORIZERS

Humidifiers and vaporizers come in different sizes and shapes, and they sell at widely different prices. Each has its advantages and disadvantages, but they are needed fairly often during the cold season when the furnace is in operation.

Usually the cool-mist (cool-moisture) humidifier and the vaporizer come in small size units to be used in a room, though there are large portable units that are designed to humidify a whole apartment.

When shall we need to use them?
Generally speaking, when a child develops a cold, an upper respiratory infection, bronchitis, croup, wheezing, pneumonia and some other respiratory problems, he or she will need additional humidity in the room. This is especially true during the seasons when the furnace of the house is in full operation. The central heating will cause the

air inside the house to lose a substantial amount of its humidity; it is not unusual for the relative humidity indoors to be as low as fifteen to twenty percent. This is too harsh and too dry for the normal respiratory tract, let alone one that is inflamed or irritated.

By putting a central humidifier on the furnace, you can raise the indoor humidity level to the "comfort zone," which is forty to forty-five percent. By so doing, there will be less chance for respiratory irritation, and this will help prevent some of the respiratory problems. This is also true of using a portable large central humidifier for apartments or houses where a fixed central humidifier on the furnace cannot be used.

But these central humidifiers do not help that much after a child develops a respiratory infection of some sorts. To soothe an inflamed mucous membrane, a child will need a higher level of humidity than the forty percent. That is the reason to use a cool-mist humidifier or vaporizer in addition to the central humidifier, to deliver more moisture to the room. Don't forget, the vaporizers or the cool-mist humidifiers are used to help in the treatment of the respiratory infections mentioned above, not for prevention.

Should I use a vaporizer or a cool-mist humidifier?

You can use either kind if you happen to have one at home. However, if you want to buy a new one, the cool-mist humidifier has some advantages over the vaporizer.

The cool-mist humidifier is relatively noisy while the vaporizer may raise the room temperature to some extent and may lead to accidental burns.

It is important not to add Vicks or other medications to the water in these units. All the sick child needs from the machine is additional humidity in the room -no more, no less. If added to the water, Vicks and other chemicals are not only of no help but they may irritate the child's respiratory tract, leading to wheezing on some rare occasions.

How and when shall I use these units?

1. Put the cool-mist humidifier or vaporizer a few feet away from the child, and put it in such a way as to direct the mist or the

steam towards the child.
2. Leave the door of the room open only slightly to allow some degree of air circulation.
3. If you want to build a tent on the bed of the child (as in cases of croup), you can use a bed sheet for that purpose, and direct the cool mist or the steam through the open side of this tent.
4. Use the above units mainly at night (eight to ten hours), about three to four nights for an average illness. However you may use them day and night in case of a severe respiratory infection.
5. Use these units for colds and upper respiratory infections, bronchitis, etc.; i.e. whenever there is dry irritating frequent cough, stuffy nose, or hoarse voice with a cough. When the child has a loose cough or a rattly chest, do not use these units since they may make the condition worse.
6. Do not overuse the units.

Overuse?

You don't need to use these units for more that three to five days at the most. You can ease them off once the cough has stopped being dry, harsh, or barking. And once the cough has become loose, you can stop using these units completely.

If you use these humidifiers or vaporizers for too long, you stand to grow some mold (fungus) on the moist windowsills. This mold may be irritating and allergenic to many children, and may in turn lead to more cough or even wheezing.

It is also to be remembered that the unit should be thoroughly cleaned often. This is to help prevent the growth of the fungus and/or bacteria on the unit itself. Please pay extra attention to the cleaning directions that come with the unit.

ELECTRONIC AIR FILTER

Having had too many colds and allergies, and having had so many respiratory problems, you may want to ask the doctor if there is any way to help reduce the incidence. After all, you think, one cannot keep going on and on with such allergies.

Your doctor will review the child's record and may come to the conclusion that an "electronic air filter" may be of help.

What is an electronic air filter?

An electronic air filter is a device that can be installed in the hot-air furnace of the house. The circulating air inside the house will pass through it. As its numerous particles pass through the electronic air filter, they become electrically charged, and can thus be attracted to the filter and electrically trapped. The air will then be "purified."

It is said that about ninety to ninety-five percent of pollutants and impurities in the air will be so removed when an electronic air filter is permanently installed in the hotair furnace of a house.

Describe the "portable unit"?

In case you live in an apartment, or you are renting a house, or if you are in a house without a system for circulating air, such as hot-water heat or electric heat, you will not be able to install a central electronic air filter. For such cases a portable unit is the answer. Portable electronic air filters come in many sizes, some for one room, others for the whole apartment. A room unit or a portable electronic air filter is less efficient than the permanently installed one, removing sixty to seventy percent of the pollutants. Their lower efficiency is related to many factors. When it is used as a room unit, the door and window must be closed most of the time, so that the purified air won't get contaminated with outside air. To be very effective, many of the electronic air filters must be in operation more or less constantly, day and night.

Do we have to clean the filters?

Yes, on a regular basis. In many cases this is needed once every four to six weeks, depending on how dirty the air is. Many makes manufacture a filter that comes in two halves and both can be put in a dishwasher. This makes it easy to maintain.

Other makes, however, require that the filter be washed and rinsed in a special large container. The uninitiated will be amazed that the resultant washwater is so dirty that it is pitch black! This indicates the unimaginable degree of contamination of the air we breathe.

What do these contaminants do?

The electronic air filter usually removes dust particles, pollen, cotton linters, smoke, cigarette or cigar odor, smell of paint, etc. Most such contaminants are irritant or allergenic to the respiratory tract. Many people with intact respiratory system can fight off such contaminants, but people whose systems are sensitive or allergic will benefit from an electronic air filter.

When the contaminants are removed from the air, the child will be breathing "pure air" while indoors. This usually accounts for more than forty to fifty percent of each twenty-four hour period. This interruption of the exposure to the contaminants can yield a good dividend.

Will an electronic air filter take the place of allergy shots?

The electronic air filter will help all respiratory tracts in offering a "purified air". Children with mild allergy will benefit greatly, and so will the whole family. If the allergy is severe enough, allergy tests and shots will have to be given, though the filter will still give an added advantage.

One final useful tidbit: if the doctor prescribes it for you, the filter can be a tax-deductible item.

Why is it preferable to keep the filter operating constantly?

If the electronic air filter operates intermittently, it will remove the contaminants from the air only when it is operating. Therefore, around-the-clock operation of the filter gives the maximum efficiency and effect for the job. This is to be observed summer and winter. The doors and windows should be closed, except when you want to let fresh air in the house. If you open the windows for a prolonged period, you better shut off the air filter until you want it in operation again.

ALLERGIES OF THE RESPIRATORY TRACT

Allergies of the respiratory system are very common and of varying degrees of severity. They occur in various forms, and they affect different ages. Allergies of the respiratory tract are a vast subject in themselves. They can be seasonal, perennial, or both seasonal and perennial in the same person.

What are seasonal allergies?

Seasonal allergies show up during three seasons of the year, in most parts of the country. The seasons are spring, midsummer, and fall.

1. During spring, we are bombarded with pollen from trees at the time when various trees pollinate. This is usually followed by pollen from grass and spores from fungus in the soil.
2. During midsumer pollen from ragweed can be quite troublesome.
3. In the fall, the leaves that fall from trees become infected with highly-allergenic fungus (molds).

What is perennial allergy?

Symptoms of perennial allergy show up during wintertime, when the central heat in the house is in full operation, especially when a forced-air furnace is used. Such allergies are caused by:

1. Dust indoors, which is circulated by the furnace's fan. This dust has a protein coating which becomes "cooked" by the heat, thus becoming allergenic. Dust in a desert or outside the home is not allergenic.
2. Mildew (fungus), mainly in wet basements, crawl spaces and cellars, or near leaky faucets. You can easily smell and see the mildew.
3. Indoor pets, be they dogs, cats, or birds. The dander on the hair of such pets is a main villain along with the feathers.

Many a person has various degrees of sensitivity to both seasonal and perennial allergic factors, and may doubly suffer.

Sufferers from perennial allergies can have the symptoms all year around. This allergy can lead to frequent respiratory infections, with occasional wheezing and the notorious stuffy nose and the postnasal drip. The hot air of the furnace during wintertime will lower the humidity indoors, making the air irritating and even more troublesome to the respiratory tree, adding insult to injury. Cigarette smoke can be quite irritating too, and it behooves us to discontinue this habit to help the suffering child.

What will happen to our respiratory tract?

Very much depends on how sensitive or allergic we are. You may not suffer at all if you happen not to be allergic, or just a bit if you happen to be a mildly allergic person. However, the suffering can be frequent, severe, and incapacitating if you happen to be very allergic.

The nose is often the first to suffer with a good deal of itchy feeling, sneezing, stuffiness, and an outpouring of clear thin mucus, just like a cold (see page 273). Many of the so-called postnasal drips can be traced to mild allergies. Not only that but also children with repeated respiratory infections, of various degrees of severity, are often of allergic basis, yet give the false impression that the child's resistance is down.

When the bronchial tubes are affected, wheezing, difficulty taking a breath, and "huffing and puffing" may occur. The child may look quite sick, needing immediate attention.

Can we prevent some of these problems?

To prevent some of these problems, a few steps are to be observed. If they control the allergies or help diminish them, you may forestall having to see an allergist for allergy tests and shots.

1. Consider installing a central humidifier and an electronic air filter (see page 290 and page 292).
2. For minor nasal allergy, use antihistamines (see page 305).
3. If there is mildew in the basement or in a crawl space, use paraformaldehyde powder. Spread about two tablespoons of this powder in an aluminum pan (make a thin layer), and keep it in the area affected with the mildew. The doors leading to that area should be closed, and if possible leave them closed for a few days. You may use two to three or more of these aluminum pans per room, depending on the size of the area. A full basement may need six to seven aluminum pans. After a few days, the treated area will smell nice and fresh.

Caution: If you have to use paraformaldehyde, make sure not to inhale it for prolonged periods, because it is somewhat irritating to the eyes and the respiratory tract. However it does not damage furniture. The lingering pungent smell left will go away slowly in a week's time. After that the basement will smell normal, the fungus will be gone, and the danger to your child will have been reduced.
KEEP IT OUT OF REACH OF CHILDREN.
4. Allergy tests and shots will be needed in the more severe cases. It is best to resort to this only after exhausting all other possibilities in your fight to subdue respiratory allergy (see page 297).
5. If the child is allergic to a pet, unfortunately you have to keep the pet away (outoors), or get rid of it, as painful as this may be.
6. Irritants such as smoke, perfume, paint smell, and cigarette smoke, should be avoided.

ALLERGY SHOTS

You have heard that allergies are very common, and that somehow they are inherited. You have also seen your little one be quite susceptible to upper respiratory infections, postnasal drip, and wheezing. You have seen the child develop wheezing attacks often, usually following these frequent colds and respiratory infections.

The frequency of these episodes are such that you are tired of doctors and medicines, and may have been suggested the use of a central humidifier and an electronic air filter. But the child continues to pick up infections and you are ready to pull out your hair.

Should the child see an allergist?
Your doctor has been borrowing time until enough evidence accumulates to send the child to the allergist. When this happens, the allergist will take detailed information about the child's history and about the family history and will conduct skin tests, from fifty to seventy-five, perhaps in two sessions. The tests are not reliable

in children under one year of age.

When all the allergy tests are done, the allergist will sit down with you and give you the details of the findings, and describe what to avoid and what to do.

Don't be surprised if the child proves to be allergic to all the the following: dust, mold, pollen from trees, pollen from grass, pollen from ragweed, dogs, cats, and birds.

Most children with allergies are at least allergic to the above and many of them prove to be allergic to more than that.

Who will give the allergy shots?

Usually the first allergy shot is given by the allergist. The rest of the shots will be given by the nurse in your doctor's office or by the doctor. It is not advisable that a nurse give the shot at your home, unless she knows how to handle reaction to the shot. Such reactions may be severe on occasions, and quite unpredictable.

How often do you give the shots?

This varies a great deal from one allergist to another. Some allergists recommend one shot twice a week in the first two months, to be followed by one shot a week for a year, then one shot every second week for two or three more years.

Most allergists will start with one shot a week, then decrease the frequency to once every second week, then to once every third week.

Some allergists prefer to give two shots at a time, one in each arm, in order to avoid mixing the serum.

Most allergists like to see that you are strict about getting shots according to their schedule. If you miss by a day or two, no harm is done. If you miss by a long period then adjustment of the dose of the shot will have to be done, and you may prove to have taken a giant step backwards.

How long does the child have to take the shots?

The minimum period is three years, for not severely allergic children who respond well to the shots. Many a child will find it necessary to take the shots for up to five years. The length of treatment depends on the severity of the allergy, on the response of the child, and on many other factors. This is one of the reasons why re-evaluation by the allergist is important at times.

What is expected of the shots?

In most cases there will be gradual improvement over a period of a few months. You will see that the number of allergy problems, with or without infection will diminish steadily, but will not stop.

Your visits to the doctor will continue to be frequent, but this will be mainly for the shots and not for exasperating diseases. Your chance of success with the shots is about eighty percent.

Isn't the cost prohibitive?

Yes and no. Instead of paying for so many office visits to check for diseases, now you pay a small charge for the shots, at a predictable pace. In the meantime you will have prevented the allergy condition from becoming very troublesome later on in the child's life, and you will have made life easier not only for you and the child, but also for your doctor as well.

Above all, the child's general condition will improve upon receiving these shots, the frequency of the allergic manifestations will decrease, and you will certainly have less cause for worry.

COUGH

A child may cough his or her head off, and may annoy everyone around; your treatment with a cough medicine may help some, or not at all. You are at a loss and would like to know more, since a cough is only a symptom of so many conditions.

Why is a cough a symptom?

Cough is not a disease by itself. It may be the only symptom or one of many symptoms of a disease.

Most children with a cough have an infection of some sort in the respiratory tract. The cough can be mild, as that of a cold or an upper respiratory infection. In such cases it is usually dry, hacky, and superficial.

When the cough is loose and seems to rattle the chest, it can be ignored, since it means no more than excess mucus in the respiratory tract; the child will eventually get rid of it through vomiting or coughing it up. Strangely enough, some parents get quite concerned when the child has a rattly cough, and they attach undue importance to such a minor symptom.

If the child has a deeper infection than the above, such as bronchitis, asthmatic bronchitis, or pneumonia, the cough will be more "barking" in nature, almost like a small dog barking. A child with the croup will have nasty-sounding croupy breathing with a barking cough; a child with asthmatic bronchitis will wheeze and have a barking cough, or only a deep heavy dry cough; a child with pneumonia may have a barking cough, but more likely will have a deep, persistent dry cough most of the time, day and night.

Other conditions can also cause troublesome coughs.

What are some examples?

The cough of postnasal drip is an example. It is more bothersome at night and especially in the early hours of the morning. It is dry, persistent and hacky, and may drive you crazy; yet when the child is up and around, he or she will hardly cough.

A child suffering from allergies may be beset with many bouts of allergic respiratory symptoms, with the troublesome hacking cough, sometimes with a good deal of mucus.

In addition to all the above, some types of cough can be caused by some serious diseases such as tuberculosis, cystic fibrosis, and whooping cough, among others.

What can I do about the cough?

If the cough is mild, occasional, and there are no associated major symptoms, you may try treating as follows:

1. For a child one to six year old , (a) offer Triaminic DM or expectorant, Benylin expectorant, or Robitussin DM (nonprescription), 1/2 teaspoon four times a day. If the condition is more of a runny nose than a cough, give Robitussin PE, or simply Novahistine or Triaminic, 1/2 teaspoon four times a day. (b) If it is in an infant six to twelve months old, use 1/4 teaspoon four times a day of the above medicines. (c) If the

child is six to twelve years old, give 3/4 teaspoon four times a day of the above medicines.
2. It is important that the child rests. This doesn't mean putting the child in bed and treating him or her like a cripple. Simply don't allow running around too much, or going outdoors. Let the child have limited activity; watching TV, enjoying jigsaw puzzles, or reading a book. This should be encouraged only while the symptoms are acute and only for a few days.
3. Use a cool-mist humidifier or a vaporizer (see page 290).
4. Use nose drops if the nose is very stuffy and the child has difficulty breathing. You can use Neosynephrine every four hours, for up to three days (see page 274).
5. If you follow the above steps and the child doesn't seem to improve in a few days, see the doctor. Don't wait too long, otherwise complications may set in.

Which coughing children should see the doctor:

1. A child whose cough is: (a) barking, (b) persistent, (c) croupy, (d) too tight, or (e) too deep,
2. A child who: (a) has a high temperature with the cough, or (b) has low-grade temperature for more than three days with the cough,
3. A child who: (a) wheezes in addition to the cough, (b) has croup in addition to the cough,
4. A child who is obviously quite sick in addition to the cough, i.e. if he or she also looks pale, has flushed cheeks, doesn't eat, is very irritable, vomits, or is nauseated,
5. A child who, in addition to the cough, has rapid, shallow respirations,
6. A child who, along with the cough, has fairly severe pains in the chest, shoulders, or abdomen,
7. A child whose cough is quite persistent at night,
8. A child who is moaning and groaning with the cough,
9. A baby troubled with cough.

What if the cough is prolonged?

A cough that goes on and on may mean many things. A good example is an allergic cough that can become quite troublesome at times and may not respond to treatment easily. Another example is the cough of the postnasal drip. Diseases not seen often any more, such as TB and whooping cough, can also lead to a persistent cough.

The specific treatment of the cause of the cough is the only way to treat the cough correctly. A good example is the decision whether to use an antibiotic or not, and if so, which one and what dosage. This is also true of the kind of cough medicine and the dosage.

What is the most frequent cause of cough?

Upper respiratory infection, or what people call chest colds, are the most frequent cause of cough. This is particularly common during wintertime and in young children between the age of one and five years.

It is worthy to note that many parents erroneously give aspirin to help a child's cough and cold. This is useless since aspirin has no action on a cough or a runny nose. Aspirin will only help the achiness and the fever that accompany a cold, no more.

Will exposure make a cough worse?

If the cough happens to be a symptom of respiratory infection, then certain forms of exposure can give trouble. A child with an upper respiratory infection should not be allowed to go outside to play. The child will run around, take off on a bicycle or do vigorous exercise with PE class in school. Such a child will strain the respiratory tree that is already inflamed, and will be more likely to develop complications like bronchitis, pneumonia, and inflamed ear, among others.

Wet feet, inadequate clothes, and exposure to cold weather, wind, rain, snow or cigarette smoke will also precipitate complications. Be cautious for a few days, until the acute condition of the sickness is behind you, and allow your child to resume normal activity only when the condition seems to have improved a lot. It is worthy of note that a child with respiratory infection can be transported from one place to another by using a warmed-up car in wintertime. In so doing, you are not taking a chance for complications.

When shall I give up treatment and ask for medical help?

1. If the child's cough doesn't improve after four or five days with your treatment,
2. If the cough becomes worse in spite of your treatment,
3. If other symptoms show up in addition to the cough, such as fever, sore throat, earache, shortness of breath, wheezing, croupiness, stiff neck, etc.
4. If the child looks sicker and acts sicker in spite of your treatment,
5. Promptly, if the child is a baby.

COUGH MEDICINES

There are oodles of cough medicines in a bewildering array, a good many of which can be bought over the counter. Many of these are highly advertised as a cure-all, but too often they prove to be of little value.

The prescription cough medicines come in all varieties too. They are usually stronger, and their specific combinations are designed to help specific forms of cough.

What about the over-the-counter cough medicines?

Over-the-counter cough medicines are milder than prescription cough medicines, and are worth a try if the cough is also mild. Often they are worth using only for a few days to see if the cough will improve.

Some are single-ingredient cough medicines like Robitussin. Some come combined with a decongestant such as Novahistine DMX, Triaminic expectorant or Robitussin PE. The latter group is good for a cough with some stuffiness of the nose, be it allergic or otherwise.

Other cough medicines contain a mild cough suppressant (Dextromethorphan). This group is slightly better than a plain cough medicine. Good examples are Triaminic DM and Robitussin DM.

What is the difference between prescription
and nonprescription cough medicines?

A nonprescription cough medicine is designed for mild coughs and is safe to take without a doctor's visit. It can be used for the child's cough on a trial basis to see if it will control the cough in a few days, thus avoiding a visit to the office.

On the other hand, a prescription cough medicine often contains certain antihistamines and/or decongestants, and/or a cough suppressant such as codeine. The quality of the child's cough will necessitate the kind of cough medicine you must use.

Examples of nonprescription cough medicines are: the Robitussins, Ambenyl-D, Benylin, Novahistine DMX, Cheracol, Triaminic expectorant, Trind DM and a host of others.

Examples of prescription cough medicines are: Actifed-C expectorant, Ambenyl expectorant, Phenergan expectorant with codeine, Robitussin AC, Triaminic expectorant with codeine, Ryna CX, etc.

How can I use the above medicines?

Though the above may be confusing to you, you can be sure that they are safe, they are mainly for mild coughs, and they vary from each other only slightly in potency and range of effectiveness.

There are numerous other over-the-counter cough medicines, some advertised and designed to attract your attention. Most of them, if not all, are no more than mild cough medicines, and none can produce miracles.

How will the doctor prescribe the cough medicine?

If you take your coughing child to the doctor, and if he or she diagnoses the cough as caused by bronchitis, asthma or pneumonia, then treatment will be concentrated on the disease causing the cough.

In the case of a loose but frequent cough with nothing but mucus, the doctor may decide to give no more than a combination of an antihistamine and a cough suppressant such as Novahistine DH. Occasionally, the doctor may even give a medicine to make the child vomit to get rid of the excess mucus!

What is a decongestant?

A decongestant is usually composed of an antihistamine, pseudoephedrine, Neosynephrine (given internally) or similar ingredient, or a combination of the above.

It is given when the child's nose becomes stuffy or somewhat runny. It will help give some relief in many cases. Please note that it will not give complete relief, neither can it help every case. The degree of relief given depends on the cause of the nasal congestion and whether or not you are treating it right.

Triaminic syrup, Actifed, Novahistine, Demazin, Chlortrimeton, Dimetane, Sudafed, and Novafed don't require a prescription, and they are good decongestants. Naldecon, Dimetapp, Rynatan, Ryna liquid, and others may require a prescription.

Please remember, if the child does not respond to a decongestant after four or five days' try, he or she may be having some infection in addition, or you probably are not using the right medicine for the trouble.

If my child coughs mainly at night, what shall I do?

Quite often the child seems O.K. during daytime, but starts to cough at bedtime, and especially in early morning. This may indicate a postnasal drip. If the cough is mild, you may elect to give the cough medicine in the evening, at midnight, and at early morning. A humidifier is a good thing to use. Neosynephrine nose drops before going to bed can be of help too (see page 274).

A stuffy nose with mucus because of allergy or a cold -with or without bacterial infection,- is the usual cause of the above. Allergies to feather pillows, stuffed animals, and pets in the same room, if leading to such trouble, should be removed.

Can I combine the cough medicine with a decongestant?

This depends on what kind of cough medicine you are using, and on whether the child needs such a combination or not.

A good many cough medicines already include a decongestant in their constitution. Therefore, adding another decongestant is likely to make the child feel sleepy and drowzy.

When shall I stop using the cough medicine?

Most cough medicines help reduce the frequency and the severity of the cough. They also help change a dry, hacky, barking cough into a loose, wet cough. The latter will sound as if there is a good deal of mucus in the child's chest. In babies you may even be able to feel some rattling in the chest.

When the cough seems to have changed to a loose cough, then it is safe to stop the medication. In most cases this comes after one or two weeks of using the cough medicine.

How often shall I give the cough medicine?

Usually one dose four times a day will be sufficient. However, you can give two extra doses through the night if need be. Most cough medicines work for four to six hours and no more.

By the way, it is important to know that doubling the dose or just plain increasing it will not help any more than giving the proper dose.

I keep using the cough medicine and the child keeps coughing:

This is common; it may mean that you are not using a strong enough cough medicine and it is time for a change. It may also mean that there might be complications of the child's condition. In both cases you may have to visit the doctor.

In some however, parents keep using cough medicine although the child has a loose, noisy cough. The cough medicine in such cases tends to increase the amount of mucus and make the cough worse. The obvious answer to this problem is to stop the cough medicine, and the cough will gradually diminish in a week's time then stop.

Should I give the cough medicine before or after meals?

The difference is small, but giving any medicine before meals by about half an hour or longer will mean faster absorption into the system. This is especially true of some antibiotics.

A faster absorption will mean a high peak of the medicine in the system, and possibly better action. This doesn't mean that giving the medicine on a full stomach (after meals) will be of little use; so don't hesitate to do so if you have forgotten to do it before a meal.

UPPER RESPIRATORY INFECTION
CHEST COLD

The child started with a cold, then began to cough. The cough is hacky, frequent, annoying, and more acute at night, yet there may not be any rise of temperature. The child looks pale and feels out of sorts; the nose keeps running and even the nostrils and the skin around them look scalded; there is a complaint of headache and/or stomachache, and a loss of appetite.

You treat the child with all the cough silencers advertised on television, but you seem to go nowhere.

What causes chest colds?

Mostly it is caused by certain viruses that have a special liking for the respiratory tract. In those who are afflicted with allergies, the tendency toward upper respiratory infection can be particularly noticeable.

Such infections are most common during the cold season; usually they show up as early as October and keep showing up until the month of May.

Is it very contagious?

Yes, so be careful about being very close. Don't let the child cough or sneeze in your face if you can avoid it, don't overcontaminate your hands with the used facial tissue, wash your hands frequently, don't use the child's nasal spray for your nose, and don't overdo it with kissing the child or putting him or her in your lap. In other words, be cautious but don't treat the child like Typhoid Mary.

Should I see the doctor too?

If you have tried your luck with over-the-counter cough medicines (see page 303), and if you haven't had much success in about four or five days, it would be wise to see your doctor.

Most mild upper respiratory infections will resolve themselves in a matter of a few days. But if the cough is still frequent, and if the child develops a fever, and still feels under the weather, there is a possibility of complications such as a superadded bacterial infection, tonsillitis, ear infection, bronchitis, pneumonitis, etc.

What would you do for an upper respiratory infection?

This depends on how old the child is, how bad the infection is, and whether or not there are complications. Most uncomplicated upper respiratory infections are self-limited, and you ought to observe certain principles:

1. Rest is important. If the child rests, the rate and depth of the respiration will decrease, and there will be less irritation of the respiratory tract. Rest doesn't mean constant lying in bed; lying down watching TV, reading a book, or the like, are adequate.
2. Have the child drink plenty of liquids in the form of carbonated beverages, water, lemonade, and/or orange juice (especially the latter two because of their citrates). Using a soft diet is also recommended.
3. Increase the humidity by using a humidifier or a vaporizer in the room. If the cough is persistent, use the humidifier day and night, but as the cough improves, use it only at night for a few nights (see page 290).
4. Use the medicines prescribed by your doctor; also use an antipyretic such as aspirin or Tylenol if the child has fever or achiness (see page 131).

Can I help prevent a chest cold?

Upper respiratory infection is frequent, especially in children under the age of four years (the average is five to six infections a year), and this is one way nature helps your child build a resistance.

(a) For the use of a central humidifier and electronic air filter (see page 290). (b) Too many clothes during wintertime will not help prevent the upper respiratory infection, it will just make the child uncomfortable. (c) Overheating the house or the school during wintertime (to temperatures beyond 72 degrees F) will lead to more frequent chest colds. An active child, who goes in and out of doors too often (when the temperature outside may be in the thirties or forties), will stand to be exposed to too much fluctuation of temperature, which will increase the chance for upper respiratory infection. (d) Last but not least, don't expose the child to others who have an upper respiratory infection.

LARYNGITIS

The child seems to have lost his or her voice, and may complain of a sore throat and some cough. The cough might be of the barking type, might be fairly frequent, and the child's temperature may be up a bit. More often than not, none of the above symptoms show up except for the loss of voice. Symptoms of a cold, or simply a bout of shouting in a ballgame, may have precipitated it.

What causes it?

Laryngitis is a form of inflammation of the larynx (voice box). Though colds can affect the larynx, leading to laryngitis, more often laryngitis occurs after straining the voice, i.e. hollering and shouting. When combined with a cold, laryngitis is quite likely. If there is a barking cough, with or without fever, it may indicate that the laryngitis is part of croup or laryngo-tracheitis. Laryngitis is fairly common, seen more often during wintertime. Rarely a youngster passes through childhood without having one or more bouts of it. Most cases of laryngitis are caused by viruses. Usually the virus affects the voice box, making the vocal cords inflamed and rendering them semi-operational. Many cases, however, are caused mechanically, i.e. when excessive shouting and screaming takes place. Besides the above, certain rare diseases can cause laryngitis, particularly if the laryngitis is of long duration or has occurred in a baby. The question is often asked whether or not the laryngitis is caused by strep. It is good news that the strep germ does not like the larynx, thank goodness, and it is exceptional for it to cause trouble in this area.

What can be done about it?

Many things can be done, depending on the type and severity of laryngitis, the age of the child, and other factors. Fortunately most bouts of laryngitis are of limited duration and tend to go away.

If the loss of voice is the only symptom and the laryngitis stands by itself, we can relax a bit. It will often mean strained vocal cords, which need rest. To rest the vocal cords, the child should be silent as much as possible, and especially refrain from shouting. He or she should not even sing! To control oneself and refrain from vocal communication is very hard, and may be beyond the capacity of the child to oblige. However, it is the only way to rest the vocal cords.

Parents may develop an alternative, e.g. trying sign language, or giving hard candy to suck. Some parents let the child watch TV or play games that require relative silence. If the means are successful, after a few days the child's voice will slowly return again, ready to fill the house with chatter.

What if the laryngitis is associated with other symptoms?

If laryngitis is part of a croup or upper respiratory infection, treatment of such diseases becomes a necessity, of course. As the child recovers from them, his or her voice will return.

Babies with such a condition should be looked at differently, however.

Why is that?

Babies less than a few months old, can suffer much more from respiratory infections than older children, especially when the voice becomes hoarse. They are more likely to have croup and croupy breathing, and this is more dangerous at this age than at other ages.

Because of all this, when the tiny baby gets this condition, you better let the doctor have a look. The voice box of such tiny babies is of different nature and may give us many problems if inflamed.

Can laryngitis be stubborn?

Yes, it can, and the lost voice or hoarse voice can go on and on. This is most likely due to continued use of the larynx while it is inflamed, i.e. a child's repeated shouting and hollering in spite of your pleading to stop. Adults, especially teachers, can be in a real fix. They have to talk to earn their living, and if they have laryngitis it is likely to continue for many weeks, if not months! Eventually you must either go through a period of complete silence or see an ear, nose and throat specialist. Either way the larynx may have to be checked to see if there have been some unwelcome changes.

Why the ear, nose, and throat specialist?

A checkup by an ear, nose, and throat specialist becomes essential once a chronic laryngitis seems not to have improved despite a "talk-less" period. The reason is that sometimes "nodules" develop on the vocal cords, or the vocal cords themselves develop problems. The ENT doctor may be able to see the larynx indirectly (with a tiny mirror) while the patient is in the office, and may be able to give the proper advice. More often however, the doctor will have to admit the young child to the hospital, administer anesthesia, and take a direct look at the larynx.

Can we prevent laryngitis?

A good preventive measure consists of not straining the vocal cords, especially while having a cold. This is also true during wintertime when the cold air has an unwelcome effect on the vocal cords; if the child has a respiratory infection and plays hard outside, laryngitis is likely and sometimes sudden.

CONGENITAL LARYNGEAL STRIDOR

Congenital laryngeal stridor is not that uncommon, and babies are the target. As its name indicates, babies with this condition have some kind of noisy breathing from birth. The noisy breathing is most evident when the baby inhales (takes the breath in), more so when upset or excited. On the other hand, when the baby is quiet or sleeping, the noisy breathing can be heard only if you are listening carefully and attentively.

What kind of noisy breathing is it?

This noisy breathing is easily differentiated from that of a croup or wheezing. It is characterized by a loose, low-pitched, noisy inhalation, and it sometimes sounds as if there is some mucus. Yet at the same time the baby seems to be otherwise in good shape, without apparent suffering; the skin color looks good, playfulness still abounds -as does the appetite- and sleep is restful despite the noisy breathing.

When does it show up, and how long will it last?

Congenital laryngeal stridor can be detected during the first few days of life. At first it is very mild, and the noise can be of a very short duration. The parents usually miss it unless it is brought to their attention by the doctor.

The condition often becomes more pronounced in a few weeks, and becomes noticeable to most people. At the age of a few months, the noisy breathing will be at its worst. However parents will have become used to it by then, and will pay little attention to it, except when someone asks about it.

As the baby reaches the age of nine months or around, the noisy breathing will become less pronounced, and will gradually continue to decrease until it disappears (in most babies) by the age of one year.

In milder ones, the noisy breathing will continue only for a few months and no more, and will not attract as much attention from people around.

What causes this condition?

The condition is a nuisance and will continue to be so until it is gone. In most babies, the different components of the larynx are held together well, but in babies with congenital laryngeal stridor, some parts of the larynx are held loosely, and they will vibrate as the air goes through. This vibration will produce the low-pitched noise of laryngeal stridor.

Should it be investigated or treated?

In most mild ones there is no need for investigation especially when the baby seems to be otherwise healthy. In severe cases, particularly the loud ones heard during the first few days of life, an investigation is worthwhile. This is mainly to rule out conditions other than laryngeal stridor.

If the noisy breathing proves to be caused by one of the rare conditions other than the usual stridor, specific treatment (usually surgery) will have to be instituted.

How is it different from a croup?

Congenital laryngeal stridor is quite different from croup, wheezing, and other conditions. As said before, quite often it is present at birth or soon after, the baby seems not to mind it, and there seems to be no trouble coming out of it at any time.

Croup can also show up in babies, but in the form of an acute attack that lasts only for a short time; it is accompanied by other symptoms. The croupy baby sounds differently and his cough tends to sound like a bark (see below).

In the case of a baby with a wheeze, usually there are respiratory symptoms of cough, perhaps fever, etc., along with the characteristic wheezing and huffing and puffing. A baby with croup or wheeze is having an acute attack, and may need immediate treatment; this is exactly opposite of the baby with congenital laryngeal stridor.

CROUP

The child wakes up at night and makes a scary loud noise, loudest when taking the breath in, and seems to labor hard to draw breath. His or her face may become pale, he or she may sweat, become scared and restless, and every once in a while an awful-sounding barking cough may follow.

Naturally you will be alarmed, especially if this happens to be your first experience with the croup. Remember, however, your alarmed attitude will be felt by your child, who may become even more scared. Therefore try to be calm and collected, or at least act that way.

Are there other symptoms besides the above?

There may be croupy breathing also upon exhalation. There may be hoarseness of voice, some rise of temperature, nausea, and even vomiting. The vomiting at times works in such a way as to stop the croup.

Croup may show up suddenly or be preceded by symptoms of a cold or an upper respiratory infection. Very rarely, if at all, is there any wheezing; however, you may feel the vibration of the croupy breathing on the chest and mistake it for a wheeze.

When does it occur?

Croup often shows up suddenly at night, and will improve a great deal after only a few hours. Some children will look almost normal next morning, to your relief and surprise!

A child who had had the croup is more likely to get it again and again, not unusually two or three times a winter. Most such children, however, will outgrow this tendency by the age of four or five years. An occasional child may continue with this tendency until much later. Older children with a croup tendency may prove to have allergies and may need allergy tests and shots.

What can I do about croup?

Since most croup cases are viral infections, the obvious treatment is the relief of the symptoms. A mildly croupy child should sit inside a "tent" made with a bedsheet covering the three sides of a crib, or some similar arrangement, with the humidity of a vaporizer or humidifier entering inside. A cough medicine may help a lot, such as Robitussin DM or others (see page 304). Remember, it will take several hours until the croup subsides and the child will then fall soundly asleep. Croup is an exhausting ordeal.

If the croup is moderately severe, sit the child in the bathroom, close the door, and run a hot shower to steam the room. Don't act alarmed, just make it seem like you are doing something fun. After the hot shower has steamed the bathroom, turn it off. When the steam seems to be going away, repeat the procedure, and keep this up for at least one hour.

When the croup is not mild, notify the doctor; the child may have to be seen right away.

What are the criteria?

1. If the croupiness is truely severe, especially with both inhalation and exhalation;
2. If the child becomes pale, restless, and unable to breathe except with marked exertion;
3. If the child becomes blue in the face, though you shouldn't have waited for this stage;
4. If the cough is very barking and persistent;
5. If the child is a few weeks to a few months old.

Call your doctor in such cases, whatever time of night it is.

If the croup is better next morning, shall I check with the doctor?

Yes, since there may be some complications. Pneumonitis, laryngotracheobronchitis (see below), inflamed ears and throats, among other things can show up with the croup or soon afterwards.

The treatment of the croup depends on many factors, but by and large cough medicine (see page 304), a humidifier (see page 290), rest and limited activity, and occasional use of an antibiotic are necessary. Avoid giving the child icy cold drinks while being croupy.

Can I prevent the croup?

You can try but your chance for success is not that high. A central humidifier on the furnace (see page 290) is of some help, and treating colds and upper respiratory infections early enough may help too. A child with allergies may need the electronic air filter (see page 292) and/or allergy studies. These measures are more useful in children who have repeated croups.

TRACHEOBRONCHITIS

Often the child starts with a cold and what sounds like a regular upper respiratory infection, but soon the course of events becomes more worrisome. The cough becomes more or less persistent, and rather than "hacking" in character, it may become barking, frequent, deep, and tight. The cough may interfere with the child's sleep, and may seem to become aggravated upon resuming activity. He or she may refer to it as a tickle, and it may come in paroxysms.

In addition to the above, the child's chest may become sore, or the area under the ribs may start to hurt because of the strain on the muscles from coughing.

Though the temperature can be normal, more often it goes up, and may even reach 104 degrees F. The child feels tired, irritable, and pale, often has a poor appetite, and may also complain of a sore throat and headache.

What causes it?

Quite often, tracheobronchitis is an extension of an upper respiratory infection, though infrequently it starts as a pure case of bronchitis. Various viruses are responsible, but in a certain percentage, bacteria can complicate the matter or be the cause. A sound respiratory tree is more resistant to tracheobronchitis, and an allergic child is more likely to suffer from it.

Exposure to sudden and wide variations of temperature and atmospheric pressure, exposure to other children with respiratory infections among others, often play a contributing part. Irritants such as cigarettes, cigar or pipe smoke, may also cause trouble.

How serious is tracheobronchitis?

Tracheobronchitis is more troublesome than upper respiratory infection, and the symptoms are usually fairly severe. Not only that, but it may take longer to clear up, may need more medication, and may also require a second visit to the doctor. Complications such as pneumonia, ear infection, etc., have to be kept in mind too.

Tracheobronchitis may take longer than expected before it clears up. This is particularly true of children with respiratory allergies, or ones living in houses where there are irritant factors such as cigarette smoke.

Is a child with tracheobronchitis prone to get it again?

A child who gets a solitary bout of tracheobronchitis is less likely to get it again for a long time. However, many children with a mild degree of respiratory allergy often end up with some degree of "susceptibility" to respiratory infections, tracheobronchitis, or asthmatic bronchitis. Such children often need to have allergy shots. Occasionally a doctor may also want to test for cystic fibrosis and other diseases.

When shall I take my child to the doctor?

If the cough is severe, frequent, interferes with the child's sleep, and is accompanied by fever or other symptoms, it is better to be checked and treated by the doctor, not only to help relieve the condition but also to prevent complications.

What can be done about it?

The doctor will check the child for the severity of the condition and see if there are any complications. Often a throat culture will be taken, and occasionally an X-ray of the chest may have to be taken.

The proper type of cough medicines will be prescribed, and perhaps an antibiotic. Rest is very important, and this means minimum activity for two to three days. This will help the respiratory tree fight the infection and get rid of it in the shortest time possible. Plenty of liquids (three to four large glasses a day), especially orange juice and lemonade, will help to thin down the mucus and make it easier for the child to spit it out. Orange juice and lemonade contain citrates, which act as an expectorant. A humidifier or a vaporizer (see page 290) will help during wintertime, but often they are not needed during summertime.

Of course, during the acute phase of the disease the child will have to forego school for a few days.

ASTHMATIC BRONCHITIS

Children with asthmatic bronchitis have difficulty taking a breath; their breathing is wheezy and labored, and they are restless.

Even their stomachs seem to work hard while they breathe. Their color is pale or perhaps faintly blue. Their coughs are tight, dry, frequent, and deep. They may have fever, though not necessarily. Their appetites are low; after all, it is difficult to eat while the breathing is so labored.

These symptoms seem to come quickly, after having had a cold and some cough for a few days.

What is asthmatic bronchitis?

It is a respiratory infection of an allergic nature, with a wheezing element. A wheeze is a prolonged whistling sound of the breath, mainly upon exhalation.

There is usually a history of allergy -be it in the form of hay fever, asthma, eczema, etc- in the family of such a child but not always so.

Some children get it quite early in life, and many keep getting it repeatedly. Even young babies may come down with it, though it is usually of a different nature (see page 79).

What will trigger asthmatic bronchitis?

A cold or an upper respiratory infection often triggers a bout of asthmatic bronchitis. It may be further exacerbated by irritants such as smoke, cold air, changes in atmospheric pressure, smog, etc. It is not unusual for allergic children to come down with it three to four times a year, if not more often.

Not every wheeze is asthma. A wheeze may be caused by other conditions not related to allergy. Some babies with pneumonitis or bronchiolitis may behave as if they have asthmatic bronchitis. Croupy breathing may seem similar to a wheeze; that is, if the parents' ears are not "trained" well enough.

A child with a "rattly" chest is not a wheezing child. The rattle is an innocuous thing, caused by excess mucus, making the chest "vibrate," and it can easily be felt by the hand.

What can be done about it?

A sick child who is wheezing ought to be seen by the doctor. Once the child is checked, a medicine to dilate the bronchial tubes along with an antibiotic will be given. For severe cases some shots may have to be given.

Using a vaporizer or a cool-mist humidifier (see page 290) during wintertime will help. Encouraging the child to drink plenty of liquids, especially orange juice and lemonade, will also be of help, since they will thin down the mucus and ease the cough.

A wheezing baby may need close medical care. If the condition is severe, or seems not to improve with medication, admission to the hospital may be in the wind.

Can we prevent these attacks?

A good deal of preventive work can be done. These steps will help reduce the chances of developing bouts of asthmatic bronchitis, sometimes substantially:

1. Have a central humidifier (see page 290).
2. Install a central electronic air filter, it will help a great deal (see page 292).
3. Try to prevent sudden exposure to extremes of temperature. The cold air is quite irritating to the respiratory tree, and so is the dry hot air in an overheated house.
4. Too many irritants indoors can be quite troublesome. Avoid them or at least reduce their intensity if possible. Examples are: cigarette, pipe, and cigar smoke, smell of fresh paint (one to two days old) kitchen fumes, etc.
5. If at all possible, avoid exposure to others who have colds and respiratory infections.

How about allergy shots?

Some severely allergic children may be sick with asthmatic bronchitis so often, that allergy tests and shots may have to be instituted as early as one-and-a-half to two years of age, if not even earlier. However, most allergic children are not that allergic. If they show bouts of asthmatic bronchitis at the rate of three to four times a year, and if they get unusually frequent upper respiratory infections, then allergy tests and shots will have to be done, between the ages of two and five years.

Less severe cases may need the allergy shots later in life. There are many people who develop their allergies late, including during adulthood. The doctor will decide at the proper time when to send the child to an allergist for allergy tests.

The allergy shots will help prevent a good deal of asthmatic bronchitis and allergic respiratory infections. The child's well-being will be much improved, and the visits to the doctor will be mostly just for administration of the shots.

FOREIGN BODY IN THE LUNG
NOT EVERY WHEEZE IS ASTHMA

A wheeze, as mentioned before, is a prolonged whistling sound heard during respiration, and it is caused by some form of obstruction in the respiratory tract. During asthma or asthmatic bronchitis you are likely to hear the best example of wheezing. It is different from croupy breathing in many ways.

What other problems cause wheezing?

In some cases wheezing is caused by aspiration of foreign bodies in the lung. This usually happens to a child who is eating. The child may be tickled, made to laugh, or provoked to the point of anger or crying. When such happens, and the child takes a deep breath to laugh or cry, a piece of food in the mouth will dislodge and go down directly to the lung. Depending on its size, it will obstruct a small or large section of a lung, sometimes even the whole respiratory tract.

What will happen then?

The child will immediately go into a severe and frequent cough that will continue on and off for some time. Wheezing and breathing trouble will often be manifested right away. This trouble will continue, and it, along with the cough, coming seemingly out of the blue, following a laugh or cry while the mouth is full, will make many parents suspect that the food has gone the wrong way.

Depending on the size of the foreign body and where it is lodged, the child may or may not become blue in color, pale as if in shock, or show signs of severe trouble inhaling.

Have you seen such cases?

Yes, and I'll never forget them:

One two-year-old child was eating peanuts when her sister tickled her. The peanut got lodged in a bronchial tube and the child needed immediate surgical intervention. A few months later, the sister of this child was eating a carrot, and ....need I say more?

A ten-year-old was playing with a plastic pistol, and he shot a plastic bullet into his mouth; it went zooming to the lung, and of course required immediate surgery.

A four-year-old swallowed a needle, and it somehow got lodged in the lung, penetrating it and resulting in immediate trouble and the need for surgery.

These are scary cases, but the children made it because of the awareness of the parents and the immediate surgical intervention in the hospital.

Not everyone is so lucky. I know of one five-year-old girl who died after a pill got caught in her larynx and completely obstructed the respiratory tract.

What can we do?

Prevention is the sweetest thing. But if you suspect a foreign body in the lung, go to the doctor right away. This is particularly true of peanuts -they tend to swell as time passes, thereby obstructing the respiratory passage more and more severely and becoming more difficult to remove.

In all such cases, admission to the hospital for bronchoscopy or other procedures will be necessary to remove the foreign body. If the foreign body is missed, it can lead to a lung abscess or other complications.

How can we prevent such problems?

Be alert and always discourage your child from laughing vigorously while he or she has food in the mouth. Do not allow the child to be provoked in that situation either. This is easier said than done, but it is still such a simple endeavor when the alternative is considered.

Once you suspect that the child has aspirated a foreign body, don't wait; get in touch with your doctor right away. If the doctor is not available, take the child to the emergency room of the nearest hospital. This is much safer than simply waiting for the doctor, even if it proves to be a false alarm.

TB (TUBERCULOSIS) AND ITS TESTS

Fortunately TB is not as common as it used to be, yet it is not that rare either. The very phrase "TB" is frightening to most parents, but take heart, efforts at detecting cases early and offering prompt treatment have helped a great deal in reducing the number and the severity of this disease.

Nowadays, the TB test is much easier to do than it used to be, and there is no excuse why it shouldn't be done routinely on every child, once a year. If it proves positive, then it means the child had already picked up the TB germ and is reacting to it.

<u>What is to be done when the TB test becomes positive?</u>

For the child who has become a "converter", i.e. who reveals for the first time a positive reaction to TB test, a chest X-ray is usually done. In many such cases chest X-ray proves to be negative, but occasionally a child shows evidence of primary tuberculosis in the lung or a calcified spot.

A concerted effort should be made to examine all the contacts of such a child: X-rays and TB tests, (for the immediate family, more than once during the ensuing year) are usually decided upon. The investigation is usually carried out by the local health department, though occasionally some doctors want to do it themselves.

Any child who has converted (i.e. developed a positive reaction) should be on medication (usually INH) for a period of one year. This ought to be given whether or not the chest X-ray proves to be normal.

<u>Why should you give medication for so long?</u>

If you don't do that, a child with a positive reaction to a TB test stands a chance for developing active tuberculosis in the lungs, or TB disease spreading to other organs such as the bones, the meninges of the brain, kidneys, etc. By giving this medication over a prolonged period of one year you can practically prevent all the above possibilities.

Doesn't the child have any symptoms?

A child who develops a positive reaction to TB test but with normal X-rays of the chest will have no symptoms. But if the lungs develop tuberculosis, there will be a persistant cough, fever, pale face, poor appetite, etc. Usually they are the symptoms of a severe prolonged respiratory infection.

How about those calcified spots in the lungs?

They usually indicate that the child had fought the TB germ well with his or her own resistance. The TB germ became confined in the lymph nodes and the body deposited some calcium on it. These are usually the silent cases, and there are no symptoms; yet you will have to use the medication anyway for a minimum of one whole year, and be under the supervision of the doctor and/or the clinic.

Why is TB becoming rare?

Tuberculosis is becoming rare because of the higher standard of living, fresh air, good balanced nutrition, exercise, and the general welfare of the society, but most important is the constant efforts to detect and treat early cases of TB.

We should not, however, accept any feeling of false security just because we know that TB is becoming rare.

Are there many forms of TB?

At the present time, most of the cases of TB are those who develop positive reaction to TB, with or without calcified spots in the lungs. However, TB can occur in the bones and joints, the meninges, and the lymph nodes and skin, among other areas. These forms do still exist in societies where the health standard continues to be lower than ours. But even in our country, poverty-stricken areas and areas with substandard health delivery stand a greater chance for TB to occur.

PNEUMONIA

After a few days of having a cold or respiratory infection, some childrens' conditions will grow worse. Their coughs will become persistent, harsh, and frequent, and will perhaps interfere with their sleep. They seem to have difficulty taking a breath, though it doesn't exactly sound like wheezing. Their breathing may be shallow and frequent, and they seem to huff and puff. Their temperatures may rise. They may have pains in the chest, and their color may be off with a sick look on the face.

In babies, the above symptoms may be more alarming, and the chest and stomach may go in and out excessively with their respiration. Their color may be dusky or slightly blue, and it is more likely that the symptoms will come more suddenly and to a greater extent than in older children.

Is that the way pneumonia always shows up?

No. The above is an average case. There are mild cases wherein the pneumonia seems to creep in and be an extention of a chest cold, and may thus escape your vigilant eyes.

On the other hand, severe ones may be sudden, cause violent coughing, a high temperature, a toxic appearance and sick look, nasty pains in the chest or even abdomen, vomiting, and restlessness. It can be very scary. There are numerous variations, since pneumonia is so multifaced.

What causes it?

Pneumonia can be caused by a number of viruses. Bacteria can also be the cause, mainly pneumococcus, which takes a special liking to the lungs. There are other causes of pneumonia, but they are rare.

Lobar pneumonia means pneumonia of one lobe of a lung; double pneumonia means the two lungs are affected; walking pneumonia is when a pneumonia seems to be resolving in a lobe of one lung, only to appear in a different lobe.

Walking pneumonia does not mean that it comes from the fact that the child was walking. It is called so because it goes slowly from one lobe to another, affecting one side or both, as if the pneumonia "walked" in its manner of spread.

When should I suspect it?

A child with upper respiratory infection, whose cough seems to become severe or persistent, who has difficulty taking the breath in, whose temperature shoots up, or who has pains in the chest or any new scary symptom, should go to see the doctor. Don't take chances, don't wait too long.

A sick baby with a cough should see the doctor, especially; don't wait for any alarming symptoms of pneumonia to show up before going to the doctor.

What will the doctor do?.

Having checked the patient thoroughly, if the doctor suspects pneumonia, chest X-rays will be taken to make sure. The X-ray will help show the area affected, the lobe involved, and the size of affected area.

Most pneumonias can be treated at home. Severe ones, however, and those affecting babies will have to be treated in the hospital for a few days. When treated at home, the child will be on an antibiotic, until the condition is over. Cough medicine will be given also. A vaporizer or cool-mist humidifier (see page 290) will have to be used during winter, but not during summer (there is too much humidity in the air during summer). Soft diet and plenty of liquids, especially orange juice and lemonade, are usually suggested, and the latter have citrates that tend to thin the mucus.

Physical rest is important, i.e. lying down to watch TV, read a book, assemble a jigsaw puzzle, and the like. Rest will help the lung do its best to fight the pneumonia. Too much movement may "tire" the lung, which is already burdened by the pneumonia.

The doctor will want to see the child several times to assess the extent and progress of the disease, the presence of complications, etc. Fortunately most pneumonias will be over in a week or so, and no more than three to four visits will be necessary.

Can we prevent pneumonia?

Since pneumonia is often a complication of upper respiratory infection, croup, and asthmatic bronchitis, treating these diseases in a prompt manner may help prevent it. Therefore, early care and prevention of exposure may go a long way in avoiding trouble. Extra vitamin C or other vitamins are useless in preventing this disease.

PLEURISY

The pleura is a sac that covers the lungs and lines the chest cavity, and it helps facilitate breathing, both during inspiration and expiration.

The term pleurisy is used when the wall of the pleura becomes inflamed. The inflammation can be acute, subacute, or chronic, and it can be wet or dry. Often pleurisy is part and parcel of an inflammation in the adjacent lung (such as pneumonia), though pleurisy can show up by itself at times.

What symptoms will be present?

Pleurisy is much rarer in children than in adults. Usually a child with pneumonia will have only the symptoms of pneumonia. But if pleurisy develops in addition, there will also be severe pain of the affected side. Inhaling will make the pain worse and the child may resort to taking shallow and frequent breaths in an attempt to avoid the pain.

With the child's coughing, sneezing, or even trying to laugh, the pain will of course increase and be quite sharp, because of the deep breathing necessary.

In some, because of certain anatomical mechanisms, the pain will also be felt in the corresponding shoulder. In others the pain will be felt in the abdomen; in the latter it may even mimic appendicitis.

What causes pleurisy?

Usually it is an extention of the disease involving the nearby lung.

Whatever is causing the pneumonia may be causing the pleurisy. This may be pneumococcus or other bacteria, mycoplasma or even on occasions various viruses.

Pleurisy can be reactive; in other words, it can show itself as a reaction to some trouble in nearby tissues.

What if pleurisy shows up by itself?

Though this is very rare in children, it can happen. Usually the point that will alarm you will be the severe pain described above, without any of the accompanying symptoms of pneumonia. The pain will be such that it will make you run with your child to the doctor.

What will the doctor do for it?

A child with pleurisy is usually a pretty sick one. He or she will have to be checked and examined, and if pleurisy is suspected then an X-ray will have to be taken. The X-ray will spot the extent of trouble in the nearby lung, and will show if any fluid has accumulated in the pleural sac.

In severe cases, admission to the hospital becomes necessary. In milder ones, treatment of the diseased lung will clear the pleurisy at the same time. This means the use of a proper antibiotic, cough medicine, rest, etc.

Can we prevent pleurisy?

Yes, you can lend a hand. As said before, pleurisy usually is an extention of the disease of the nearby lung. If there is pneumonia, early and energetic treatment of the pneumonia may prevent pleurisy.

This is not always true, however; sometimes pleurisy shows up along with the pneumonia almost from the start, in severe cases or special forms of pneumonia. A good example of the latter is pneumonia caused by the staph germ in babies.

Can pleurisy be a serious disease?

Yes it can be, since on many occasions wet pleurisy (the one with fluid) may reveal certain nasty bacteria. Usually the fluid of the wet pleurisy has to be aspirated (withdrawn), not only to relieve the distress of the child, but also to culture it. The bacteria that show up in the culture will often dictate the method of treatment.

On rare occasions, the wall of the lung can be involved in such a way as to lead to a communication between the pleural cavity and the lung itself; allowing air to enter the pleural cavity, in addition to the fluid of the pleurisy itself. This is called pneumohydrothorax, or pneumopyothorax; it can be life-threatenting, and it often requires immediate intervention.

CHAPTER TWELVE

THE DIGESTIVE TRACT

what is the digestive tract?
appetite
vitamins
the "balanced diet"
they are cute, they are chubby
cholesterol and our diet
food allergy
stomachache
what is a normal stool?
acute constipation in children
chronic constipation
vomiting
gastroenteritis
diarrhea
dehydration
the bloody stool
inguinal hernia
appendicits
round worms
pin worms
infectious hepatitis
diabetes

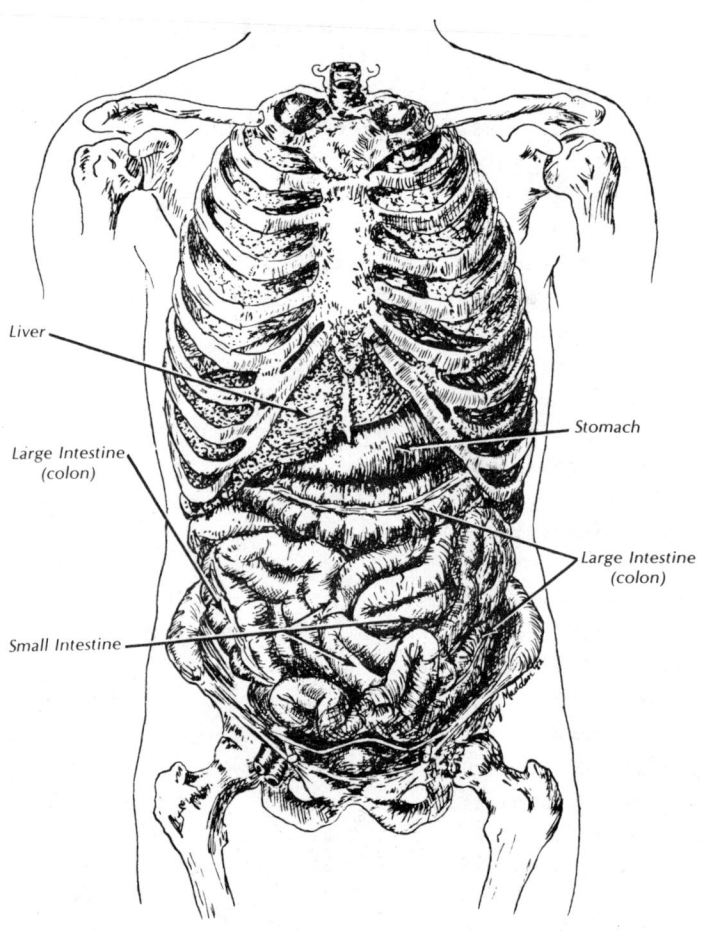

Redrawn from Gray's anatomy, p 79, fig 71, 26th Ed
Coutesy Dycleshymer and Jones
Written permission from the publisher, Lea & Febiger, Philadelphia

WHAT IS THE DIGESTIVE TRACT?

The digestive tract is the tube that handles the food from the time we eat it until we expel the remnants in the form of a bowel movement. The digestive tract is unique indeed. It is juicy and complex in certain parts, as in the mouth, lips, teeth, tongue, palate, and the salivary glands. It is straight in other areas, such as the esophagus, or gullet. It bulges almost like a football to form the stomach, and it curves on itself like a boa constrictor to form the small intestine, then it curves like an upside down U-shape to form the large intestine. Finally, the tract ends up in the rectum and anus for the disposal.

The juice that helps digest the food is manufactured by certain organs and glands, such as the liver and pancreas.

<u>What happens to the food?</u>

As you suspect already, the food becomes chewed, lubricated and mixed in the mouth. It is then known as a bolus of food; it will go down to the stomach, where churning, mixing, and kneading will take place. This way, the food particles will break down to a fine degree, and will be prepared for the finer process of digestion that lies ahead.

Upon entering the small intestine, the food will be further mixed and churned with the juices of the liver and pancreas. After so many hours of hard work on the part of the intestine, the minute food nourishing particles will be absorbed. This will take them even a step further for chemical and other changes and will help make the food suitable for use by the body.

The roughage and the remnant of the food, mixed with a fantastic number of bacteria (in the billions), will form the bulk of the bowel movement.

Because of its size and complexity, so many things can go wrong with the digestive tract. The teeth can suffer, the tongue can be bitten or burned, the throat can be inflamed, and so on "down the line."

The organs further down can get inflamed with viruses leading to gastroenteritis (inflammation of the stomach and intestine), or by bacteria leading to some fairly serious trouble.

The various parts of the digestive tract may not function in perfect unison, thus creating special problems of their own, or they may become blocked at certain areas, posing a threat to life. Part of the intestine may push through certain weak points in the wall of the abdomen, thus leading to a hernia.

The rectum has its own problems too. A baby's anus can crack leading to a fissure causing notoriously painful bowel movements. The rectum can also have some congenital anomalies necessitating surgery.

The knowledge of these gloomy facts will make us grateful that our child's digestive tract is healthy and sound. And that the occasional episode of gas pains, indigestion and other upsets are simply minor episodes in such an incredibly complex factory.

We still have to be on the alert though, because our job is to correct any problems and bring them to a positive healthy condition.

Will diseases of the digestive tract differ in babies as compared to children?

Because the baby's stomach and intestine are still slightly "immature," and because of the nature of food requirement, many diseases quite unique to the baby's stomach and intestine may show up. Milk allergy, colicky pains, and spitting up are but a few examples. Many special surgical conditions may also affect babies in particular. In addition, the same diseases often behave differently in babies as compared to older children. Good examples are gastroenteritis and many of its aftermaths.

There are many diseases that affect the stomach and intestine in older children but very rarely affect babies. Our aim here is to cooperate and work with nature in such a way as to preserve the integrity and function of the child's digestive tract.

APPETITE

Appetite is a major concern for many parents. After all, you could hardly fill the child up when he or she was a baby; milk, cereals, fruits, meats, etc., were devoured with gusto. But now that the baby has grown to be two years old, he or she seems to treat food like a poison!

Why is that?

During the first eighteen to twenty-four months of life, the rate of growth is quite fast. To supply nourishment for such fast growth, the child has no choice but to keep demanding more and more to eat.

But after that and beyond, the rate of growth will slow down a great deal. Actually, in a period of a whole year between the age of three years and four years, a gain of only three pounds is regarded as very good.

The growth will continue at a slow rate until the child is around five to seven years of age, when he or she will take off again, relatively speaking.

During adolescence the growth is again quite fast, and the child will certainly raid the refrigerator time and time again because food is needed to support the rapid growth.

Does this mean I don't have to worry about the child's appetite?

If the child is between the age of two and six years, and seems to be growing as expected, then your worries will certainly be in vain. Being strict about what to eat and what not to eat won't help at all. The child may oblige, and I have seen such a case in which a child kept a piece of chewed meat between his cheek and teeth and went to sleep, just to spit it out the next morning! In this particular case, I felt that the mother wasn't being fair to her child, and the poor fellow thought he was being nice and obedient to her!

Since two to three year-old children are about one third your size, and since their growth rate is slow at this age, they will need about one third of what you usually eat in a day. Since you eat three meals a day, they will need one big meal a day, and most of them will eat just that.

I still worry, can you help me improve the child's food intake?

O.K., let's try. Take a look at what the child eats each day:

1. If the child takes too much milk, this will supply too great of a proportion of the calories needed. Reduce the amount of milk to

one pint a day (measure it), and give it in the form of one or two percent skim milk. Given this way, you will drastically reduce the amount of calories from the milk, yet you will still be giving the child the usual nourishment of protein and calcium. By so doing, you will have made it necessary for the child to have solid meals for his or her calories.
2. Cookies, candy, pretzels, potato chips and other junk foods must be avoided. Do not fool yourself; simply stop buying them so that they will not be available at home. They are murder for a child's appetite, offer only "empty" calories, and are bad for the teeth.
3. Avoid too much orange juice, coke, pepsi, and other liquids; they block the appetite, since they are rich in calories too.

By following the above guidelines, the child's appetite for solid food will improve.

<u>Can medicines improve the child's appetite?</u>

In most cases, medicines are useless as stimulants for appetite, and this is especially true in the case of children. Some of these medicines even contain a good helping of alcohol! Vitamins will help correct vitamin deficiencies, but they don't help the appetite much.

However, if your child is pale, have the blood tested and if anemia is confirmed, then treat this condition. By so doing, the child's appetite will improve.

If the child's appetite is poor because he or she is chronically sick with some disease, your doctor will treat those conditions, and your child's appetite will improve.

<u>How can I know the child is eating enough?</u>

This is the crucial question. Have your doctor see if your child's weight is right for the height. If the weight is too low for the height then your doctor will offer advice gladly. Generally speaking and strangely enough, a child whose ribs can be seen through the skin seems to be among the healthiest most of the time.

<u>Will exercise help the appetite?</u>

Good healthy exercise, usually in the form of active play, will certainly help, especially when it takes place in fresh air. But don't overdo it during wintertime if it is very cold outside.

If the child eats nothing but one kind of meat, is that okay for the system!

Yes, it is okay. Meat is meat, be it chicken, hamburger, fish, or hot dogs. It is the protein of the meat that the body needs, and to the body the protein's content of the meat is just about the same.

My child hates milk and eggs; shall I worry?

No, don't worry. Your child's constitution may be telling you something; the child may be potentially allergic to these foods, so don't push your luck.

My child doesn't even want to touch green vegetables:

Fruits can easily take the place of vegetables, and you will usually see that such a child takes a good helping of fruits. It is true that green vegetables have some protein, but the protein of the meats, milk, eggs, and peanut butter is far superior to that of the green vegetables. So, don't make a scene about him or her being repulsed by the green vegetables, it is not worth worrying about. Vegetables and fruits are important for their minerals, vitamins, roughage, and small measure of amino acids, carbohydrates among other things.

My teenager loves milkshakes:

If the teenager's weight is reasonable compared to the height, milkshakes and dairy products are fine. They will supply calcium and proteins. If he or she is suffering from a "midriff bulge," then be cautious and help reduce this food intake.

My child is hard to please, his or her likes are way out!

All families, sooner or later, will suffer from such syndromes. Don't be disgusted, and keep your cool. Prepare what the child wants at certain times and what you like on other occasions. Teach the art of reciprocity and don't bend backwards to please.

AN APPROXIMATE GUIDELINE:

When your child's height is:	the weight should be around:
34 inches	27 pounds
37 inches	32 pounds
40 inches	36 pounds
43 inches	40 pounds
45 inches	44 pounds
47 inches	49 pounds
49 inches	54 pounds
52 inches	62 pounds
54 inches	68 pounds
56 inches	75 pounds
58 inches	84 pounds
61 inches	98 pounds

VITAMINS

Vitamins are essential components of our food and come in various forms. Many are subdivided into different groups, such as the vitamin B complex. Some are poorly stored in the body and tend to be eliminated when taken in excess (e.g. vitamin C or B). Others are stored in our systems for some time (e.g. vitamins A and D). They keep our system in good working order, but if they are in excess or are deficient, they cause trouble. Many companies add extra vitamins to foods during processing. That, along with the vitamins already present in food and the vitamin D produced by the skin upon exposure to sunlight, usually insures a more than adequate supply of vitamins in our usual diet. However, if our food variety is not well balanced, supplemental vitamins may be needed.

You mean we don't need to take vitamins?

Not usually, because of the adequate amount of vitamins in our food. There are certain situations, however, in which giving vitamins may be desirable.

A good many people take vitamins they don't need, thinking vitamins will prevent infection or improve the appetite. This, of course is a fallacy, except when there is a vitamin deficiency. Such deficiency is not common in America. As a matter of fact, culturally we are quite vitamin oriented. It is said that the American urine is the most vitaminized urine in the world! Congratulations.

Who will need vitamins, then?

During periods of fast growth, when the body's demands are greater than usual, an extra helping of vitamins may be desirable. For this and other situations they may be taken, specifically the following:

1. During the first two years of life, when the baby is growing very fast,
2. During the growth spurt of adolescence, usually between eleven and

eighteen years of age,
3. During pregnancy and nursing,
4. During and after a prolonged illness,
5. During late middle age and old age.

Vitamin drops can be given to babies, syrups or chewables to older children, tablets or capsules to adults. One dose a day usually suffices. Most such vitamin preparations have well-balanced components as suggested by the F.D.A., and they are suitable and satisfactory for most situations.

Which vitamins would you suggest?
For babies, Tri-Vi-Sol, Abdec, Poly-Vi-Sol, ADC, etc., will do. They come with or without iron, and with or without fluoride. Vitamins with fluoride can be given to breastfed babies, and to those who do not drink from a fluorinated water supply. Vitamins with fluoride require prescription.

Vitamin drops can be given directly in the mouth or mixed with the milk. Babies take them well, even though the drops smell. Chewable vitamins are made to taste like candy, though their taste leaves much to be desired. Several varieties are available, and you can pick the ones your child likes best.

Of the tablets, One-A-Day vitamins with or without iron is as good as any, and may be used when the occasion arises. None of these preparations needs a prescription except the ones with fluoride. They are safe to take, but not to be overused or abused. The vitamin syrups and chewables must not be kept within reach of children, to avoid an accidental overdose of them, especially those containing iron which can be toxic in large amounts.

How about the "big" dose vitamins?
There are numerous vitamin combinations, of various concentrations, presented in many different ways. Some have a very high content of a particular vitamin component, others have certain minerals, and some only a combination of three or four vitamins in high proportion. Rarely if ever do we need such vitamins. If taken, most of the excess vitamin will be excreted in the urine.

Overuse of vitamins, which is common, is a waste of money and effort, and in a way it is an abuse of the body, too.

How about vitamins with iron?
Iron is needed when there is anemia of the iron-deficiency type, or when there is a chance or likelihood for such an anemia. Therefore, formula with iron (i.e. Similac with iron), Tri-Vi-Sol with iron, etc. may be used in babies whose diet may be deficient in iron, whose mothers had anemia during pregnancy, twins, prematures, and other special situations.

What types of vitamins are there?
The main ones are vitamin A, vitamin B complex, Vitamin D, and vitamin C. The worth, value, advantages, and side effects of such vitamins are well established, and widely talked about. Standards for vitamins, such as vitamin E, are less well established.

Each of these vitamins has special functions, and when it is deficient in the body, specific symptoms may show up. On the other hand, when vitamins are given in excess, symptoms of toxicity can appear. Symptoms of vitamin D and vitamin A toxicity are well documented and can be quite troublesome.

Vitamins do not prevent infection. Infection is a matter of the mobilization of the body's defence mechanisms versus viruses and germs, and the role that vitamins play in such a war is of only limited value.

THE "BALANCED DIET"

A "balanced diet" represents the relative amounts of food components for the best nourishment your child needs for sustenance and growth, depending on the age. Needed are proteins, fats, carbohydrates, vitamins, essential minerals, and water.

Why does balanced diet "depend on his or her age"?
A fast-growing baby will require more calories, vitamins, minerals, etc. for his or her specific size, compared to an adult who needs them only for sustenance. The same applies for a fast-growing adolescent. A child who grows slowly, say between ages two and five

years, will not need as many calories; yet it is good to emphasize the balance and quality of the intake.

What are proteins?

Proteins are the body's building blocks, more so in a fast-growing child. They should constitute about fifteen percent of the caloric intake; more during periods of fast growth.

Foods that have lots of protein are: (a) meats, (b) fish, (c) liver, (d) eggs, (e) milk and cheese, (f) some green vegetables, such as beans and peas, (g) peanuts, (h) and some fruits, such as bananas.

Are we a protein-oriented culture?

To an extent, yes. Too much advertisement about proteins has clouded the picture. Some families consume as much as sixty to seventy percent of their calorie requirement in the form of proteins. This is certainly one extreme. The opposite extreme, eating mainly carbohydrates, can lead to obesity by taking in too many of those fast but empty calories. Neither extreme is good.

What about the fats?

The fats are an important and concentrated store of calories, and should constitute about thirty-five percent of our calorie intake.

Animal fats are seen in the form of butter, milk, eggs, and other dairy products. Too much fat may give us trouble later in life, mainly in the form of "fat" deposits in the arteries; this can lead to hardening of the arteries, thus a likelihood for heart attacks, strokes, and other dreadful consequences.

The vegetable (unsaturated) fats are present in various vegetable oils such as margarine and shortening like Crisco. They are less troublesome than the animal fats, as far as our future health is concerned.

What are the carbohydrates?

Almost 50% of our calorie intake should come from this component. Abundance of carbohydrate is found in bread, rice, cereals, potatoes, and in almost all the sweets that contain oodles of sugar and flour.

Tell us about vitamins and minerals:

They are essential, as you well know, especially (as with other food components) in a growing child. They are present in most foods, particularly in fresh fruits and vegetables. By the way, most fruits and vegetables have plenty of fiber, water, vitamins, and minerals, but not much in the way of calories (see page 337).

What then is a balanced diet?

A balanced diet consists of the proper mixture of the above components of food, in the proper percentages, i.e. fifteen percent proteins, thirty-five percent fats, and fifty percent carbohydrates.

A baby who gets the usual milk supply, an egg or two a week when old enough, meats and vegetables once a day after the age of five or six months, and cereals and fruits when few months old, will do very well indeed.

Adolescents who live on apple pies and milkshakes are cheating themselves. The ravenous appetite should be counteracted by offering the essential foods listed above, and not predominantly the coke, cakes, cookies, and other forms of empty calories.

Our bodies will adjust to the appetite peculiarities of our cultural tendencies. However, this will be at a price: obesity. This will lead to unhappy cosmetic results, fat deposits, high blood pressure, and many other obesity-associated problems.

It is strange that in such a land of plenty, there is so much calorie affluence in the wrong direction. Trust the call of your child's stomach, and give gentle guidance. A child who relies on hunger instinct is more likely to get a balanced diet. You may guide the child gently to the variety of food he or she takes, but don't overdo it. Many of the diet problems arise when parents are eager beavers and try to encourage the obliging child to eat and eat. The food intake pattern in the family is also a major determining factor as to what the child will take. So take a look at your family's pattern of eating and adjust accordingly.

Shall I, then get rid of the cookies and cakes?

No, don't go to this extreme. Serve pies, cakes, cookies, or ice cream on occasions, but not routinely. Avoid buying cookies, so you won't have them at home all the time, in case your child is cookie-crazy.

THEY ARE CUTE AND THEY ARE CHUBBY

We all agree, the child does look cute. He or she has been overfed, and many parents think this leads to a healthier, happier child. But there are potential dangers that may not show up until much later in life. The social trend goes in that direction, we also agree, but there ought to be an acute awareness about this problem. After all, it is well known that one out of every three Americans suffers from being overweight to a small or large degree.

<u>When shall we be concerned about this problem?</u>

The time to be concerned about it is from birth through the teenage period, especially during the first year of life. You see, when a baby is overfed, the number of fat cells in the body will increase, sometimes at an alarming rate, and will become almost constant once he or she becomes a young adult. Not only that, but the size of the fat cells will also increase, although this increase may vary from one person to another.

This means that if the child becomes overweight, he or she will fill with an abnormally large number of fat cells, which of course must be filled with fat to a varying degree. This is particularly true in the first year of life, and maybe up to the sixth or seventh year. When such children grow up to adulthood, they will be stuck with this large number of fat cells for the rest of their life: meaning obesity. This will then lead to the necessity to "crash-diet" during adulthood, but mostly with disappointing results. If the child is left "lean" during early childhood, he or she will not have to suffer that much during adulthood.

<u>What kind of health problems will obesity lead to?</u>

Other than appearance problems, an obese person may have high cholesterol and lipids (fats) in the blood. This can lead to hardening of the arteries, trouble with heart attacks, and strokes. It may also lead to trouble with diabetes, because of the load put on the insulin secretion by the body. As if that is not enough, an overweight person is more prone to develop high blood pressure, trouble with the gall bladder and the joints among other things.

Does this mean that a child should be skinny?

It is better for the child to have the proper weight for his or her specific height. If we do our preventive work during childhood, he or she will reap a tremendous dividend as an adult.

Our work should start from babyhood and last all the way through the teenage period. It is fine for a baby to be reasonably chubby but not fat, and after a few years he or she should look lean. It is normal and good to see a few ribs through the skin, and not to see the bellybutton sinking or surrounded by a layer of fat.

What if the child is already chubby?

The sooner you start to help the better. When baby's or child's weight is too high in proportion to the height, it ought to be controlled. The more you wait, the bigger the number of fat cells will grow, and the more difficult it becomes to overcome the problem.

The guideline is simple. Don't let the child lose weight, instead try to hold it where it is long enough until the height catches up with it. Don't put the child or baby on a strict diet; instead, serve proportionately less at mealtime. Don't let the child take seconds, offer less dessert or none, and please stop the snacks. It is as simple as that.

Most of the studies done indicate that better than four out of five obese adolescents will continue their obesity into adulthood! Not only that, but when their obesity continues into adulthood, it becomes more stubborn and persistent.

As you can see, won't you rather have a lean healthy child, than a chubby child who will have to cope with such a problem all through life. And the problems of the child will have been started by the parents.

What shall I do?

Meats are nourishing and not too fatening. Offer them in reasonable amounts. Fruits and vegetables have small amount of calories, therefore, be liberal with them.

Your enemy is the excessive intake of the "empty calories," i.e. too many potatoes, especially french fries and potato chips; too much bread, toast, and too many sandwiches; too much rice; too many pies, cakes and milkshakes; too much milk, ice cream, coke, cookies, candies, pretzels, etc.

Sometimes the child doesn't take too much of any of the above, but nevertheless he or she takes two or three helpings at a meal. In such cases, his or her midriff bulge will continue to spread until it forces you to put the leash on!

But the child wants to keep eating:

That is true of most of them. More likely than not, they eat because of "boredom and habit" rather than real hunger. When the child is bored and doesn't know what to do, he or she will raid the refrigerator mercilessly.

Sometimes it is the mother or father or even the whole family that is overweight. They have simply slipped into the habit of overfilling the poor stomach. Much of these problems will be behind us if we eat when we are really hungry, and make sure when we eat not to overdistend our stomachs with too much food.

But I cannot always keep my child away from the food:

Welcome to the club. There are a few tricks however:

1. Don't serve french fries, potato chips, or broiled potatoes too often, or in too large quantity.
2. Don't serve a lot of toast, sandwiches, rice or other foods rich in carbohydrates.
3. Don't bake or buy cakes and pies; instead, serve fresh fruits for dessert.
4. Let the child drink one pint of one or two percent skim milk in a whole day; regular milk has too many calories.
5. Don't buy cookies, candies, pretzels, etc.

6. Diet soft drinks may be used instead of regular ones. Even better is water, or lemonade.
7. Avoid too much spaghetti, macaroni, and pizzas.

What shall I serve then?

The combination of meats, fruits, and vegetables on the one hand, and less fats and starchy foods on the other, can make a well-balanced diet; not so high in calories, yet very nourishing. Be careful with dairy products to some extent. Heavily fried foods are to be avoided in favor of broiled foods.

Don't you think the child will be skin and bones?

It may be because of the fear of "being skin and bones" that our population suffers so much from overweight. As long as the child has the proper weight according to his or her size, then there is no reason to worry.

Children who are four years old and who "show" three to four ribs through the skin are not undernourished. They are supposed to look that way. They are not supposed to have a double tire of fat on their abdomens.

Help prevent the overweight problem in the first year of life, and you will have saved yourself and your child a great deal of trouble. If the child is older, then don't push him or her into being a "glutton." Please remember, it is the "fear" of being skin and bones, i.e. the mental attitude of the family, that is so very harmful.

Why not give the child some pills?

Reducing pills don't work well. It is better to use them according to your doctor's advice and only in rare circumstances if at all. The child quite often becomes pill-dependent, instead of depending on his or her own will and the will of the family, which are so much better. Some pills have side effects too.

How about the glands?

Most families try to put the blame for obesity on "glands" rather than on themselves.

Most of the overweight children, on being studied, prove to have perfectly normal endocrine glands. Such studies prove to be normal so often that we rarely waste the families' effort and money for such tests. Only in a tiny percentage of obesity do we suspect trouble with the endocrine glands, and in such cases the necessary tests will have to be done.

<u>Therefore you mean reducing obesity is nothing more than hard work?</u>
The thing that counts is hard work and persistent emphasis on the quantity, quality, and variety of food taken, with full intention to "contain" the weight or reduce it.

It is a tough job. That is why there are so many failures. That is also why there are so many gimmicks and so many books that promise the secret for reducing. It is only the earnest endeavors of the parents that can be of any real help. And the younger the child is, the better is your chance for success in controlling his or her weight.

A good many "mildly" overweight children will benefit successfully if you follow the recommendations above. Forget about how many calories are in this piece of food or that. This may be okay for you, since you are not growing in height, and your weight must come down if you happen to be overweight. But your child is growing in height, and the height can catch up with the weight, i.e. you have to contain the weight until the height catches up.

Following a strict regime for your child is more likely to be a failure than a success. The child will disobey you and cheat you by eating when and where possible.

A liberal attitude of modifying the meals you fix, providing fruits for dessert or when the child is hungry, is very important, and simply restraining from making fattening foods, will help a great, great deal.

<u>How about exercise?</u>
Exercise is very good in stimulating your child's constitution, it uses up calories but at the same time it stimulates the appetite. Therefore, if the child exerçises to contain the weight, he or she should restrain from overeating in the mean time.

So often though, an exercising child gets hungry and eats even more than his or her usual amount of food-intake. In so doing, rather than losing weight as intended, the exercising child may even gain more weight!

Please observe the following:

1. Let the child exercise, but
2. restrain the amount of the eating, while
3. feeding him or her a well-balanced nourishing diet,
4. but not excessively so
5. and avoid those foods with too many empty calories.

Good luck!

CHOLESTEROL AND OUR DIET

A lot of emphasis is put on blood cholesterol and lipids (fats), and a good many adults know that a high cholesterol level is not good.

A good many cases of hardening of the arteries (atherosclerosis) can be traced not only to a high level of cholesterol and/or lipids, but also to obesity, smoking, etc. Hardening of the arteries can lead to heart attacks and strokes and many other gruesome problems, and such diseases of adulthood are the plague of this society at the present time.

However, if we start early enough, we can work on the factors that lead to hardening of the arteries, and help prevent some of its complications later on.

Since we are dealing with children, why should we bother?

The process of hardening of the arteries is a very prolonged one, and it takes many, many years before it is bad enough to give trouble. It is said that this process starts in early childhood, it gradually gathers steam, and by adulthood it may emerge as a major problem. By then, injury will already have taken place, and potential complications such as heart attacks and strokes can be disasterous.

You can help your child in three ways:

1. Help reduce obesity, since sometimes this is associated with relatively high levels of cholesterol and/or lipids in the blood. Better still, help prevent obesity.
2. Offer fewer of the foods that are loaded with cholesterol and fats.
3. Help detect the presence of high blood pressure and take care of it. This is usually picked up during routine checkups.

In an adult, in addition to the above, smoking and stressful living are two major risk factors for heart attacks, along with lack of exercise.

What foods are high in cholesterol?

1. Egg yolk (not egg white) is loaded with these lipids. A breakfast of two eggs a day, with or without other fried foods, contains too many lipids and too much cholesterol to be healthy. It is obviously better to cut down on such an intake to one to two eggs per week, either for breakfast or in cooking.
2. Butter is also loaded with saturated fats. It is better to use margarine or vegetable oils as a replacement to some extent. Remember, solid margarine is also full of cholesterol since it is comprised of hydrogenated fats. This is not the case with vegetable oil. Chocolate and coconut oil are also high in cholesterol, so watch it.
3. Homogenized milk has a certain degree of saturated fats also. It is better to use one percent or two percent skim milk instead.
4. Baked goods cooked with egg yolk or butter, e.g. lemon pie, certain kinds of cakes, greasy food, etc., can be full of cholesterol and lipids.
5. Shellfish (crabs, lobster, clams, etc.) have their very high share of cholesterol and fats also.
6. The organ meats such as the liver and heart also have a lot.
7. Pork, bacon and related products.

Does this mean that our children ought to avoid these foods?

No it doesn't. All it means is to offer the above foods in moderation, so that the children are less exposed to high levels of cholesterol and lipids through the years.

It is better to start the children on healthy habits even when they are babies. Remember, so far there is no proof that these precautions are going to prove a health bonanza later on, but common sense dictates that it is better not to play with fire.

How about blood tests for cholesterol?

It is not necessary for them to be done routinely in children. However, if there are members in the family who have had heart attacks before they have reached the age of fifty years, then it is good to do the tests on the children. This is because there are certain inherited diseases that cause the cholesterol and/or lipid level to be very high, thus posing potentially serious trouble.

For a cholesterol test, all that needs to be done is to draw blood from a vein of the children. Usually this is done when they are five years old and up. Such determinations might prove to be invaluable, because these inherited lipid diseases are controllable and their complications can be prevented.

Remember please, not all people react alike to the high intake of fats, some do, others don't. Many people seem to be able to eat all the eggs and high-lipid foods they want, and they come out of this battle unscathed.

FOOD ALLERGY

Food allergies are not rare. They can not only show up at different ages, but the symptoms an allergy creates for babies may be quite different from those in older children.

As with all other allergies, children with a family history of allergy are more prone to come down with this form of trouble.

How will food allergy show up in babies?

Babies with food allergy are likely to have some stomachache not unlike that of a grinding colic; they are likely to have gas pains, to spit up more than usual, and to have trouble with their bowel movements. Some children may have diarrhea, which may be prolonged and contain mucus or even blood.

Besides the above symptoms, many allergic babies may prove to have stuffy or runny noses, many bouts of respiratory infections (some with wheezing), many ear infections, or even some trouble with postnasal drip (see page 290).

In addition to the above or exclusive of it, the baby may show trouble with his or her skin in the form of dermatitis, hives, or occasionally just some ulcerative irritation around the anus.

The above symptoms show up in varying degrees of severity and keep recurring for a long time.

How do we know that this is caused by food allergy?

1. If some or all of the above symptoms keep coming on and off for a long period,
2. If there is a history of allergies in the family especially involving siblings, parents, or other immediate members, and
3. If avoidance of a suspected allergy-causing food relieves the symptoms, and the symptoms reappear upon eating the food again later on,

then there is reasonable evidence to conclude that food allergy is the culprit.

What kind of food can a small baby be allergic to?

In babies the biggest villain is cow's milk. When this is suspected, we shift the baby to a soybean formula. Eggs are well known for being allergenic and so is wheat and wheat products, orange juice and other citrus products.

Other kinds of food are less troublesome at this age, so the food control in such situations is not difficult.

How about older children?

As children grow beyond the age of one year, their exposure to many kinds of food becomes bigger and more varied. Not only that, but the trouble resulting from food allergy shows up differently.

In mild cases of food allergy, the main symptoms will be hives of varying degrees. The hives may show up only as a few spots and for a few days, or be more severe as to cover the child all over and take a good many days before going away. Occasionally this may show up in addition to an already existing eczema or dermatitis of some sort.

Food allergy in a child beyond the age of one year is less likely to produce respiratory trouble as it does in a baby, but stomach symptoms are not infrequent. In such cases, stomachache, gas pains, vomiting, or diarrhea may be the result. Again, the severity of these symptoms depends on the severity of the allergy.

What kind of food can a child be allergic to?

It can be any kind of food, though some foods are more prone to produce allergy than others. Certain groups of food stand out in this regard: milk, eggs, wheat, fish, peanuts, citrus, and tomatoes.

The above and their products can give a wide range of trouble, depending on the severity of the allergy. There are certainly many, many other foods that can produce allergy but they are not as notorious as the seven categories of food listed above.

To find out which food your child is allergic to, you and your doctor may have to investigate many possibilities and you may be lucky enough to come out with the right answer. But please don't be disappointed if you cannot find the one, because this can be very difficult to do in many instances.

Will allergy tests help?

Unfortunately, the allergy tests are least reliable in regard to food allergy. They are only of minor help, whereas their ability to determine inhalant allergies, such as pollen, pet animals, dust, and mold is very good.

Can we use soybean formula to prevent milk allergy?

If there is strong evidence of allergy in the siblings and the immediate family, you may consider giving soybean formula to the newborn right from the start. This should be continued until about the age of nine to twelve months. It may help prevent a good deal of would-be sickness. Better still is breast feeding.

In other words, rather than wait for the baby to develop the symptoms of allergy, such babies of severely allergic families may be even started on soybean formula right out if bottle feeding has to be used.

By the way, there are a few anti-allergenic formulas other than soybean formulas. They may be tried if soybean formula doesn't agree.

Another preventive measure is to delay giving highly allergenic foods until the baby is nine to twelve months old.

STOMACHACHE

Stomachache is a fairly common occurrence in children. The child complains once or twice a day of a stomachache which seems to be mild but fairly annoying. Upon further questioning, you may learn that the pain is ill-defined, more or less in and around the area of the bellybutton, not bad enough as to double the child up, and often is not associated with nausea, vomiting, fever, or other noticeable symptoms. The pain may be related to eating or may show up at any time during the day.

This kind of stomachache seems to be fairly persistent and may continue for a few weeks if not months. Sooner or later you will start worrying about it.

What causes it?

This kind of stomachache is different from the acute stomachache that has to be investigated right away. The stomachache we are interested in here is the one that is mild, vague, and recurrent, and without any accompanying symptoms.

You may find out that such a stomachache is caused by some degree of constipation in many children. This will also produce gas.

In some children, the stomachache may be caused by dairy products, especially milk. The main reason is that there may be an intolerance to the lactose of the milk, or a mild degree of allergy to the dairy product itself, or merely the constipating effect of the milk.

Yet, in some other children the stomachache may prove to be caused by hunger, mild colitis, or eating too much of some particular foods. The last example may mean too many apples a day, raisins, chocolate or chocolate milk, onions, spicy food, and the like.

In a small percentage of children, worms, parasites, an ulcer, or low-grade urinary tract infection may prove to be the villain. Other ill-defined, vague causes of stomachache are psychogenic, or expressions of the child's tension and pressure. The cause of the tension may prove to be too many commitments, too much discord in the family, too much competition, school trouble, etc.

What can be done about stomachache?

If the cause of the stomachache is discovered, then correct it. If it is caused by constipation, you may want to use a high fiber diet (see page 358).

If the child likes raisin bran cereal and in addition eats lots of raisins, stop giving him or her the extra raisins, to see if they are the cause of the trouble. This is also true of an excess of chocolate milk, apples, other fruits, onions, spicy foods, etc. In other words, stop giving the suspected food to see if the child improves, and if so, discontinue that item. You may have many food items under suspicion.

How about dairy products?

If the above measures don't work, you may want to stop all dairy products for about two weeks. If the stomachache disappears during that period but reappears again when the dairy products are offered, then you have something to investigate. What you do is to stop the dairy products for two more weeks, then offer one item at a time, perhaps for a week or so. If milk is given and there is no stomachache for one week, it is safe to say that milk is not the cause of the pain. Then eliminate and add eggs, and once more observe the child for pain, and if it develops, the child can be regarded as sensitive to eggs. If not, then eggs are O.K., and you may try another food and continue this line of observation.

When shall we investigate further?

If the above measures seem to be of no help, the stool should be checked for parasites and worms, and a urinalysis done. A urine culture may also be needed for a female.

If all these tests are negative, and the pain continues beyond a period of several months, an X-ray of the stomach and intestine may be indicated to look for ulcers and other rare conditions.

WHAT IS A NORMAL STOOL?

A bowel movement is the product eliminated from the bowels; it usually occurs every day. A bowel movement of a baby behaves differently than that of a child or a grown-up. In most cases there are no problems, but when they arise, they can affect the character of the stools and their frequency, and can lead to different consequences.

What is normal stool for a baby?

A breast-fed baby often has several bowel movements a day. Three to four are not unusual, though at times they may have as few as one or two a day, or as many as six or seven. The stool will be soft, if not seedy and slightly liquid. It may smell slightly sweetish. If a breast-fed baby has one or two firm or hard stools a day, it is good to bring this to the attention of the doctor.

On the other hand, a bottle-fed baby is more likely to have one or two bowel movements a day. Often they are not soft but firm and formed, and the baby may grunt more before elimination. It may also smell and be offensive to the nose. A baby on the bottle who has six to seven movements a day, of a soft nature, may be heralding the onset of diarrhea. Babies on whole milk (which is not used that often before the age of one year), are more likely to suffer from constipation than those on formula, since whole milk has tough curds because of the nature of cow's milk.

How about stools in older children?

One movement a day is usual, though occasionally they may have as many as two or even three a day, or as few as one every second or even third day. In rare circumstances we are confronted with a child who has only one bowel movement every five to seven days, even though there appears to be no suffering. These are variations of the norm, and will be with the child through life.

A child's stool should be well-formed, not too hard, and yellowish-brown. A large, hard stool which is unusually wide can lead to trouble. This is more true in children who have infrequent bowel movements.

What problems can wide stools lead to?

A wide stool usually results from too much of a refined diet, i.e. a diet that is deficient in fiber. Such a diet is easily absorbable by the efficient intestine, but will be without the moisture-holding properties of fiber.

When this happens, the large intestine will accommodate itself to the situation by enlarging, but at the same time will lose its responsiveness to the urge of evacuation. This trouble will then build on itself, leading to enlargement of the abdomen, trouble with chronic constipation, soiling of the underpants with passage of mucus, the child's urge to "hold in" the stool (because it hurts to pass it through), and even a crack in the anus.

This is why it is important to treat constipation problems early, before the tonicity of the wall of the intestine gives way.

How can we add fiber to the diet?

Milk, cheese, rice, bananas as well as some other foods are constipating; therefore, they should be given in smaller amounts to children with constipation problems.

Added dietary fiber increases the water content of the stools by about ten percent. One or two tablespoons of "Bran buds" cereal added to the regular cereal every day, and if refused, bran cereals of any kind may be tried. If still refused, use Fiber Med, two wafers a day (they come fruit flavored too). Metamucil (nonprescription) can be given in a glass of orange juice once a day. Salads are helpful, and so are fruits and vegetables. Malt-soup extract (maltsupex), prunes, and raisins may be of help in milder cases. Naturally, drinking a lot of liquids every day can be of help too.

These simple measures correct both the trouble of the large stools and their oft-resulting stomachaches. In fact, a large percentage of children's stomachaches can be corrected this way.

What if the stool has a different color?

A green stool rarely means much, unless the child is having a severe diarrhea. The condition becomes more important if there is mucus in the stool. If such is the case with your child, get in touch with your doctor.

If the stool is dark or tarry, or if the child has stomachache and some other symptoms, it may mean that there is digested blood in the stool, i.e. there is bleeding in some parts of the intestine.

A child on iron medication will have black stools, and one who is on Povan for pinworms may have red ones. These are expected, so don't worry about them. But a child who passes bright red blood with the stools may have a polyp, a fissure in ano or any of several other important diseases of the lower intestines. In such cases, see the doctor right away.

ACUTE CONSTIPATION IN CHILDREN

There may be several underlying causes of acute constipation in children, so it should be treated accordingly. Let us give some examples:

1. If the child tends to be regular, but all of a sudden becomes constipated:
   It is best to use a Fleet enema, child size (nonprescription), and if you follow the instructions on the package, you will see that in a few minutes the child will evacuate nicely. Or you may want to use a soap suds enema, about a pint of water with a little soap suds in it. Draw the liquid into an enema bulb, insert the nozzle of the enema bulb into the anus and squirt the contents into the rectum. Evacuation is usually immediate.

2. If the child had had trouble with constipation in the last few weeks or months, look at the diet:
   Too much homogenized milk, or cheese can be the reason, or too little roughage. Roughage means fruits, salads, vegetables and certain forms of cereal and bread. Balance the child's diet; offer less milk and more roughage. If this doesn't help much, offer four to five prunes a day, or some raisins on a daily basis, and you may become successful.

How about laxatives?

They are okay for occasional use, mainly for acute constipation, but use them sparingly. Milk of Magnesia and Castoria are okay, but follow the instructions on the bottle. Usually laxatives take almost twelve hours or longer before they work. Some laxatives may move the bowels, but bring constipation again afterwards.

My child became constipated after a bloody bowel movement:

If at some time you saw a line of blood on the surface of a hard bowel movement, this will mean that the bowel movement has produced a "Fissure" in the anus (see page 81). This will make having a bowel movement a painful experience, and the child will tend to hold the movement in, being petrified of the pain that is associated with it. This in turn will lead to more and more trouble with constipation. Early treatment of such a case will help save you much worry and headache.

CHRONIC CONSTIPATION

Constipation can be acute, but more often it is chronic and quite troublesome at that. A child with chronic constipation will, of course, have trouble passing a stool; but more importantly, the stool will be wide and large, and the child may be able to pass one only every two or three days if not less often.

However, your concern will increase if the child keeps complaining of stomachache or starts having problems messing himself or herself around the anal area.

Why does leakage happen?

A small number of children with chronic constipation will ooze almost liquid stools from the anus, often without the child even feeling it. But in the process, the bottom becomes quite messy, the child (especially in school) becomes embarrassed, and the area involved may even become infected. On top of that, the case may erroneouly be misinterpreted as diarrhea.

The problem arises because of this: as the chronic constipation continues for a long time, the rectum responds less and less energetically to it, and the wall of the intestine and rectum becomes less adept at its duties. Then, the rectal wall starts secreting a lot of mucus to lubricate the passage of the stools (which is a form of self-defence for the rectum). When this happens, the mucus, mixed with some bowel movement material, will ooze around the blockage and through the anus. This shows us what happens if chronic constipation is left uncorrected for a long time. In addition to that, chronic constipation can cause stomachache, gas, gas pains, bad breath, discomfort, etc.

How about those who have one bowel movement a week?

This is rare, but it does happen. If these children have a normal-sized and normal-looking stool, with no stomachache, gas or other symptoms, and if they seem healthy, then their tendency for the infrequent movements can be regarded as a normal part of their nature. They probably will have this tendency for the rest of their life. They probably will need no treatment or interference, and they should be left alone. It is important to keep in mind, however, that such cases are quite rare and that the majority are cases of the usually chronic constipation.

What can I do for chronic constipation?

Milk and certain foods such as cheese, rice, bananas, etc., tend to make the constipation worse. Therefore it is better to eat less of these foods or avoid them until the constipation is corrected.

Most cases of chronic constipation are related not only to our highly refined food, but also to not having enough fluids. Therefore, to increase the bulk intake, roughage in the form of fruits, vegetables and salads should be eaten in greater amounts. In addition, "Bran Buds" cereal can be added to the regular cereal every morning, and if refused, any bran-containing cereal can be tried. If the child does not like that (and a few don't), give Metamucil, one or more teaspoons a day, to be mixed with orange juice or milk.

Along with all the above, the child will have to be urged to take more fluids, be it in the form of water, juice, soups, etc. In so doing, the roughage will hold the water and this will make the stools softer and more easily manageable by the intestine.

You may become amazed at the speed of your success and at the regularity of the child's bowel. Comfort will be restored and embarrassment prevented.

Medicines may be used, but most of them can be avoided with the above natural methods of control. Milk of Magnesia and the like are more helpful with acute episodes of constipation, while Modane bulk or Modane regular, Peri-colace, Milkinol (all nonprescription) can be given for the chronic one.

How about the child who "holds in" bowel movements?

This is not common, and it shows up in young children, usually under five years of age. Many are scared of having a bowel movement in the toilet, or remember some degree of pain upon moving the bowels after having developed a crack in the anus before. In most, the stools look normal, but they are eventually deposited in the underpants instead of the toilet, usually when the child is standing up.

The difference between these stools and those related to constipation is that the stools usually look normal, are deposited intentionally, and affect mainly young children. Most of these children will hold the bowel movements for as long as possible, will squirm and squirm, often go to a corner in the room, under the bed, or somewhere else, and intentionally but as if unwillingly, deposit their long-awaited stools in their underpants.

In practically all such cases the doctor should be consulted for advice and treatment, since the treatment may be quite involved.

VOMITING

Suddenly the child starts to vomit, and keeps vomiting. At first the stuff consists of food material, tastes terrible, and smells strong and pungent. Later on, the stuff is liquid, may be yellowish in color or even bile-stained. Then the child keeps heaving, but nothing comes out. He or she may become wet with sweat, complain of a pretty bad stomachache, and seems to involve just about every muscle of the body with each episode of vomiting.

Of course, he or she already might have messed up the bed, the floor, or your clothing if you happened to have been near the "gush" of vomitus.

How can I help?

If the child is eighteen months old or older, and has no symptoms other than the vomiting and the stomachache, it might mean the beginning of viral gastroenteritis, or perhaps the flu.

The best thing to do initially is not to give the child anything by mouth, either to drink or to eat, for about four hours after the last time he or she has vomited. If the child vomits again, you better time it anew. The little sufferer may plead for something to drink, water or otherwise, but don't succumb. If you do, you may irritate the stomach and make the child vomit again, thus making the condition worse.

When the four-hour period is over, you may start the child on crushed ice or Popsicles, off and on for a period of one hour. If this is kept down, then give Coke, Pepsi, 7-up or orange juice using small amounts (one-half to one ounce) at frequent intervals (fifteen to thirty minutes). The next day, you may start the child on clear soups, then a soft diet.

What if the child keeps vomiting?

Vomiting three to five times a day is not regarded as very severe, but if the child vomits more often, then there will be real danger of dehydration. Medication may have to be used by your doctor, or special treatment be instituted.

What causes vomiting?

Vomiting can be one of the symptoms of a good many diseases, and those symptoms will help you decide if the child should be seen by the doctor or not.

In a number of cases with frequent loose cough, the child may vomit a few times. Thick mucus will come out, thus clearing the chest, and the cough will have improved a lot. This is one of the few times when vomiting is a welcome sign.

Vomiting can also be a sign of appendicitis.

Tell me about appendicitis:

Briefly stated, the poor little one starts with a stomachache. The pain is usually around the navel or above. A few hours afterwards, the pain shifts to the right lower quarter of the abdomen. The pain is usually fairly severe, but can be mild. Often there is some rise of temperature, but not very high. The child will also have some nausea and may vomit once or a few times. In some, the bowels will not have moved in the last day or so.

The area of the pain may be tender to the touch, and if you press there, the child may jump with pain and try to stop you.

Of course, there are other varieties of symptoms of appendicitis; most of them are enough warning for the alert parent.

Please don't give a laxative if you suspect appedicitis. If the child has symptoms that make you suspect appendicitis, an enema or a laxative can lead to a ruptured appendix. This is more difficult to treat surgically than non-ruptured appendix (see page 372).

How about vomiting in babies?

The younger the baby, the more you have to be careful about vomiting and consult with the doctor. They may vomit because of a viral gastroenteritis or other common causes, but some diseases with vomiting, common at this age, involve an obstruction somewhere in the stomach and intestine. If this proves to be the case, special treatment, including surgery, may be in the horizon (see page 80).

GASTROENTERITIS

The child feels queasy, may be quite pale, and may complain of some stomachache. Suddenly he or she rushes to the bathroom to vomit, and this may be repeated a few times. The vomiting may come in episodes, and after the child seems to have nothing left, there may still be a few "dry" heaving episodes afterwards.

It is not unusual to have stomachache severe enough as to double the child up. The temperature may go up, often to around 103 or 104 degrees F.

Along with the vomiting -more often a day or so afterwards- the child may begin to have diarrhea. The diarrhea may be a matter of a few loose bowel movements a day; in more severe cases, they may be quite frequent (six or seven times a day or more) and liquid. By then the vomiting will have stopped. The diarrhea often lasts a day or two if not longer, after which things seem to come under control gradually and the child will be back to normal again.

What causes such a trouble?

By far the commonest cause of gastroenteritis is a viral infection. This is very common in children, especially in babies. But viral infection is not the whole story. Sometimes the trouble can be caused by such nasty bacteria as shigella (dysentry), salmonella, and the bad E. coli. There are other causes besides, and they can be determined through different tests and cultures.

How dangerous is gastroenteritis?

The mild ones are not dangerous at all; the child may have no more than two or three liquid bowel movements a day, he or she may vomit once or twice, and in a day or two it quietly ends.

But if the child has more than a mild case, he or she may vomit four or five times or even more, the diarrhea may be in the order of four or five times a day, and there may be a rise of temperature and a fairly nasty stomachache.

Such cases should be stopped before they cause major problems such as dehydration. This is more true in babies, who are quite prone to this trouble.

Therefore, cases of moderate to severe gastroenteritis should see the doctor for careful evaluation, management and preventive treatment, before the illness goes too far.

Is it contagious?

Yes, but to a variable extent, depending on whether or not those in contact have developed immunity against the causative agent from a previous exposure. It is not unusual to see gastroenteritis going from one member of the family to the other, or even everyone in the family coming down with this trouble at the same time! It is also not rare to see many children with gastroenteritis in the same neighborhood or community in one season.

To help prevent the spread of this disease in the family, it is wise to wash the hands after handling the soiled area.

What would you do to treat it?

For mild gastroenteritis, it is quite adequate to simply put the child on liquids for one day, to be followed by soups and soft diet the next day. This is enough to rest the stomach and intestine and to help get rid of the disease. For average gastroenteritis, you may try the same technique, a little more gradually. Put the child on nothing but liquids for the first day. Next day, you may feed the child clear soups, with bread, toast, or crackers, but without using butter. The day after, you may add jello, pudding, applesauce, cottage cheese, bananas, yogurt, rice, etc. If this treatment is not successful, consult your doctor.

Of course, when a baby gets this disease, take him or her to the doctor before dehydration can develop.

Kaopectate (nonprescription) is popular and so are other medicines. It may be used when needed. It is probably better to stick to the diet technique described above than to jump to medication, initially.

As for the stomachache, if it is tolerable and seems to go away, you may choose to wait and see. However, if it is quite severe, it may indicate some problems other than gastroenteritis, some of which are quite serious. If this is the case, you will need the doctors help. There are two clever tricks you ought to remember, however.

What are they?

When there is vomiting, don't give anything by mouth for about four hours from the time the child had vomited last. Try to strictly time this period. When you want to start the liquids, try Popsicles or crushed ice first, and keep offering them for one hour. If the child seems to hold them well, you may then start the liquids as suggested above (see page 360).

When the child has diarrhea, avoid offering ice-cold liquids (be it Coke, Pepsi or others) which are taken directly out of the refrigerator. Very cold drinks tend to make the diarrhea worse. Take the chill off the liquid first then offer it.

DIARRHEA

All of a sudden the child's bowel movements become frequent, smelly, and watery, and he or she may complain of stomachache that may even cause doubling up. There may be vomiting, two to three times or so, but it is the diarrhea that seems to be particularly troublesome. The child's temperature at times goes up to 103 or 104 degrees F, yet in others there seems to be nothing but the diarrhea.

In mild diarrhea there may be four to five bowel movements a day, in moderate ones perhaps nine to ten, and in severe ones up to twenty a day!

The stool can be loose, but more likely than not it is the consistency of water.

What causes diarrhea?

Mostly it is caused by viruses, i.e. it is part of gastroenteritis. Rarely, however, bacteria or other factors can be the cause. If the child passes a lot of mucus and/or blood in the stools, then a stool culture should be done. In some children food allergies can also be the cause of the diarrhea; for babies, this is more true of allergy to milk and eggs than anything else (see page 75).

What can I do about it?

For mild diarrhea, you simply feed the child liquids for the first day; use soft drinks such as Coke, Pepsi, orange juice, weak tea, etc. Don't offer any solid food yet. Next day, if there has been improvement in the outlook, in addition to the liquids offer clear soups such as tomato soup, bouillon, or clear broth, with toast, bread, and crackers -don't use butter. By the day after, if the child has continued to improve, in addition to the above, offer jello, pudding, applesauce, cottage cheese, mashed potatoes, bananas, etc. (no eggs yet, please).

After a day or so, you cautiously put the child back on regular food, including eggs and regular milk. But even so, don't offer fresh fruits and vegetables, nor heavily fried food for a few more days, since they may irritate the intestine.

How about babies?

Babies, especially tiny ones, who develop diarrhea, should be seen by the doctor. The treatment they need is different and they are more likely to develop dehydration (see page 366).

Can diarrhea become prolonged?

Certain diseases can lead to chronic and prolonged diarrhea. Salmonella, shigella, certain E. coli, and other diseases (usually rare), can play havoc with a child's intestines. Allergies to food, especially milk, can do the same thing. A good many tests may have to be done.

Important: when there is diarrhea don't be too rough on the baby's sore bottom. Don't use force to clean the area as you wipe; better still, dab the area with a piece of wet cotton and clean it gently. Then use A & D ointment, Desitin, or even Vaseline to protect it, and wash your hands afterwards.

Most mild diarrheas don't need medicines, and only a few need Kaopectate or other medications. Many parents rush to such medicines unnecessarily, yet pay no attention to the diet. This is a backward treatment. Putting the child on the above diet will help stop the diarrhea in most children, and there will be no need for medication. However, in moderately severe cases of diarrhea, medication will have to be used in addition to the diet.

DEHYDRATION

The child has been having severe vomiting, and the stools have been frequent, runny, and watery. The child refuses to eat, looks slightly greyish, is sluggish, fretful and may have a fever.

It is at this juncture that the parents start to have suspicions that their child is dehydrating, and rightly so.

What is dehydration anyway?

To function properly, the body has to have its proper amount of fluids. When vomiting and/or diarrhea occur, there will be loss of some of the fluids of the body; the amount of loss depends on the frequency and the amount of the vomitus or the diarrhea stools.

When a significant amount of fluid is lost from the body, dehydration or "drying" of the tissues will take place, and this can often become quite dangerous for the proper functioning of the body.

Who is more likely to become dehydrated?

The smaller the child, the more it is likely for dehydration to develop. Therefore, a baby is far more likely to become dehydrated than an older child exposed to the same degree of fluid loss. This is because the system of the baby is still quite labile, and the baby's constitution is somewhat different from that of an older child. This contributes to a faster fluid loss and more dehydration in babies.

When is dehydration likely to appear?

By and large, dehydration results from excessive and frequent vomiting, or from copious and frequent diarrhea stools, or from both. This is more so if the baby or child refuses to take fluids orally or has fever in addition. This means he or she is not replenishing the fluids orally, or when feverish, in addition he or she is losing more fluids by sweating.

The key to this question is, "What is meant by:

1. Excessive and frequent vomiting?"
2. Copious and frequent diarrhea stools?"

    Many parents become alarmed if the baby or child vomits two or three times and they think that dehydration has set in already. This is also true of their concern in case the child has about two or three liquid bowel movements. The truth of the matter is that most such situations are way too mild to lead to any dehydration, and it is better for the parents not to become concerned at all at such an early stage of gastroenteritis (see page 362).

    If the child has vomited a large amount of liquids, seven to ten times a day, or has had ten to twelve or more large liquid bowel movements; and in addition has refused to take anything by mouth, then the parents ought to become concerned about possible dehydration.

    This is a general assessment, and there are exceptions depending on the baby's or child's condition.

<u>What can be done about it?</u>

    Since dehydration is dangerous, it is good to get in touch with the doctor if the baby vomits more than a few times, or has a few liquid bowel movements, or if an older child has vomited many times (six to seven times) or has many liquid bowel movements. The doctor can evaluate this condition in the office or even over the phone, and he may be able to suggest some remedial measures to prevent the progress of the vomiting and diarrhea into dehydration.

    If you see the doctor when the dehydration has become already established, the doctor will usually admit the child to the hospital. An intravenous feeding will usually be necessary, which may have to be given for several days. Special tests on the blood will have to be done several times, and measures to stop the vomiting and diarrhea may have to be taken too.

    Usually, during such treatment, the dehydrated baby and child will improve dramatically over a period of a day or two if not sooner.

Can we prevent dehydration?

A lot can be done to ameliorate the factors leading to dehydration in their early stages, and if successful, dehydration will be prevented.

Prompt and proper treatment of vomiting and/or diarrhea in their early stages can go a long way to help prevent dehydration.

THE BLOODY STOOL

The parent discovers that the child's stool is bloody; he or she correctly assumes this will need a doctor's visit. The doctor asks for a specimen of the bloody stool, be it in a diaper or in a jar after being recovered from the toilet.

What causes a bloody stool?

There are numerous causes, but certain ones stand out. To facilitate describing them, stools that have become bloody can be divided into two groups: soft or liquid, and normal or hard.

What if it is a soft (or liquid) stool but bloody?

In the case of ordinary diarrhea, it is not rare to see mucus mixed with the stools. But when blood shows up too, be it in a few spots or in good amount, it will usually necessitate that a culture of the stools be taken. The doctor will try to determine through the culture if there exists any of three certain nasty diseases, each needing different treatment. They are salmonella, shigella, and pathogenic E. coli. The latter usually appears in babies. Stool analysis may also show rare forms of parasites indicating certain forms of dysentry.

In babies, chronic bloody diarrhea, along with mucus, fussing, stomachache and gas can also be caused by milk allergy.

Your doctor may have a look at the stool to confirm seeing the blood, and may want a stool analysis and a stool culture on at least three separate stool specimens. The treatment will almost entirely depend on the result of these tests.

What if it is a normal (or hard) stool but bloody?

The first thing you look for is whether it is bright red blood (fresh), or whether it is dark red blood (digested), and whether it is mixed with the stool, or on top of it like a red streak, or has dripped out after the stool had already passed through. All these observations are of importance.

If the blood is bright red, and if it shows up as a line on the surface of the stools of a baby, it may mean a cracked anus or fissure in ano (see page 81). For this kind the blood may also show up after the hard stool has passed, on the anus itself or on the toilet paper. In addition to the above, there is usually a good deal of pain upon moving the bowels. Having a bowel movement through a cracked anus becomes a painful ordeal, and the poor baby will scream bloody murder because it hurts so much!

If the child passes bright red blood, usually following a bowel movement, and if it is without pain, it may mean the presence of a polyp. A polyp is a growth into the inside of the intestine and it can cause a good deal of trouble at times. If a polyp is suspected, the child is usually sent to a surgeon for proctoscopy and perhaps sigmoidoscopy (a look at the insides of the rectum and nearby intestine); even a special X-ray may have to be taken. A polyp that shows up must be removed surgically.

Please keep in mind that children are not as likely to suffer from hemorrhoids as adults are.

Describe some other causes of bloody stools:

It is well known that peptic ulcers do show up in children every once in a while. Also a condition called Meckel's diverticulum, a congenital extra "tube" coming out of the small intestine, not very rare, can on occasions cause bloody stools needing immediate surgery. Rarely, a child may have ulcerative colitis. More common however is a child with anaphylactoid purpura (see page 403). This latter disease is not that common, and in such a case, the child will develop "bloody" pinpoint spots under the skin (called petechii), mainly on the legs and ankles. In about a third of such cases there will be stomachache with bloody stools. In cases of intussusception, a young child develops severe abdominal pain and repeated vomiting, and will pass bloody mucus through the rectum, resembling red currant jelly. The latter is a very important sign in the diagnosis of intussusception.

All the above diseases and many, many more can show up as bloody stools, along with other combination of signs and symptoms. Extensive investigation may be needed at times. All this means that if you see blood in your child's stool, don't get rid of the specimen; get in touch with the doctor for a visit, and take the specimen with you.

INGUINAL HERNIA

You may discover an inguinal hernia accidentally, after you have given him a bath; or he may complain of some pain in the groin area. A bulge, of variable size, may show itself now, disappear later on, and reappear again. Usually it is above the crease of the middle of the groin by about half an inch. This is a spot of weakness in the wall of the abdomen, and when he coughs, it may bulge or swell to be the size of an egg or even bigger.

If he is older, he may ask your opinion and complain of some pain. The sneaky hernia may even be on both sides, puffing itself to a temporary bigger size upon coughing, sneezing, grunting or blowing the nose.

Why do you keep saying "he"?

Most inguinal hernias affect boys. At each side of the wall of the abdomen, there is a particular spot that is weaker in males than in females. Such a spot can develop a hernia, whereby the wall is pushed by the contents of the abdomen (such as the intestine); in so doing, the area bulges on and off depending on how much pressure there is from inside.

Of course, there are a number of other kinds of hernias, but they are not as common as the inguinal hernia.

What can be done about this?

You will be scared, of course, when you see the hernia, and you must call the doctor to confirm your suspicions, even if the hernia has already disappeared by the time you have gone to the office.

If the suspicion is confirmed, then the child must have an operation. The operation is not that complicated, and the child will have to be in the hospital only for a few days. An operation done early enough on a hernia is much simpler to perform than one done on a hernia that has been neglected.

Why should a hernia not be neglected?

A hernia that is left uncorrected for a few months or longer, can gradually become bigger and bigger. Its sporadic appearances will be more frequent and for longer periods of time, and it will disappear less often. It can gradually descend to the testicular sac (scrotum), at which point it can be as big as a golf ball or a grapefruit!

There can be other problems too, if the hernia is neglected. It can become incarcerated, or even strangulated. Such complications can even endanger the life of your boy. In such situations the treatment is an emergency surgery, and the operation is more difficult to perform.

Can babies get hernias too?

Yes babies can get hernias too. In fact, even congenital hernias exist. The weak spot in the wall of the abdomen can have an open communication between the cavity of the abdomen and that around the testicle. It can also be on one side or both sides of the abdomen.

What should I do?

If your baby or child has a bulge or a lump in the area above the groin or in the groin itself, and the bulge disappears, don't assume that the trouble has gone away. If the testicular sac (scrotum) has become big, then it is spelling trouble. If there is pain in the groin area, have it checked. Though girls are much less likely to get a hernia, it can occasionally happen.

How is a hernia in a girl different?

The bulge above the groin may be more towards the middle line, and is called a direct hernia. Usually the bulge is not as big as that in boys. Another point is that the hernia will make one side of the female genitalia bulge at the top. When you try to push it back you may even feel the gurgles of the intestine.

APPENDICITIS

You have heard about appendicitis, perhaps you have had it, and it is quite an unwelcome problem. The appendix is an extra projection from a special area of the large intestine, and it can become inflamed, thus leading to further trouble.

What symptoms shall I expect?

In a child or an adult, there is usually some pain, more or less around the umbilicus at first. A few hours after that, the pain may shift to the right lower quarter of the abdomen. The pain can be severe, though not necessarily so, but the important point is its area of distribution. It is common for the temperature to go up, but usually not to a high level. In addition there is some nausea and perhaps vomiting, once or twice.

If you try to feel the stomach, you will discover that the right lower quarter of the abdomen is tender and the child may flinch when you press. You may also be able to feel some stiffness in the painful area.

Does appendicitis always show up in this way?

Usually but not always. The symptoms usually depend on the location of the appendix, the degree of the inflammation, and some other factors. Most likely the symptoms are enough to make you seek medical advice.

Please remember that even babies can develop appendicitis. Not only are the symptoms in babies different from the above, but they may also be alarming at times. Fortunately this is very rare.

When shall I call the doctor?

Don't be lulled into false security, and don't think the symptoms will go away if given more time. Appendicitis is a disease that cannot wait; you ought to call the doctor and explain the symptoms. He or she may want to look at the child right away. If the symptoms are quite obvious, the doctor may refer you to a surgeon.

Waiting too long may lead to a ruptured appendix. When this

happens, the operation becomes quite risky and more difficult to perform than a simple appendectomy operation.

Are there any differences between appendicitis in children and adults?

Yes there are, and they may be important. Cases of appendicitis in children are more likely to rupture early, more so in children under the age of four years.

Not only that but the symptoms can fool you too, since the young child will have difficulty describing them. Be on the alert for these possibilities.

Quite often a child will have constipation in addition to the symptoms mentioned before. A good many well-meaning parents will give the child an enema or a laxative. An enema or a laxative given to a child with appendicitis will help speed up the rupture of the appendix and give more trouble to everyone.

How long will the child be in the hospital?

If it is an average case of appendicitis, the child will have the operation and be in the hospital for only a few days. If the appendix has already ruptured, the stay in the hospital will be longer, and the treatment will be more involved. There might be a chance for some complicatons too, and if so, the child's stay in the hospital will be longer, and the treatment will be more complicated.

Is it easy to diagnose appendicitis?

Usually it is, but at times it may be quite difficult. There are other diseases which mimic appendicitis, and they may even fool a well-seasoned doctor. This is one of the reasons why at times a child may have to be observed carefully for a day or two, and some blood tests and urinalysis may have to be done. Such possible cases of appendicitis may prove to be nothing but false alarms; the trouble may be caused by other diseases not needing surgery.

I have heard of chronic appendicitis; does it affect children?

Children usually don't get chronic appendicitis.

Please remember that not every stomachache means appendicitis. Watch out for the symptoms as they progress, give them enough time, and if they make you suspicious of appendicitis, then call the doctor. Fortunately, appendicitis is a disease that can be cured with a simple operation if it is discovered early, and even if it has ruptured, the treatment is not that difficult.

ROUNDWORMS

No parent can remain calm and collected upon seeing the child pass a wiggly giant round worm (ascaris). The whole scene may be quite unnerving, and it may make us wonder as to what is going on in the tummy.

There are a good many varieties of roundworms, from the very small to the very big. Good examples are:

1. The giant roundworm (ascaris), as big as a pencil (ten to twelve inches long);
2. The whipworm (trichuris), only about 1/4 inch in length and barely visible.
3. The threadworm (strongloides), longer than the whipworm.
4. The pinworm (oxyuris), about 1/4 inch in length and familiar to many people.
5. The hookworm (ancylostoma), a small worm (1/3 inch), that can give a lot of trouble.

How can these worms get into a child?

These worms don't enter the stomach in their mature state. They usually enter the body in their larval stage of development. Some worms (piworms, for example), however, do enter in the egg stage.

Some of them enter through the mouth of the child when he or she plays in infested soil (this is true of the giant roundworm and the whipworm). This soil becomes infested when someone with the worm infestation has had a bowel movement in that area. The eggs of the worms will hatch in the soil and progress to the larval stage. The larval stage remains in the soil, ready to infest, for weeks or even months, depending on the kind of worm.

The eggs of the giant roundworm prefer hard clay soil, while the eggs of the hookworm and some others prefer rich moist sandy humus, such as the soil near lakes or banks of streams. Each female giant roundworm deposits an average of 200,000 eggs a day.

The eggs of the pinworms, on the other hand, enter through the mouth when the child's hands become contaminated by playing with other children who have pinworms, or by scratching or wiping his or her own bottom. The contaminated hands will then transfer the eggs to the mouth.

Some worms enter through the skin, such as the hookworm or the threadworm. The larva usually pricks the skin and goes through the blood to the lungs, and from the lungs up to the throat to be swallowed. They will then mature to be adults, to live in various parts of the intestines. It is quite a journey, but they all do it without getting lost on the way!

What trouble can worms produce?

It all depends on which kind of worms the child has. Most roundworms cause stomachache, which may be of the nagging type that comes and goes, on and off; it is usually mild but may be severe at times.

They also cause some loss of appetite, with some degree of nausea and even vomiting at times. The bowel movements may become irregular too. Pinworms are well known for the good deal of itching they produce in the pant's area, and they are the commonest of the round worms.

Often a child with roundworms will have a sallow complexion and will lack vigor in general, be it mental or physical. This is especially true if the infestation is heavy, as quite often happens with hookworm infestation. Hookworms are mean and they do lead to a good degree of blood loss resulting in iron deficiency anemia, because they suck the blood from the intestinal wall for their needs.

Roundworms can occasionally produce many symptoms other than the above. Heavy infestations can be more troublesome; I have seen one person who passed about 650 ascaris worms. The abdomen shrunk to normal size after having looked like a pregnancy!

How common is this infestation?

Infestation is more common in warm, humid climate areas, especially in the southern states and in the Gulf area.

Sanitary conditions are of utmost importance, and an infested child who deposits a bowel movement outside is likely to be the very source of passing along worms to others.

The innocent victims who come either to play in the area, to fish, or to work the field, can easily pick up the infestation. Going barefoot in such infested areas is an open invitation for the worm infestation.

Can we prevent such an infestation?

There are a few points which ought to be followed. Don't let your child play with dirt when you suspect that the area may have been infested, i.e. in certain rural areas, or in some fields where you suspect poor sanitary conditions.

Let the children wear shoes when they are near lakes, banks of streams or in fields. This is especially true if you are vacationing in the south, or you are camping in areas where sanitary conditons are suspect.

There are specific medications for each kind of roundworm, but first the doctor may have to do a few stool analyses or other tests, not only before but also after the treatment.

PINWORMS

The child may scratch his or her bottom persistently, especially around the anal area. This occurs more often in the early morning hours, particularly around 5:00 to 7:00. The intensity of the itching varies according to how heavy the pinworm infestation is. In very heavy infestation, the child may be itching day and night.

Pinworms reside in the large intestine, from the area near the appendix down to the rectum. Heavy infestation means the presence of literally thousands of these worms.

Other than the discomfort it causes, the intense itching in the pants area can interfere with sleep, and it may make the child irritable, cranky, and quite restless. Other than that, pinworms rarely produce other symptoms.

No others?

Many people think that pinworms may be the cause of stomachache, but this is not true. Other kinds of worms can cause stomachache but not pinworms. Symptoms erroneously blamed on pinworms by people include gritting teeth, slobbering, poor appetite, looking pale, not gaining weight, or even having a big tummy. All these symptoms are related not to pinworms but to other things.

How does my child get pinworms?

Pinworms are usually transmitted from child to child. This often happens during play or other forms of contact. Not only that, but a child with pinworms can self-transmit the worm infestation via the "bottom-to-hand-to mouth" route. The female pinworm will deposit its eggs in the area around the anus. When the child touches that area after moving the bowels, during a bath or at other times, the eggs will stick to the fingers, and from there they will be transmitted to the mouth.

How common is pinworms?

It is very common. Often the infestation is mild, and it may hardly produce any symptoms. It is an easily transmissible disease, and it is not easy to prevent. For each child with a hefty dose of pinworms, there are dozens who have very mild infestation. It is more common however in certain sections of the population, more so in children than in adults.

What shall I do upon suspecting pinworms?

If the child seems to scratch his or her bottom often, there may be a cause for suspecting pinworms. It may be a good idea to start looking for them. Take a flashlight and take a good look at the area around the anus. Do that when the itching is most intense, i.e., in the early hours of the morning. If you don't see any pinworms, don't give up, keep looking for them daily for seven to ten days, and you may be able to see them.

They look transparent, slightly milky, and about one third inch long. They are thin and they move slowly. Once you see them you cannot mistake them. If they appear in the bowel movement, the infestation is very heavy. It is not unusual to have 10,000 worms or more in an average case!

Upon seeing the worms, call the doctor for treatment and advice. If you cannot see the worms, and the itching cannot be ignored, the doctor can do special tests, such as the scotch-tape test or some similar one. These tests are more accurate than checking the stool under the microscope.

What will the doctor do?

Fortunately, by now there are medicines that can eradicate pinworms with only a single dose, Vermox or Povan, (prescription). The doctor will prescribe one of these medicines not only for the child but also for everyone in the family, because pinworms are highly contagious.

It may be advisable to use a second dose of the medicine for a child who has the pinworm infestation, to get rid of the remnant of the pinworms completely. The second dose is usually given ten to fourteen days after the first dose.

The doctor may also advise you about washing the hands, care of the bedsheets, toilet seats, underpants, etc. These measures are of some importance to help prevent the infestation from coming back.

How can we prevent pinworms?

Other than treating the whole family when infestation shows up, there are no reliable methods for preventing pinworms. There are lots of children who have them, and through contact in school, during play, etc., transmission can be very easy and hard to prevent.

Pinworms are troublesome but usually they don't cause major problems. On rare occasions they can cause vaginitis by crawling into the vagina, or appendicitis by entering the appendix.

INFECTIOUS HEPATITIS

Infectious hepatitis is a contagious disease that affects the liver in particular. It is caused by a virus and usually the symptoms show up a relatively long time after exposure, perhaps a few weeks or longer.

Infectious hepatitis may not be easy to suspect at first: you may not take the child to the doctor because you think it is the flu. The child becomes tired and achy, with some stomachache, headache, maybe some rise of temperature, nausea or vomiting, and poor appetite. Some of these symptoms may show up for a few days or longer. Usually the patient becomes progressively sicker, and may develop jaundice, in which the skin and the white of the eye look yellow in color. The color of the urine may become unusually dark, and the color of the stools may become pale, almost white.

Because the early symptoms are so variable and because some people wait so long before they see the doctor, some valuable time may pass before the disease is discovered. In the mean time, a good many people will have been exposed to it, and there is a good chance that they will develop the disease also.

What would you do for those exposed?

There is a shot called gamma globulin that can help prevent the disease. It ought to be given within the first few days of the exposure. The amount to be given varies according to the weight of the person.

By the way, an exposure is when there is close contact with the patient suffering from the infectious hepatitis, for a significant time period, such as a person living in the same household or a regular baby sitter.

The gamma globulin shot gives good protection, but not 100%. It also gives better protection to a child than to an adult.

Is gamma globulin helpful when we travel abroad?

Many authorities suggest giving the gamma globulin shot before you travel abroad, mainly to countries other than western Europe and Canada. This is particularly true if you plan to go to Africa or Asia.

The immunity offered will last for an average of about six weeks. If you plan to stay longer than that, another shot may have to be given once every six weeks or so. Of course, if you do plan a long stay, frequent shots of gamma globulin may not be practical.

Is it true that hepatitis is more common in children?

Yes, and it affects children of school age more frequently than younger ones. Fortunately, however, the disease is mild compared to its effect on adults, and it may not last as long. Not infrequently, the symptoms disappear a few days after the jaundice shows up, and in three weeks or so the patient seems to be over the predicament. In mild cases, the course can last only a week or two, but in severe ones it can take as long as three months before going away! Fortunately, infectious hepatitis is only rarely fulminant or fatal.

DIABETES

Diabetes is not as common in children as it is in adults. More often than not, the child seems to be ill for a few days, then suddenly and unexpectedly, he or she completely loses consciousness or becomes semiconcious. This is an explosive beginning of diabetes, and it shows up this way in some. If the diabetes shows in a slower manner, you will notice that the child will drink a lot of liquids, and often eat a good deal, but will not gain weight. You will also notice that the child urinates much more than usual. You may notice some degree of weight loss. Occasionally a child who has been well trained for some time may start wetting the bed.

Not all the above symptoms appear in every child, but if several do, see the doctor immediately. If the child happens to have diabetes and you wait, you will be risking the chance of a diabetic coma, which is a grave emergency requiring immediate admission to the hospital for diagnosis and treatment.

How will the doctor diagnose diabetes?

If the child develops one or all of the aforementioned symptoms, a checkup and a urinalysis will suffice. The urine may show sugar and acetone. Fasting blood sugar or the full glucose tolerance tests will also have to be done.

What is diabetes caused by?

    Diabetes is caused mainly by insufficient production of insulin by the pancreas. Since insulin is essential in regulating sugar in the blood, the liver, and the muscles, its absence or ineffectiveness will play havoc not only with the regulation of blood sugar, but also with other blood chemistries. This can lead to numerous problems if not controlled, some immediate and others (like eye problems) years later.

    Most cases of diabetes in children are hereditary, and about one in every twenty-four cases of all diabetics happens to be a child. Unfortunately, diabetes is usually more severe in children than in adults, and the need for daily shots is necessary for life. If there is a strong family history of diabetes, it is worth checking the child's urine every year, even if there are no symptoms to indicate any trouble.

How is diabetes treated?

    Most children with diabetes will usually need daily insulin shots. Not only that, but keeping a record of the amount of sugar and acetone in the urine is very important. The tests for these are simple, consisting of dipping a specially-treated paper in the urine and reading the results after fifteen to thirty seconds.

    Care about what to eat and how much is important; the doctor will explain that in detail. Naturally, limiting sweets is mandatory. But the diet does not have to be too strict; it must be good enough to allow for growth, must make the child feel normal, and at the same time not raise the blood sugar much.

    The insulin shots are usually given once (and occasionally twice) a day. There are certain types and sizes of disposable syringes for that. Once the proper dose is determined, it will have to be given regularly, with a slight increase or decrease depending on the urine or blood tests. Once the child is old enough, he or she will be trained to give the shots to himself or herself. Believe it or not most children will agree to this; the trouble is that when they become teenagers, they may balk or stop taking the shots.

    Taking one shot a day for life may seem an almost impossible task, but the child and the family will get used to it. A child may resent or even rebel against all this. However, by fully knowing what may happen if he or she does not take the insulin, or even by experiencing some of the consequences, the child may think twice before rebelling.

What will happen if the child takes too much or too little insulin?

The doctor will try to determine the best dose of insulin the child needs, and will prescribe the kind and amount to be taken every day. However, the child's need for insulin is also affected by the degree of activity, the amount of food intake, the kind of food, health condition, etc. Therefore, on certain occasions the same amount of insulin may prove to be insufficient or too much.

An insufficient amount of insulin will lead to more sugar in the urine, with some acetone (sugar level shows better in blood tests). This is the reason for testing the urine (or the blood) so often during daytime. Once insufficient dosage becomes obvious, an adjustment in the dose of insulin will have to be made, otherwise high blood sugar will lead to trouble.

If the dose of insulin seems to be excessive, symptoms of low blood sugar (hypoglycemia) will show up. The child might become pale, feel hungry, somewhat dizzy, and shaky. If the hypoglycemia is severe, he or she may even convulse or pass out. All diabetics should know about such a possibility, and be aware about what to do in such a situation. Some will take candy, orange juice, or other high sugar foods that the doctor advices, and within a short time, the symptoms of hypoglycemia will disappear.

There are numerous pamphlets, booklets, and books about the subject, and within a short time diabetics and their parents can become experts in this subject.

CHAPTER THIRTEEN

CHEST, HEART AND BLOOD

the chest
tidbits about the breasts
chest pains
heart rate
heart murmur
high blood pressure
the child bruises easily
the blood
low blood (iron-deficiency anemia)
purpura
anaphylactoid purpura
sickle cell disease

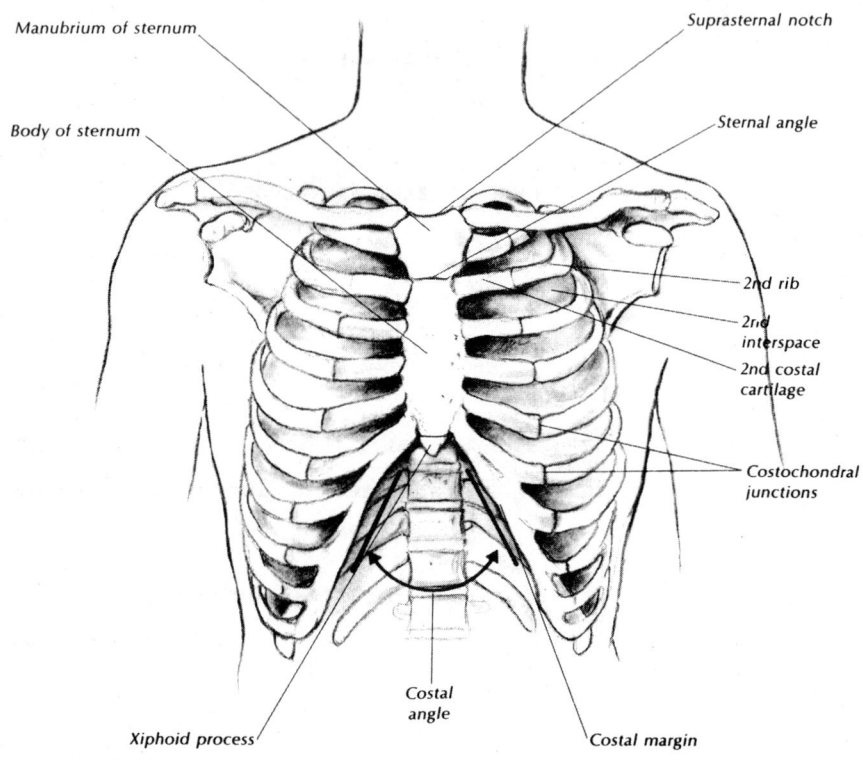

Courtesy Barbara Bates, M.D.
from a Guide to Physical Examination, p 112
Written permission from the publisher, J. B. Lippincott Co.

THE CHEST

Not unlike a barrel, the chest protects the heart and the lungs inside. It is shaped that way because of the twelve ribs on each side, which are connected to the spine in the back, and partly to the breastbone (sternum) in front. The shape and malleability of the chest are slightly different in babies and children than in adults.

How does the shape of the chest differ from children to adults?

The sternum (breastbone) is the central flat bone to which many of the ribs are attached. It tapers to a point at its lower part, not unlike an elongated wedge. In children, the end of the sternum (breastbone) often protrudes as a hard lump sticking out at the upper part of the abdomen. This is normal and should not cause parental concern. To many uninitiated mothers and grandmothers, the protruding end of the breastbone evokes surprise, fear, and apprehension. After rushing to the doctor, they give a sigh of relief when they find out that it is nothing but the tail end of this innocent bone.

Some babies have a "funnel chest". This is a depression at the end of the sternum and its nearby ribs, varying in size. When it is large, or if there is a good deal of sensitivity on the part of the child, an operation to correct the defect may be necessary.

How about the insides?

The heart and the two lungs, along with other organs, all lie protected inside the chest. The heart is somewhat to the left of the middle connected to the upper and lower part of the body with large blood vessels. The blood vessels will bring "stale" blood (unoxygenated) to the heart and take away "purified" or oxygenated blood (which has detoured through the lungs) to the rest of the body. These blood vessels are contained in the mediastinum.

The heart is a remarkable pump, and it is in a delicate mechanical balance with its large network of vessels. Sometimes, however, things can go wrong.

What can go wrong?

You have heard of congenital heart diseases (those that children are born with.) There are oodles of them, and they show up in various combinations. Some affect the valves of the heart, others the size of the vessels, and others involve holes between the various chambers of the heart. Quite often combinations of such defects take place, and different signs and symptoms will be the result.

Other diseases can show up too, rheumatic heart disease being one that occurs more often in children. This disease is related to strep infection that has been left undetected, or treated improperly.

What would you do about congenital heart diseases?

A good percentage of children with congenital heart disease will need extensive investigation and surgery to correct the defect. Operations such as heart surgery, are quite successful in many children, thanks to startling advances in the art of medicine. On the other hand, certain diseases of the heart will not need surgery, and special medicines and careful medical attention by the pediatrician or the cardiologist is more than sufficient.

How about the lungs?

Besides the heart and mediastinum, the lungs fill the rest of the chest cavity. They are remarkably resiliant, hugging the heart on each side.

The right lung consists of three lobes, while the left lung consists of two lobes. There are also fine partitions within each lung to produce further subdivisions.

On the outside, the lungs are covered with a thin layer called the pleura, which rubs itself against its continuation that forms the lining of the chest cavity. The pleura has a smooth lubricated surface, to make the movements of inflation and deflation of the lungs painless and trouble-free.

Are the lungs likely to have trouble?

Yes, more so in children than in others. The lungs get affected to various degrees when the heart suffers from diseases, as well as when the blood vessels of the heart are affected.

Besides that, the lungs more often develop diseases of their own since they are directly open to the air and atmosphere. Respiratory infections (see page 306), bronchitis (see page 315), asthmatic bronchitis (see page 317), and pneumonias (see page 324), are examples.

THE BREASTS

The baby is only a few weeks old, but his or her breasts seem to be large as if there is a walnut sized lump beneath the nipple. It is not painful and it is not tender. The question is whether you should worry about it or not.

What causes this enlargement?

Enlargement of the breast tissue in a newborn is caused by the mother's female hormones during pregnancy. It is a common occurrence and is nothing to worry about. When left alone, the breast tissue will gradually shrink to normal after a number of weeks, and the baby's chest will look fully normal when he or she is about three months old if not before.

One point to be emphasized though; don't massage it or keep handling it since this can lead to inflammation of the breast tissue and create problems.

The breasts will remain dormant during childhood until after the age of ten years in most children.

Are there any exceptions?

At times we see girls whose breasts do enlarge to some extent, before they have reached the usual expected age. In many this does not mean much, yet it is essential that the doctor sees such a child and keeps her under "observation". Usually the breasts will recede back to normal after a number of months. Pre-adolescent budding of the breasts can take place before the age of nine years, but this may happen occasionally. The familiar adolescent development of the breast usually shows up along with other signs of maturing, in both males and females.

What do you mean in males?

It is quite common to see adolescent boys with a lump beneath the nipple. This lump may be as big as a walnut and tender to the touch. Quite often, it shows up more on one side than the other, and may be followed by a similar lump on the other side a few months later.

It is important that the breasts be left alone in such circumstances. They will gradually go back to normal in a year or two.

How about girls?

Naturally, as the breasts develop and assume their adult shape, it is good for the girl to learn to feel for lumps regularly. This is a healthy habit if started during adolescence and continued throughout life.

It is very rare for tumors to show up in the breasts during adolescence. Mother is more likely than daughter to worry about small lumps showing up in the girl's undeveloped breasts, and understandably so. But mostly these turn out to be nothing but the breast tissue itself, which can be slightly larger than usual at times.

How often shall we check them?

It is a good habit to check the breasts every time the female takes a bath. Look for the lump in the breast tissue, up to the junction of the breast with the armpit.

As said before, lumps in the breasts are very rare during adolescence. But if the girl makes it a habit to check for them, she may one day prove to have prevented serious problems. This healthy habit should be practiced by all females from adolescence onward.

Do we have to see the doctor in case of any breast enlargement?

Perhaps it is good to do so, even if only for parental peace of mind. Furthermore, there are some diseases that lead to premature enlargement of the breast. Many such diseases have to do with the endocrine glands, ovaries, etc. The doctor will be able to suspect such diseases if there are enough signs at hand. If the doctor sees nothing, you will at least feel reassured.

What are the endocrine glands?

They are ductless glands that secrete their material internally. Some of them control certain aspects of the breast tissue and secondary sexual characteristics. That's why if there is premature or unusual development of the breasts, with or without secondary sexual characteristics (pubic hair, axillary hair, changes in voice, etc.), a doctor should be consulted early.

CHEST PAINS

The child may complain to you of some pains in the chest. It may be in the area of the heart, and it may be sharp, intermittent, yet not incapacitating. He or she may have had this pain every so often for the last few weeks.

The child is usually of school age, more likely of high school age. Aside from the bouts of pains, the child doesn't seem to suffer from other symptoms, such as excessive sweating, vomiting, shooting pain to the left arm, etc. Nevertheless, although no one mentions it, the possibility of a heart attack lingers.

Doesn't it sound like a heart attack?

No, it doesn't. Such pains are not rare, regardless of whether the child belongs to a family with a history of heart attacks or not. Not only does the child have no associated symptoms that may implicate the heart, but heart attacks are just about nonexistent in children anyway.

Then what causes such pains?

These pains are usually muscular in origin, probably related to muscular strain, viral infection of the muscles of the chest wall, or perhaps to some degree of indigestion or stomach upset.

Other causes might be pleurisy or coxsackievirus infection of the chest muscles, or cases of respiratory infections of various severity.

What can we do about chest pains?

By simply having a complete checkup, including blood pressure measurement, and by simply being told that the heart sounds good, the child's chest pain will seem to fade away gradually! Often these occasional pains are exaggerated to a great extent in the minds of children.

However, in some children the doctor may find it necessary to treat the actual cause of the pain, depending on the findings.

Will special tests be needed?

An EKG, X-rays, blood tests, and similar things will rarely be needed to supplement the checkup. However, if pleurisy is suspected, or another disease, the doctor may have to do some special investigation.

What about other kinds of pain in the chest?

There are a number of diseases that can cause pain in the chest, each having its own characteristics.

Pain caused by pleurisy is usually sharp and severe, and it may become worse not only upon taking a deep breath, but also upon coughing or sneezing. There is usually associated trouble with pleurisy, such as pneumonia.

With tracheobronchitis and severe upper respiratory infection, the pain is often behind the breastbone, and is dull and heavy. Coughing may make it worse but not as much as in the case of pleurisy.

HEART RATE

You can count the rate of the heartbeat wherever there is a pulsating artery, but the artery immediately above the wrist, on the inner side of the arm on the same side as the thumb, is the easiest to locate. By putting gentle pressure on this artery with your fingers, you can feel the pulse easily, and you will be able to count the pulse rate (beats per minute).

What is a normal heart rate?

The rate varies because of many conditions. If a normal adult is resting, lying down and relaxed, the heart rate is around 72 beats a minute. This varies a good deal depending on certain conditions.

Do not be alarmed if your child's pulse rate is 85 to 95. A normal baby has a faster heart rate than a child, and a child has a faster heart rate than an adult, therefore age is a factor. An athlete may have a somewhat slower heart rate, because an athlete's heart can push the blood more effectively.

What does a fast rate mean?

A person with a fast heart rate during rest usually has a condition, e.g. certain disease, that makes it necessary for the heart to speed up.

When the child exercises, runs, jumps, etc., the heart rate will increase. This will supply the body with a greater blood supply to meet the demand for oxygen and other nourishment the body needs during exercise.

A person with fever will have a fast heart rate too. The heart responds by contracting at a faster rate when the temperature of the person goes higher. The higher the temperature, the higher the pulse rate will be up to a certain limit.

It is important to keep in mind that for each degree Fahrenheit that the person's temperature rises, the pulse rate will rise by ten. If the child's temperature is 103 degrees F, for example, then the pulse rate will have increased by an extra 45 beats, i.e. it will be around 125 (80+45=125). This might scare many parents, thinking that the heart is beating unduly fast, but it is an expected phenomenon and there should be no cause for alarm.

Will a very fast heart rate be dangerous?

Yes, because this will overtax the capacity of the heart. A "very fast rate" is 150 and up.

This is likely to be the case in a special disease of the heart called paroxysmal tachycardia. This is a rare disease in children, but more common in adults. Quite often it is even difficult to count the heart rate because it is so fast, and an EKG and other tests are mandatory to help in the matter. A cardiologist will usually be consulted and treatment instituted accordingly.

Will a slow heart rate be dangerous?

Except in trained athletes, a very slow heart rate may indicate trouble too, especially if the rate is around 50 or less. Some diseases can cause such a condition, notably heart block, which is a blockage in the pathway of the electrical impulse that travels in the wall of the heart to make the heart contract. An EKG is also mandatory and it will help a good deal (along with other tests) to elucidate the cause. Heart block is rare in children, however. It is more likely to be congenital or associated with some kind of congenital heart disease.

How valuable is it to take the pulse rate?

Usually it is not that valuable. Children with fever will have a faster heart rate than usual, of course depending on the level of the temperature. We can get far more mileage out of taking the child's temperature than the pulse rate.

There are rare situations, though, in which it does become very important to take the pulse rate, to see if it is too fast, too slow, or if it is irregular. Such conditions, however, are rare and their diagnoses require the help of the physician.

HEART MURMUR

The heart sounds are usually clear and regular. A murmur manifests itself as a vibrating sound that shows up along with the otherwise normal heart sound, or replacing them. There are two groups of murmurs, innocent and organic.

It is said that one out of every three children develops an innocent murmur at some time during childhood. It shows up at times, then it will disappear spontaneously, and may even show up again; that is to say it will come and go.

What is an innocent murmur?

As the name indicates, it is a murmur of no significance. It only needs investigation in the rare case that it shows suspicious signs of being like an organic murmur.

An innocent murmur is also called hemic or physiologic murmur. It may sound louder when there is fever, after an exercise, or if there is anemia. The doctor's experience is vital in differentiating the organic from the innocent murmur.

As a matter of fact, many doctors don't even bother to mention the presence of an innocent murmur to the parents, to avoid needless worry. However, your doctor will tell you if the murmur should be checked every year or so.

What is an organic murmur?

An organic murmur is of a completely different breed. It is usually caused by some trouble with the valves of the heart, the arteries or the veins that lead to or away from the heart, or some major trouble of the heart wall itself.

An organic murmur may be a result of a rheumatic heart, or some other serious heart problems.

Are there different kinds of organic murmurs?

The experienced ear of the doctor is of utmost importance, especially when it comes to murmur differentiation. The character of the murmur itself, its location, relationship to the other heart sounds, length, loudness, etc. are very important clues. Of course other signs and symptoms in the child, the use of EKG and other specialized procedures, X-rays, etc., will all help in the diagnosis.

If there is rheumatic heart disease or congenital heart disease it is best if the child is followed by a pediatric cardiologist, if there is one in your area. Such a heart specialist will go a long way in offering the best advice and treatment, and will keep an eye on the child's condition.

Will some organic murmurs disappear?

They may change character and strength from time to time. Occasionally, murmurs caused by rheumatic fever or congenital heart disease may disappear completely, and the lesion may heal and be gone for good. However, the majority of congenital heart diseases and those caused by rheumatic heart may need heart surgery sooner or later, and not once but twice or more at other times.

HIGH BLOOD PRESSURE

If you have thought that high blood pressure is an adult's affliction guess again. High blood pressure can affect children, though in a different way than it affects adults.

Blood pressure is recorded in two readings, the first is called systolic, and the second diastolic. More attention is paid to the diastolic pressure because it is more meaningful and less changeable than the systolic. In other words, if someone says my blood pressure is 120, it does not mean half as much as saying my blood pressure is 120/80. The second reading is more meaningful and valuable, being less likely to change with excitement, temperament, exercise, or other parameters.

How does blood pressure behave in children?

Blood pressures of children differ from those in adults, being somewhat dependent on age. The level is also generally lower than adults. Not only that, but we have to use a smaller cuff for the reading, depending on the size of the arm of the child or even on the baby.

Children who are discovered to have high blood pressure may need a good deal of investigation. A large percentage prove to have trouble elsewhere.

What kind of trouble causes high blood pressure?

Trouble with the arteries of the kidneys, trouble with the substance of one or both kidneys, or chronic infection of one or both kidneys, can be important causes of high blood pressure, especially in children. At times, trouble, congenital or otherwise, with certain glands in the system or certain organs (including the heart), may also lead to high blood pressure.

However there are also a number of children with high blood

pressure who prove to have no known cause for it. This is called essential hypertension.

What about these cases?
They also behave in a unique manner in children. To have an average reading, your doctor might ask you to bring the child back weekly for three times for taking blood pressure.

If the blood pressure proves not to be very high, the blood pressure readings may gradually and spontaneously go back to normal in a year or two. This actually happens in about one out of every three children with "essential" hypertension, and it needs no special treatment. The remaining two out of three will persist, and their pressure may need to be controlled.

How do you control high blood pressure in children?
There are a good many medicines on the market. A medicine or two (prescription), taken once a day, may suffice. In more severe cases, a number of medications may have to be used, and hospitalization may be needed too.

High blood pressure can be dangerous since it can lead to heart failure and many other problems. Most children who have high blood pressure have no symptoms and no complaints. The problem will simply be discovered by the doctor during the yearly checkups, or during other visits to the office; if not, the case might be missed, or detected late in the game.

How will I know my child needs the reading?
Blood pressure readings for the child are important if there are members in the family with high blood pressure. The same thing applies too if the child happens to be overweight, since an obese child is more likely to have high blood pressure than others.

It is good to check the blood pressure routinely when the child is around the age of three years and up; this is especially true in teenagers. However, under certain circumstances, even a baby may have to have a blood pressure reading taken.

Is high blood pressure curable?

Sometimes high blood pressure is caused by trouble in a kidney, a gland, or an organ such as the heart. Treating the cause often brings the blood pressure down to normal. A heart disease called coarctation of the aorta is a good example. When this is the cause of the hypertension, and when it is corrected surgically, the blood pressure often comes down to normal.

Prevention of a kidney infection (pyelonephritis), by prompt recognition and treatment of urinary tract infection, will indirectly help prevent a possible future cause for high blood pressure. As stated before, although one out of three cases of essential hypertension will revert to normal in a few years, the other two are likely to continue into adulthood, and usually can get consistent control only with medication.

THE BLOOD

The blood is the "red gold" which can give a store of information to the doctor when the proper tests are done. It consists of red blood cells, white cells, and platelets. They all bathe in a special fluid called plasma which is loaded with various forms of proteins, fats, carbohydrates, enzymes, hormones, various forms of electrolytes, and rare elements.

The functions of the blood are numerous indeed; it is the transport mechanism of oxygen, carbon dioxide, nourishment, and some waste material, among other things. The tissues of all the organs depend on the blood to keep them well-functioning.

Pumped by the heart, the blood rushes quickly inside the blood vessels. It purifies itself in the lungs, gets rid of much of its waste through the kidneys, and transports nourishment from the intestines to various parts of the body. The blood has a fighting capacity; it fends off intruding germs to the body via white cells and other material, wherever the germs find an access into the system.

When the blood shows up in areas where it is not supposed to, it will give a signal to children, parents, and doctors of a possible source of trouble. Good examples are blood in the urine or in the stools, or blood that does not clot fast enough (as in hemophilia), among many other possibilities.

What tests are usually done on the blood?

These are numerous and each test or group of tests is designed to give information for a specific disease or diseases. The search for newer and more refined tests will continue into the foreseeable future. The amount of blood needed for a test depends on that specific test. Numerous tests can be done on one or several drops of blood. Examples of such tests are the CBC (complete blood count), hemoglobin and hematocrit tests for common anemias, bilirubin test for jaundiced babies, PKU, thyroid and other metabolic tests for babies, infectious mono test, and sickle cell anemia test.

What is the hemoglobin or hematocrit test for?

Through these simple tests, anemia can be discovered, but these tests don't inform us of the kind of anemia. When there is anemia in a child or an infant, it usually is an iron-deficiency anemia. However, every once in a while a different form of anemia may be suspected, and further tests may be needed.

If the above tests are done routinely with the yearly checkup, an average pediatric office will pick up four or five cases a year, and every once in a while a rare kind of anemia may be detected. However, in low socioeconomic areas, the number can be much higher.

How about the bilirubin test?

During the first few days of life, some babies become jaundiced (see page 103). This jaundice has to be kept under close observation with frequent bilirubin tests. If the bilirubin goes to a certain level, it is likely to cause grave problems to the baby, and preventive measures must be taken before the dangerous level is reached. That is why bilirubin tests are done frequently, sometimes twice a day or even more often.

How about the PKU and thyroid tests?

PKU, thyroid and a host of other tests are done on a heel stick to draw blood. They are now done routinely on all newborns, to make sure the baby is not going to have PKU disease, low thyroid function, or other rare but preventable diseases. Some states recommend repeating these tests when the baby is one month old too. If such diseases are discovered early in life, much can be done in the way of preventive treatment, to help stop permanent damage.

How about the mono and sickle cell tests?

These are useful tests that can easily be done on one drop of blood. This is an office procedure and it is to be done when the doctor suspects such diseases. The mono spot test is to rule out infectious mononucleosis.

The same thing applies to sickle cell tests. Sickle cell disease or traits are common in black people, and it is a good idea for all black people to have this test done (see page 405).

How about the CBC?

CBC, or complete blood count, is important for certain diseases or certain situations. A good example is in case of appendicitis; the high white count helps in the diagnosis. Through the CBC, a doctor can have a better picture of the red cells, white cells, platelets, and the cell indices.

Therefore, a CBC can give information about the red cells, their shape and condition, thus it can help in diagnosing the form of anemia. A CBC can also tell the different kinds of the white cells, their count, kinds, proportion, and whether they are normal or not. This helps to show (a) if there is infection, (b) the kind of infection, and (c) if there is trouble with the white cells themselves. The platelet count also helps in diagnosing certain diseases having to do with frank bleeding (bleeding under the skin or in the tissues).

LOW BLOOD
IRON-DEFICIENCY ANEMIA

The child is fretful and pale, prefers to drink milk rather than eat solids, may look chubby; this may have been going on for some time. You take a good look and notice that the child's lips look pale and the ears seem to be waxy colored. You take the child to the doctor, who will give him or her a checkup and a blood test. The doctor tells you that the baby has low blood, or iron-deficiency anemia.

What kind of anemia is this?

Iron-deficiency anemia is caused by a low iron supply and it is fairly common. It usually shows up in a baby who is approaching the first birthday, though it may show up earlier. After the age of three to four years, however, it becomes rare unless there are special forms of anemia or special reasons for it, such as chronic blood loss.

During adolescence, a girl whose periods are heavy and prolonged is likely to develop this kind of anemia too. A teenager who decides to be a vegetarian but does not maintain a well-balanced diet may also develop this type of anemia. If so, the teenager will become pale and tired.

In short, any time the iron blood supply seems to be less than what the body demands, "low blood" or iron-deficiency anemia will insidiously show up.

What causes this anemia in a baby?

A fast-growing baby during the first two years of life will need a good constant supply of iron. After having depended on the iron supply of the mother during pregnancy, which lasts for only a few months, the baby will need the proper iron supply in his or her food. Because of the baby's fast growth, the demands for iron are high. Some foods are iron-poor, like milk, potatoes, bread, and starchy foods. Others are iron-rich like meats, egg yolk, liver, enriched baby cereal, and certain fruits and vegetables.

If the baby's demand for iron is much greater than the amount in the food, anemia will develop. That is one major reason many doctors put emphasis on nutritious food supply. It is also the reason why iron-fortified baby cereal, meats, eggs, and other iron-rich foods are given at certain times, along with advice to stop giving the baby large amounts of milk. A variety of foods, well-chosen and given at the proper age, is a good preventive measure for iron-deficiency anemia.

Are there any other causes?

Yes, there are many besides the above. The common ones are premature babies, twins, and babies whose mothers have been pregnant frequently and closely spaced.

Quite often formulas with added iron (e.g. Similac with iron), and vitamins with iron (e.g. Tri-Vi-Sol with iron) will have to be given to prevent the expected anemia in these babies. This has to be done knowing that these babies need more iron than usual and more frequent blood checks. Some doctors use such formulas and/or vitamins routinely on all babies, in an attempt to prevent anemia. Others prefer to tailor the iron supply according to the baby's need.

If my baby is iron deficient, what will the doctor do?

Once sure that the anemia is due to iron deficiency, an infant is put on iron medication. This comes in the form of drops, and when the dropper is filled to the proper level, it is put deep into the mouth of the infant to bypass the taste buds (this way the metallic taste is avoided). The medicine is squirted slowly so that the infant swallows as much as possible without spitting it out. If the infant spits it out, the teeth may stain dark, but this is temporary. The stools will be dark too because of the iron. A drink of orange juice (not milk) to follow the dose of medicine is often suggested, since the vitamin C increases iron absorption. Offer the medicine between meals for better absorption.

Medicines frequently used are Fer-in-Sol drops or Mol-Iron liquid (nonprescription). They have to be given three to four times a day and for a prolonged time, depending on how severe the anemia is. Two to three months of medication is not unusual, since the anemic child needs not only the blood level brought back to normal, but the iron store replenished too.

Along with the iron intake, it is advised to lower the amount of milk consumption and increase the amount of meats, liver, eggs, and other iron-rich foods.

Besides all this, you will have to check the blood at fairly regular intervals until it becomes normal. You will see that over a period of two to three months, if not before, the blood level will be up to normal. The infant in the meantime will "pink up", and regain red lips, vigor and vitality, and an appetite for solid food.

Are there any other causes for anemia?

Anemia is a vast subject, and there are numerous types, each with its specific cause or causes. Because of the multicolored face of anemia, the treatment will vary greatly. Even the same kind of anemia at two different ages may require two different forms of approach.

How about anemia in older children?

For a teenager who is found to be anemic, iron pills can be given three to four times a day for one to three months, until the anemia is gone. The diet will have to improve too, and if he or she insists on a vegetarian diet, it may have to be modified as to a better balance per the doctor's or nutritionist's advice.

PURPURA

Purpura is a disease that affects the platelet component of the blood. The platelets, along with red and white blood corpuscles, are carried in the plasma. The platelets are microscopic bodies essential for blood clotting.

In purpura, the number of the platelets decreases to a very low level, giving rise to certain symptoms.

What kind of symptoms does purpura give?

The most obvious symptom is the presence of tiny pinpoint-sized hemorrhages under the skin. Such pinpoint spots (petechii) show up all over, not only on the face and trunk, but on the arms and legs too. When you press on the skin to see if these petechii fade (as do other rashes), you will see that they do not.

Another possible symptom is the occurrence of fairly severe nosebleeds, but fortunately this is not so common. Fever and other symptoms will be absent, and rarely if ever will you see bleeding in the intestinal or urinary tract.

What causes such a disease?

In most purpuras, the body for some unknown reason builds up some kind of mechanism whereby it destroys the platelets, or affects their production mechanism in the bone marrow. When the platelet count falls to a very low level, the symptoms of this disease will show up.

In some children, however, other serious blood diseases can cause similar symptoms. That is why a good many blood tests, and bone marrow tests among others, will become essential for the diagnosis.

If there are symptoms of fever, vomiting, and severe headache along with the petechii, it may indicate something else.

Like what?

Meningitis often shows petechii, with high fluctuating temperature, sleepiness, vomiting, stiff neck, and a number of other symptoms (see page 503).

What all this means is that if you see petechii call the doctor.

In some occasions fine petechii show up on the face only after vomiting or severe cough; this is not serious. If the petechii are present all over, however, they mean serious trouble, and they require full investigation.

And what if it turns out to be purpura?

Most cases of primary purpura are self-limiting. The condition lasts for a long time -weeks, if not months. A certain percentage goes on for even a year or longer. Blood tests are to be done frequently to monitor the progress of the disease. The child will have to be protected to a great extent, because bleeding might endanger his or her life. This is one of the reasons a child with this disease is often admitted to the hospital.

Why the hospital?

Other than investigating his condition in the hospital, the doctor will recommend limited activity, to protect the child from complications, or undue bleeding.

If the case is chronic and seems to last for a year or longer, it is not unusual that removing the spleen will solve the problem. The spleen can "eat" more than its share of platelets.

What is the moral to the story?

If you see any unexplained lesions on the child's skin, be they petechii or not, give the doctor a call. A false alarm is better than missing an important disease or not finding out about it until quite late.

Rashes in general are difficult to diagnose on the phone, and there are so many kinds of them. But generalized petechii, be they associated with fever or not, should never be ignored. Such lesions may look to the untrained eye as some kind of a rash, but to the eye of the doctor they are something else.

ANAPHYLACTOID PURPURA

The child has some pain in the ankles; you notice that there is perhaps some swelling of not only one ankle but both. Not only that, but you also notice some rash in that area, which goes up the legs, almost to the area of the knees.

You may also see a similar rash in the buttock area. Rarely do you see this rash anywhere else, including on any other joint.

The rash will look bright red and seem slightly raised. Later on it becomes purplish brown and "recedes" under the skin, as if there have been tiny spots of bleeding under the skin.

Other symptoms such as fever may be there, but not commonly.

What causes such a problem?

Many theories have been advanced to explain this problem, but none are acceptable by all. Fortunately the condition is not that common, but when it shows up, we must look out for certain consequences and symptoms.

What are the consequences and symptoms?

We have to keep an eye on the urine and stools, since in about one out of three cases, if not more, the kidneys become involved. A form of nephritis will be the result. When this happens, the urine becomes smokey or bloody, and the doctor will have to keep a close check on the blood pressure, the amount of urine the child passes, and the condition of the kidneys. Also in about one out of three of such cases the intestines become involved, causing a stomachache, often severe. The child may pass blood in the bowel movement; the blood may be openly visible or microscopic in amount.

Every once in a while a child with this affliction may develop a complication called intussusception. This is a form of intestinal obstruction, and it will need immediate surgical intervention.

What we are saying here is that anaphylactoid purpura is a generalized disease; although to your eyes it shows up around the ankles, it actually affects important organs of the body in an unwelcomed manner.

What can be done about it?

When mild, usually you take the child home to rest, and the condition will go away by itself. The doctor will probably want to see the child several times to evaluate the condition. In the meantime you will keep an eye on the urine and stools; they might even have to be checked a few times by the laboratory.

If the kidneys or intestines are quite involved, the child will need to go to the hospital. He or she may not be there for a prolonged period, but mainly during the very dangerous period, and if the intestine becomes obstructed, then an operation will have to be done right away.

Certain medications can be used, but the decision on whether and when to use them depends on your doctor.

What shall we expect?

Anaphylactoid purpura usually takes two to three weeks before it subsides and goes away. The swelling and discomfort in the ankle area will gradually go away over a few days. The entire rash will undergo changes in color, and will eventually fade away.

As the acute stage of this disease passes by, so will the changes in the kidneys and intestine. The urine will gradually clear up, and the abdominal condition will also show improvement.

When this condition is over, it will be gone for good. In most cases there will be no aftereffects and no permanent trouble in the kidneys or intestine.

Unfortunately, there is no way to prevent this disease, at least as of this date.

Can this disease be very serious?
Anaphylactoid purpura is usually a benign disease. However, in rare cases the kidney involvement may become chronic for a few years.

The intestinal bleeding can be quite severe on rare occasions, thus needing immediate proper therapy. This is also true of the intussusception and intestinal obstruction.

SICKLE CELL DISEASE

Sickle cell is a disease resulting from an inheritance of certain types of hemoglobin (the red matter in the red blood cell, which carries the oxygen to the tissues). When this inherited condition is discovered, it will help the parents and the doctor to be on the alert, so that they will be able to take the appropriate measures when the child needs them.

How prevalent is sickle cell disease?
Sickle cell disease proper is primarily a disease of the Blacks. It affects one out of each nine American Blacks in the form of sickle cell trait. However, only one in four hundred will show sickle cell anemia. Sickle cell anemia varies in intensity from one person to another, and the child can have various degrees of symptoms.

What is the difference between the trait and the anemia?
The sickle cell trait often goes unnoticed since it rarely causes symptoms in children under ordinary circumstances. It can, however, cause symptoms later on, so it is important to detect it.

Sickle cell anemia is a severe form of the trait, and symptoms show up in children and babies as young as three to four months of age. These symptoms may prove to be extreme and most troublesome.

Other aberrant types of hemoglobin do exist, and often the symptoms are not as severe as in sickle cell anemia. These conditions can affect not only Blacks but also Caucasians and Orientals.

How can we find out about it?

A blood test can be done to determine the type of hemoglobin the child has, and once this is done, you will be able to tell if the child has a normal hemoglobin, the sickle cell trait, the sickle cell anemia, etc. Let us take examples: If the hemoglobin turns out to be type SA, then the child has sickle trait; and if it turns out to be type SS, then the child has sickle cell anemia; and if it turns out to be type SC, then the child has sickle cell hemoglobin C disease.

Is it worth doing this test on all Blacks?

Yes, and also on all Oriental children. Orientals can inherit certain kinds of hemoglobin too, as can people from the Middle East, and although this is not common, it is not a bad idea to do the hemoglobin type-determination test if the child proves to have anemia.

What symptoms shall we expect?

Sickle cell anemia shows as various degrees of pallor; the presence of jaundice indicates the chronic anemia, which can lead to other symptoms. But what worries everyone so much is the so-called "crisis" that can show up rarely but ferociously.

The crisis may include a severe stomachache that may double up the child, making the wall of the abdomen as stiff as a board, thereby mimicking what is called a surgical abdomen. It is not unusual either to have pains and swelling in the bones and joints. The central nervous system may become affected too, leading to convulsions, paralysis, and even coma.

However, by understanding the crises above and by discussing them with the doctor, prompt measures can be taken to make them pass with little if any damage. When infections are treated early and promptly, and plenty of liquids are given orally, even prevention of a crisis can be accomplished.

How long do these crises last?

A crisis may take two to three days, and hospitalization is often necessary. When the crisis is over, it is quite likely that jaundice will show up, indicating the disintegration of a goodly amount of the red blood corpusles.

CHAPTER FOURTEEN

GENITOURINARY SYSTEM

the urinary tract
urine
urinalysis, urine culture, IVP, etc.
the case of the bloody urine
urinary tract infection
glomerulonephritis
bedwetting
meatal stenosis
hydrocele
undescended testicle
vulvovaginits

The Urinary System

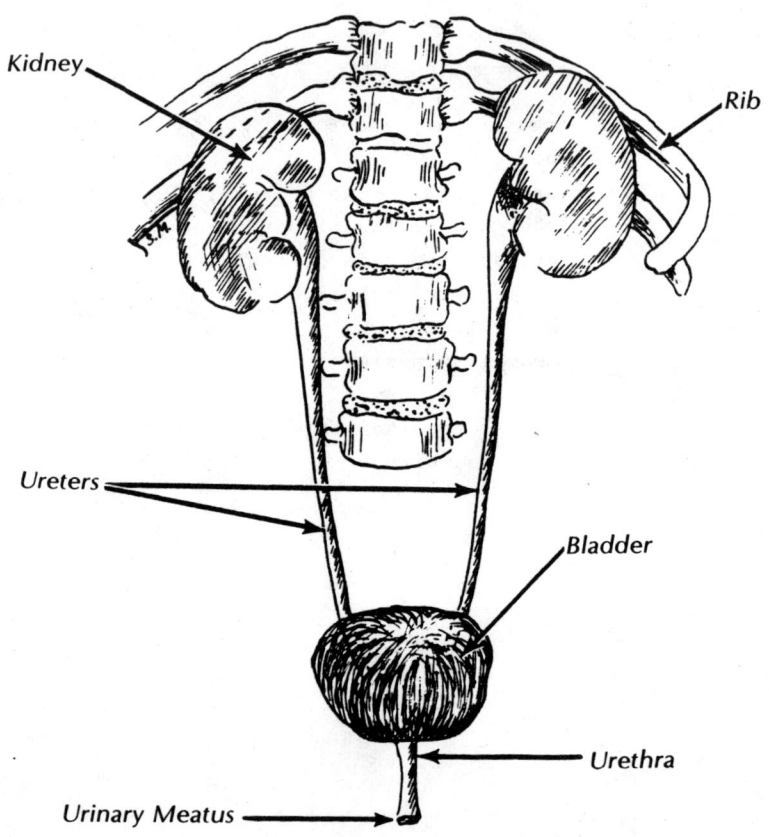

THE URINARY TRACT

Securely seated in the abdomen are the two kidneys. They are up in the lumbar area, one on each side. As the urine is manufactured by the kidneys, it has to drain to a storage area. Therefore, each kidney is connected to a long slender tube (ureter) that empties its content into the bladder. The bladder holds the urine until it becomes too full. Then, it empties its content through a tube called the urethra. This whole system constitutes the urinary tract.

The kidneys are a complex manufacturing organ that performs a magnificent job of "cleaning and purifying" the circulating blood of its waste material. They will play a vital role in keeping intact the various chemical necessities of the blood, and in so doing will indirectly protect the integrity of the organs and the tissues of the body.

In the process, the kidneys, bladder, and the tubes can be involved in various diseases. They can also develop diseases due to their individual peculiarities.

Like what?

Congenital diseases are not a rarity. A good example is a horseshoe kidney, whereby the two kidneys are fused together into one mass. Another example is the occurrence of three kidneys -two on one side and one on the other side. In other instances the child may have one kidney on one side and none on the other. Naturally, the ureter, too, may end up with problems because of such abnormalities, or have specific congenital problems of its own. A good example of the latter is narrowing of the ureter at certain spots, leading to grave damage to the kidneys.

Having three orifices (openings), the bladder stands to have many peculiar conditions, many of which will lead to repeated infections, distention of the bladder itself, or backward passage of the urine upon urinating.

What other diseases can affect the urinary tract?

The list is very long. Some diseases may be quite dangerous, some even devastating.

Kidney stones, rare as they may be, show up mainly in adults, and may prove to be troublesome, painful, worrisome, and may need surgery. Glomerulonephritis is a disease of the kidneys that may go into subacute or chronic condition. It is related mainly to strep infection that has been left without treatment.

The kidneys can malfunction and produce a peculiar disease called nephrosis. Once recognized, this disease ought to be treated promptly and methodically by someone who specializes in it.

Besides that, tumors may occur, though that is rare. Tumors of the kidneys, mainly in the form of Wilm's tumor, show up far more in children than in adults. If discovered early and treated promptly, there is as high as an eighty percent chance of recovery.

Why do doctors frequently check the urine?

Being a waste product, the urine may vary a great deal in amount, frequency, smell, or color.

If the urine shows blood, prompt investigation and treatment will have to be started. Cloudy urine with putrid or fishy smell may mean infection of the urinary tract.

Variation in urine consistency associated with troublesome symptoms of the urinary tract often mean some kind of disease of the urinary tract. They may show up at any age. Keen observation by parents and early diagnosis by the doctor often prompts early energetic treatment, and prevention of a heap of trouble.

What are the common ways of investigation?

When trouble with the urinary tract arises, urinalysis may be the first thing to do. Often, this is followed by a urine culture if there is suspicion of urinary tract infection. To visualize the urinary tract, an X-ray (IVP) of the urinary tract itself will have to be done. Various other forms of investigation (cystoscopy, voiding cystourethrogram etc.) are available, but they are not performed as often.

URINE

A child usually urinates several times a day, but if the frequency drops to only two or three times a day, assess the strength of the stream of urine. If the stream seems weak or interrupted, it may mean some form of obstruction in the urinary passages. If the stream seems strong, ask if it hurts to urinate. If this is the case, especially with girls, it may mean an infected urinary tract.

The shape of the female genitalia, the short urethra, and many other important factors make girls far more susceptible to urinary tract infection than boys are.

A healthy child who tends to drink a small amount of liquids, will of course urinate less, and this obvious point ought to be remembered.

What if the child urinates often?

If he or she urinates often and has some accompanying pain, it often means there is some degree of infection of the urinary tract. This is far more common in girls than boys. There are three important symptoms to watch for in such cases: (a) frequent urination, (b) pain upon urinating, (c) passing only a small amount of urine along with the above symptoms. Any child who has these symptoms ought to be checked by the doctor, and to have the urine looked at.

Of course, there are other causes for frequent urination, such as diabetes, some forms of kidney diseases, etc.

Sometimes excessive drinking of liquids may make the child go to the bathroom often, though not on a chronic basis.

You ought to observe not only the symptoms associated with urinating but also the urine itself.

Why should the urine be observed?

As you know, urine ought to be amber in color, clear, and have its familiar smell.

If it changes color, it may be telling us something. If it is the color of iced tea, there may be a possibility for glomerulonephritis. Dark urine may mean trouble with infectious hepatitis. Bloody urine may mean trouble with nephritis or obstruction. A hazy urine may mean infection of the urinary tract. A change in the color of the urine may also reflect the intake of certain medicines by the child at the time.

Sometimes the urine is clear when passed, but will form a sediment when it cools down, such as when it is put in a refrigerator. As strange as this sounds, such a urine is usually O.K., but it may mean that certain crystals are present. A urinalysis ought to be done anyway, to rule out possible problems.

What if the urine smells different?

Apart from the usual smell, minor changes in the smell of the urine are still within normal limits. This depends on the child's diet to some extent. However, the urine can sometimes smell fishy or putrid. When this happens, it may indicate infection of the urinary tract.

When will a urinalysis and a checkup be important?

1. If the child urinates too frequently, especially if the urine volume is small;
2. If the child (mainly a girl) urinates infrequently and has pain upon urinating;
3. If the child (mainly a boy) urinates infrequently and has a weak or interrupted stream;
4. If he or she has a burning feeling upon urinating;
5. If the urine looks bloody, or if some blood comes after he or she has urinated;
6. If the urine has changed in color to a good extent;
7. If the urine smells "rotten" or "fishy";
8. If the urine is not clear and at the same time the child has some urinary symptoms;
9. If the child passes excessive amounts of urine, and this persists more than a few days;
10. If the child is well toilet trained but starts with frequent "wetting" accidents.

If you seek advice for the above conditions early, the treatment will not be as complicated, nor will the chance for damage be as big.

URINALYSIS, URINE CULTURE, IVP, ETC.

For the investigation of the urinary tract, urinalysis, urine culture, IVP (X-ray of the urinary tract), voiding cystourethrogram and cystoscopy stand out as first tests to choose. They are mentioned in their order of importance and priority, in the minds of most doctors.

Urinalysis gives information in regard to the character of the urine: its concentration (specific gravity), albumin content, sugar content (for sugar diabetes), pus cells (for infection), red cells (for rare conditions), pH (reaction), crystals, etc. Because doctors can get a good deal of information through urinalysis, it is usually done yearly with checkups, and is often done when there is suspicion of certain diseases.

How about urine cultures?

Urine cultures are done for the purpose of detecting the presence of bacteria in the urine. The urine is supposed to be sterile, but when culture of the urine proves to be positive, it will mean infection of some parts of the urinary tract. Urine cultures are rarely needed in males, because they do not tend to get infection of the urinary tract.

Because of the anatomy of their genitalia, females are quite likely to pick up urinary tract infections.

More insidiously, females can be spilling bacteria in the urine without even knowing it, i.e. without having any symptoms. This can be dangerous, since a smoldering low-grade "infection" of their urinary tract can produce a number of serious problems later on in life. This is the reason why cultures of the urine are so important in females.

Why is a non-symptomatic urinary tract infection of concern?

Because a certain percentage of females spill bacteria in the urine without having any symptoms, they will risk damage to the urinary system if they don't discover the problem and treat it. Since there are no symptoms to alert them to it, the only way to discover this condition is to do a screening urine culture once every one to three years for females. If the culture proves positive, the proper treatment can be instituted.

When there are symptoms of urinary tract infection, a definitive urine culture, colony count, and sensitivity are mandatory: In a definitive urine culture, the kind of bacteria can be discovered and identified. A colony count is done along with it, to determine whether the culture has enough bacteria to render it positive (more than 100,000), or suspicious (between 10,000 and 100,000), or negative (less than 10,000). For a definitive urine culture to be complete, a sensitivity test on the bacteria is done. For this test, the bacteria in the urine are exposed to tiny concentrations of certain medicines to see if the medicine can kill them promptly. This test, therefore, will give us a good idea about which medicine should be used for treating the urinary tract infection.

Are there different kinds of cultures, and when should they be done?

Males rarely need to have their urine cultured. Females are to have screening urine cultures with checkups every one to three years. If there are symptoms raising suspicion of urinary tract infection, a definitive urine culture has to be done, as described above.

What is an IVP?

An IVP (intravenous pyelogram) is a series of X-rays of the urinary tract. This test is done after injecting contrast material in the vein, then several X-rays at certain intervals are taken. An IVP can be done at any age, even in tiny babies. It is done if there is suspicion that there is damage to a part of the urinary tract. It can tell a doctor lots of things, from the presence of a stone, to dilatation or disfigurement of the urinary tract, to spots of damage, abnormalities, growths, kinks, etc.

What is a voiding cystourethrogram or cytoscopy?

Simply said, voiding cystourethrogram is a test to show if there is backup pressure of the urine in the bladder upon urinating. It is not needed as often as an IVP, but when it is indicated, it can yield a good deal of useful information. In cystoscopy, a patient is put under anesthesia, and a special instrument is passed through the urethra to the bladder, to take a look at the wall of the bladder.

If a child has repeated infections of the urinary tract, all the above tests will have to be done, i.e. urinalysis, urine culture, colony count, sensitivity, IVP, voiding cystourethrogram, cystoscopy, and possibly even a few others.

THE CASE OF THE BLOODY URINE

The child may discover that the color of his or her urine is red. There may or may not be symptoms of pain upon urinating, an abnormal frequency of urinating (every fifteen to thirty minutes), or fever, but the fact remains that showing blood in the urine is not normal. In some the blood may show up when urinating is almost finished. Some girls may see blood in their underpants. Whenever blood shows up in any of these ways, it ought to be investigated.

What is to be done if my child passes blood in the urine?

Observe carefully the manner in which the blood comes out. Is it mixed with the urine, does it come as bright red drop after the child finishes urinating, are there any other symptoms such as pain, abnormal frequency of urinating, joint swelling, fever, rash, etc? Your doctor will need detailed information of the symptoms.

Most likely the doctor will want a clean-catch urine specimen (see page 417) in a sterile container, so that he or she will be able to do a urine culture and colony count.

If these tests are negative, your doctor may want to recommend an IVP (X-ray of the urinary tract), and a voiding cystourethrogram. If the X-rays show trouble, then the doctor will explain the problem and how to treat it.

But if the X-rays are negative, the next step might be what is called cystoscopy to be done by the urologist. From now on the investigation can become quite involved, to the point where it might be very confusing to the parent.

If my girl shows blood in her underpants, where does it come from?

The blood may come from the female external genitalia. The doctor will check the female genitalia, the urinary tract, and the female organs. He or she will look for any discharge from and any possible points of trouble in the external genitalia, and may want the girl to be checked by a gynecologist for further investigation.

Of course, if the blood in her underpants does not seem to be connected with the urine at all, the doctor may concentrate on the genital organs.

In a baby boy who has some blood on the diapers, the cause may easily be traced to an ulcer on the opening of the tip of his penis. This is not rare and is easily correctable.

Sometimes a baby passes urine that stains the diaper an unusual pink color. It is often mistaken for blood by the parents, but to the trained eyes of the doctor it is easily discernible as being caused by urate crystals that are sometimes present in the urine. These show up in perfectly normal children, and parents don't have to worry about it.

URINARY TRACT INFECTION

She rushes to the bathroom often, perhaps as often as every fifteen minutes or so. She says it burns upon urinating, and she may cross her legs as if trying to hold back her urine. Her temperature may be up, she may be grouchy and cross, and may have a poor appetite. Sometimes there may even be vague abdominal pains. Her parents start suspecting some trouble with the bladder, or a urinary tract infection.

Why do you say "she"?

As stated before, urinary tract infections are far more common in females than in males; the cause and effect are probably due to the particular anatomy of the female genitalia. It is easy for the germs to ascend through the short urethra of the female to the bladder, and on through the rest of the urinary tract. These infections can affect females of all ages, from babyhood to adulthood. It is not unusual for a girl to have these infections a number of times.

It is quite rare for a boy to get it. If a boy shows up with signs of urinary tract infection, he should be investigated thoroughly to see if he has abnormalities of the urinary tract. If such is the case, he may need surgical correction.

How do you investigate the girls?

By the time a girl gets her second or third bout of urinary tract infection, we administer a battery of tests and X-rays (see page 413). Some doctors start the investigation earlier. If anatomical abnormalities show up through these investigations, then a urologist will take over.

Sometimes there is infection but there are no symptoms whatsoever.

How can I find out about the infection if my child has no symptoms?

Urinalysis is usually of some help. A screening urine culture is better (see page 413). To have a clean-catch urine, do the following:

Get the first urine specimen in the morning if possible. Make sure you do the following: (1) Clean the genitalia from front to back with soap and water, then rinse well; (2) Collect the specimen in a clean well-rinsed-sterilized jar; (3) Collect a mid-stream urine specimen (interrupt the urine stream with the jar); (4) If the specimen is collected the night before, keep it in the refrigerator; (5) Leave the specimen in the refrigerator until you are ready to come to the office, and (6) bring the specimen inside a plastic bag full of ice chips.

How long will she have to be treated?

If she has an acute infection, she should be on the medicine for a short period of time, maybe for two weeks or less. The doses should be given regularly without fail. If not, there will be a good chance for a relapse, especially during the first six to twelve months after the infection.

The symptoms often disappear in three to four days, but the child should continue on the medicine for the course of treatment; some doctors even recommend using the medicine for as long as three to six weeks.

The urine should be cultured after the treatment is finished to make sure the infection is gone.

Are there different forms of urinary tract infections?

A urinary tract infection with symptoms (as opposed to the silent form) can be mild, severe, recurrent, chronic, etc. Babies can suffer from it, though it is not that common in them.

The biggest trouble with urinary tract infection is that it tends to recur, often for many times. In these situations, investigation has to be done, and frequent courses of medications may have to be given, with cultures, colony count, and sensitivity tests. When relapses are frequent, it is not unusual to put the poor child on a tedious prolonged course of medication, for six to twelve months or longer!

Are there any preventive measures?

Yes, and they are well worth observing.

1. Upon having a bowel movement, let the child wipe herself from the front to the back (this is often forgotten).
2. Practice good hygiene of the bottom.
3. Let the child take showers instead of baths.
4. Avoid bubble baths.
5. Let her use cotton pants, and make sure they are not too tight. (avoid nylon or polyester pants.)
6. Do screening urine cultures, preferably yearly.
7. Have urinary tract infections treated promptly once symptoms show up.
8. Urine cultures will guide the doctor during treating the infection and after it is controlled. Many such cultures will have to be taken.

GLOMERULONEPHRITIS

The child may have been irritable lately, somewhat feverish, and may have been complaining of a headache or some stomachache, particularly in the flank area. His or her color is also slightly "off" if not pale.

You look more closely and you will see that there is some degree

of swelling under the eyes, mainly in the lower eyelids. The child
may volunteer to say that it hurts to urinate. You notice the urine
looks dark, like iced tea.

What does all this mean?
It may mean that the child's two kidneys are affected with this
disease. A urinalysis is needed, and a series of blood tests may have
to be done. The doctor will check the child thoroughly, paying
special attention not only to the blood pressure which often becomes
high, but also to the child's legs, to see if there is any swelling.

In mild cases the symptoms are often not that severe. In severe
cases, however, a high blood pressure, trouble urinating, possible
convulsions and other scary symptoms can be severe and even life
threatening.

What causes glomerulonephritis?
This is a disease that is an aftermath of certain types of strep
infections that have been left without treatment. It usually follows
such infections by about one to two weeks, and it is likely to show up
in a small percentage of such cases.

The strep infection may have been in the form of a sore throat or
an upper respiratory infection that has been ignored, or in the form
of impetigo that has been ignored or treated improperly.

What will the doctor do?
In a good many, if not the majority of cases, the child will
have to be admitted to the hospital. It may take one to two weeks of
hospitalization if not longer. Close observation will be paid to the
patient's blood pressure, the degree of swelling, and the amount of
urine passed. A good many tests will have to be done to assess the
progress of the disease. The child will also be required to stay in
bed for some time and may be given a special diet.

What will happen to the child afterwards?
Glomerulonephritis can be very troublesome in the acute stage,
i.e. while the child is still in the hospital. That is the reason for
all the tests and the energetic treatment. Fortunately, when the
acute condition is over, the recovery will progress smoothly in most

cases. The urine (and perhaps the child too) are to be rechecked on several occasions, though.

Can we prevent this disease?

You stand a better-than-fifty-percent chance of preventing glomerulonephritis if you keep treating and eradicating strep infections. This is as true of strep throats as it is of impetigo, and is the reason why throat cultures and cultures on impetigo are taken so frequently. Strep is the villain in this game.

If someone has an iced-tea-colored urine, does it necessarily indicate this disease?

No; the color of the urine is only one of the manifestations of glomerulonephritis. There have to be other signs and symptoms (as mentioned at the start of this section) for a diagnosis.

That color, by the way, is caused by red blood cells in the urine, along with other components. However, if it is not associated with other signs and symptoms of glomerulonephritis, it might mean a different disease or problem. Of course, when any urine looks odd to you, have it checked, be it in the presence of symptoms or not.

Will the blood pressure come down to normal too?

Yes in practically all cases, as will the swelling of the eyelids, the iced-tea-color urine, the stomachache, the headache, and all other symptoms. When the glomerulonephritis is over, and the child seems to be normal to you, he or she should still continue to be under the supervision of the doctor.

BEDWETTING

The child wakes up in the morning soaking wet, smelling of urine, feeling bad because of what had happened, and the parent feels exasperated, yet helpless.

Bedwetting may be regular -almost every night and even twice a night- but in milder cases it may occur only occasionally. This seems to go on and on, and the parents have tried punishing, ignoring, screaming, lecturing, waking the child up, restricting fluids, but alas, nothing seems to have helped.

What causes bedwetting?

No one really knows for sure, that is why it is so difficult to control. Children whose parents were bed-wetters, who are under emotional tension, or have trouble of the urinary tract itself, are more likely to suffer.

Whatever the alleged cause may be, an important question is when to attempt to remedy this nasty situation. Occasional wetting before the age of about four years is certainly to be tolerated, and you don't have to do anything about it yet.

What would you do after the child is four?

A child that old, who wets the bed only occasionally (one or two times a month), can still be accepted as normal. Patience, offering less to drink after dinner, and avoiding pressuring the child too much, may be all that you need.

If the child wets the bed more often than that, especially if it happens every night, then there are a few steps to be taken.

What will the doctor do?

Have the child checked first, especially the genitalia. The urine ought to be checked too to make sure there is no urinary tract infection. If the child is six or seven years old or older, an X-ray of the urinary tract may even be advisable, to spot any possible abnormalities there.

If all the above are normal, a medicine by the name of Tofranil (prescription) may be given internally, and it can help in a good percentage of cases. A full three-month course should be tried if the medicine proves to be successful. A second or even third course might be needed if the wetting starts again after the medicine is stopped. Many an older child will need no more than one course in most cases.

However, if the medicine doesn't seem to work within two weeks, you might as well stop it, and assume that the child didn't respond to it.

Concomitant with the medicine, do not offer anything to drink after dinner, and make sure that the child goes to the bathroom before going to bed. When he or she wakes up and the bed feels dry, offer your good approval to boost the morale.

In case the medicine doesn't help, there is a machine that can be of some help.

What kind of machine?

You can purchase such a machine through your local drug store or places like Sears, Roebuck & Co.

The machine works on the principle of conditioning. There is a special pad to be put on the bed. When the child passes only a tiny amount of urine, the machine will be activated. A bright light will turn on immediately, a loud noisy bell will ring, and the child and many others at home will wake up instantly. It is important that the child becomes fully awake, and some authorities say that he or she should change the bed at that time of night too.

This method of treatment may sound cruel, but as a last resort it is worth a try. The machine has to be used for several months.

Lately a modification of the above apparatus has become available, and probably will soon replace it. It uses the same principle but is much easier to use (the sensor is attached to the child's underpants). Wet-stop can be ordered through Palco Laboratories, 5026 Scotts Valley Dr, CA 95066. Another good devise is by the name of Nytone. It can be ordered though Medical Products, Inc., Salt Lake City, UT 84119.

There is also a theory that a wetter's bladder cannot hold as much urine as a non-wetter's can. When the child grows up, the bladder will also become bigger and by adolescence, the size will be adequate.

Yet, there are ways to stretch the bladder:

1. Most four to six-year-old children will tend to hold themselves from urinating. You will see them squirming, moving their legs this way and that, yet they would rather do this than go to the bathroom. This is nature's way to stretch the bladder so that the child will not wet the bed. Many parents mistakenly tell the child to go to the bathroom rather than keep twisting and twirling, so be aware of this and don't let the squirming annoy you.
2. For a proven bed-wetter, you may want to start a regime to stretch

his or her bladder. Offer the child a great deal of liquids to drink during daytime, especially before noon. This will make him or her want to urinate more often. At the same time, encourage the child to hold the urine as much as possible, even to the point of pain. You may even encourage self competition by letting the child urinate in a bottle and see if he or she can urinate a bigger amount than previously. If the child cooperates, then the bladder will gradually become bigger over a period of three to four months, and you will stand a fair chance of stopping the wetting.

All the methods described above are exasperating, but bed-wetting in itself is more so.

How about the bed-wetter who is under stress?
This happens when the family moves to a new neighborhood, or upon the arrival of a new baby, or if there is a stressful situation in the family or in the school.

Most such cases of bed-wetting ought to be accepted with patience and calmness. Don't get too mad, just try to see what is bothering the child. You and the pediatrician will help find out what is causing the problem.

The child may have insecure feelings and stressful circumstances around that cause them to not respond to any of the above treatment. The child may show signs of trouble discernible to the pediatrician, who may recommend specialized action. Fortunately this is quite rare.

How about those who wet themselves during daytime?
Some such children may need full investigation of the urinary tract including urinalysis, urine culture, X-ray, etc. Yet many others can be ignored, especially if the child is five or six years old, since often it is caused by laziness and by an intense interest in playing.

MEATAL STENOSIS

Meatal stenosis shows up mainly in males, is a fairly common condition, and it can easily be detected. The term meatal stenosis means narrowing of the opening through which the urine is passed to the outside. (If a male is not circumcised, norrowing of the opening of the prepuce is called phimosis.)

What can this condition cause?

With meatal stenosis, there will be partial obstruction of urinary flow. In other words the urine stream will not pass freely or with ease. If this continues for a long time, i.e. years, it can gradually affect the integrity of the urinary tract. The degree of trouble will depend on the degree of the stenosis and its duration.

Therefore, there will be a chance for the backed-up urine to affect the bladder, and in rare cases this will lead to some untoward effect to the ureters and even the kidneys. While this aftereffect is not that common, when it occurs it can be serious or devastating, posing a potential danger to the health of the growing child. The changes are insidious and can be almost imperceptible.

Can we tell if the child has meatal stenosis?

There are a few visible indications. Watch the stream of the urine and see how strong it is. If the boy urinates with a strong urine stream, he is O.K. If he urinates with a weak urine stream, or with an intermittent stream, especially if he grunts or pushes upon urinating, then mention that to the doctor. Also check the size of the meatus and see if it is small; and ask the doctor to check it too.

What can be done about it?

In some cases of meatal stenosis, the meatus can be enlarged in the doctor's office with forceps. In more advanced ones, the child will have to have a small operation. The operation, called meatotomy, consists simply of surgically enlarging the small opening, making it easy for the urine stream to pass through.

Is it common to see damage to the urinary system?

Fortunately this is rare. Most cases of meatal stenosis are easily detectible and correctable, and often they are mild. Therefore the urinary system will be less likely to be subject to the effect of the urine back-pressure for a prolonged period.

This doesn't suggest to ignore the condition. On the contrary, since it is an easy thing to diagnose, every parent should be on the alert if it occurs, and see the doctor.

In some cases of mild hypospadias (whereby the meatus is not at the tip of the penis, and instead it will be in the underneath surface of the penis) the chance for meatal stenosis is increased. This means that both the doctor and parent should look for such a possibility and take the usual measures to correct it.

HYDROCELE

You notice that the sac of your boy's testicles is full, usually on one side. The fullness varies in size, but certainly it looks and feels as if there is some fluid or water within. This hydrocele is called "water on the testicle" by some people, and is not very common. It is not painful or tender and the baby or child seems not to mind it. To your surprise, however, you may notice that the size varies from time to time, and becomes slightly bigger when he is standing up or screaming.

What causes such a problem?

The testicles lie in the sac designed for them (scrotum). Each testicle is covered by a special sac communicating with the cavity of the abdomen by a thin narrow tube before birth. In most cases, this tube is closed and obliterated by the time the boy is born. In a few, however, this tube remains open. When it remains open, it can lead to hernia formation, and quite often a hydrocele.

A hydrocele can develop without a hernia, and if not treated it can become quite big. Hydroceles on both sides are not unusual. But the importance of the hydrocele is its potential to lead to a hernia, if not now, then perhaps in the months or even years ahead (see page 370). If a hernia develops, an operation will have to be done to fix it, and the sooner this is done the better.

In many, however, a hydrocele may show up by itself and no matter how hard you look for a hernia, you will not be able to find one.

What is to be done about it?

In case there is a hydrocele with a hernia, when the hernia is operated on the hydrocele will disappear. On the other hand, if the hydrocele is small in size and if it is not associated with a hernia, it may gradually be absorbed and go away. No surgical treatment is needed, but the process may take several months or even years.

If the hydrocele is large, a surgeon will have to handle the problem.

Will a hydrocele affect reproduction?

Although a hydrocele is an accumulation of fluid in the sac that surrounds a testicle, the fluid distends the sac to the outside. Thus the testicle will not be compressed or undergo any damage, and it will function as usual when the child reaches maturity. This is the rule in practically all cases.

Is this the only kind of hydrocele?

The hydrocele described above is the most common type; however, hydrocele of the spermatic cord may also occur. This may even be mistaken for a hernia. It usually shows up as a firm, nonpainful, nontender mass along the course of the spermatic cord, usually the size of a small walnut. In other words, it usually shows up in areas where you expect to detect a hernia. When this kind of hydrocele is discovered, an operation will have to be done to remove it. A hydrocele of the cord does not go away by itself and if left unoperated on, it may lead to complications.

UNDESCENDED TESTICLE

One side of the scrotum seems small and shrivelled, and upon feeling the area one testicle doesn't seem to be there. This is more difficult to detect if he happens to be a tiny baby.

Is this common?

A truly undescended testicle is not that common. More often, however, the testicle temporarily hides up in a receptacle (inguinal canal), leaving its usual place empty and forlorn. This "hiding testicle" is very common, and is the usual case when the baby is cold, thereby the scrotum is contracted and shriveled on itself.

In tiny babies -and especially in prematures- one or both testicles may not be completely descended. It takes some time, perhaps months, before they come down completely. They can be felt almost at the junction of the scrotum with the tissues of the pubis.

Why are normal testicles in a sac anyway?

The reason is that the temperature in the scrotum (sac of the testicle) is lower than body temperature, and for the testicles to function normally, they require this lower temperature. A truly undescended testicle may hide in the lower part of the abdomen or inside the abdomen. If it remains there for many years, especially longer than two or three years, its function will suffer and it will not produce as many sperms in the future as it usually would, thus becoming less fertile.

Are there other concerns if they are not in place?

Yes, there are two dangers besides the lowered fertility. An undescended testicle that is not corrected is more likely to develop cancer of the testicle. This is rare, but needless to say, quite serious.

More often than that, an undescended testicle left in its place suffers from the likelihood of physical injury. Most undescended testicles hide in a canal, while on the way down from the abdomen, during the development of the baby before being born. The area where it hides is the same as that of an inguinal hernia, i.e. the lower part of the abdomen above the groin. The testicle may show as a firm bulge and can easily be felt and even moved slightly from side to side. The child, being as active as he is, may expose himself to a hit, a fall, or some other physical injury to that area. If this happens, then the testicle may receive some damage.

A doctor's diagnosis is important about whether or not the testicle is undescended.

Why should the doctor evaluate it?

It is not always easy to decide if the testicle is truly undescended or not, especially in a small baby. A few months may be needed until the baby is a little bigger before such decisions can be agreed upon. In some, undescended testicle may be quite obvious, yet in others there are conditions that can mimic this problem and cause difficulty in diagnosis.

A truly undescended testicle may be on one side or (less often) both. Either way, we have to wait until the child is one to three years old before the condition is corrected by surgery.

Do we have to operate?

The majority of true undescended testicles need an operation. The surgeon will have to bring the testicle down to its sac, and this usually requires a few days in the hospital. The difficulty and extent of the operation depend on the location of the testicle. More important, however, is the timing of the operation. Most surgeons agree now that the operation is to be done before the child is three years old (preferably around one year), to avoid as early as possible the potential problems mentioned above.

Not all undescended testicles need an operation. There are hormone shots that can be given for a short period of time and they may enable the testicle to come down; these work if the location of the problem testicle is near the opening to the scrotum. There is only a certain measure of success with the shots, and if they don't work, then an operation will have to be done.

A number of years back, many surgeons waited until the child became an adolescent before they tackled the problem. This proved to be far inferior and more dangerous than tackling the problem before the age of three years. When done at the proper time, the testicles usually function and behave in a normal manner.

What is the reason for the testicles to "get stuck"?

For all males during development inside the womb, the testicles are shaped and molded inside their abdomen. These testicles slowly travel along a certain course to come down to the scrotum by the time of birth or before that. In some babies, for special reasons (known and unknown), the testicle gets stopped along its way.

The "hiding testicle" mentioned above is far more common, and if the baby is given a bath or warmed up, you will see that the testicle will come down to its usual spot. You will see and feel the testicle in the scrotum when the weather is warm or upon giving a bath to the baby, since the testicular sac will not be contracted.

VULVOVAGINITIS

She complains that her bottom hurts and it may be itchy. It may hurt only on some occasions, or continually. Occasionally it hurts when she urinates, when she has bowel movement, or while walking or sitting.

There may also be a discharge. This discharge may be scant, just enough to stain her underpants a few times a day, or it may be profuse. The discharge may be smelly at times, and it may even be bloody.

The little girl, restless and irritable, may attempt to scratch herself or rub the area against furniture. She may be scolded for that, but the poor girl is only trying to relieve her discomfort.

When mother looks at the child's genitalia, she may see a somewhat red inflamed area, or it may have a dry, chapped appearance.

What causes vulvovaginitis?

The above condition is fairly common. It has many causes, the commonest being inadequate hygiene of the area. The area is soiled easily, and after having a bowel movement, many a girl will wipe herself from the back forward, thus carrying the germs toward the vagina. This will then lead to infection of the genitalia, especially in younger girls.

Tight-fitting underpants, especially when made of fiber other than cotton, are an important cause too. The underpants will be soiled by the area, and along with the sweat they can be a good medium to transfer the infection (cotton absorbs the sweat, thus it is not as bad as synthetic fiber).

Another source of infection can occur if the child plays with herself often. When she develops a respiratory infection, her fingers may become contaminated upon blowing her nose, or simply by sucking her thumb. These contaminated fingers can become a means of infecting her genitalia. Another cause is when the child puts a foreign body in the vagina, and that is not as rare as you may think.

There are other specific causes too, such as local fungus infection, gonorrhea (yes, even in little ones; it comes from soiled linens, from adults with gonorrhea, and not always from sexual contact), and many others.

Pinworms can sometimes be the source too. The worm comes out of the anus, and it may wiggle its way into the vagina. In such cases, the itching can be troublesome and even severe at times, and the vaginitis won't clear up unless the worms are eradicated (see page 376).

If she has some discharge, shall I be concerned about it?

That depends on many factors. If a milky or even bloody discharge shows up in a baby who is a few days old, it should be regarded as normal. Such a discharge is the result of the effect of the female hormones from the mother during pregnancy.

If the girls' underpants get soiled more than two or three times a day -especially if the discharge has a yellowish tinge- have it checked. This is particularly true if there are other symptoms, or if the genitalia looks red and inflamed. In a pre-adolescent girl, a thin mucousy discharge is not unusual, but if it looks pussy or becomes profuse, then consult the doctor.

What will the doctor do?

Aside from a checkup with close attention to the female organs, a culture may have to be taken and a test for pinworms done. The type of treatment will depend on the cause of the trouble. Sometimes the girl may have to be referred to a gynecologist.

Can we prevent vulvovaginitis?

In many you certainly can. Teach the girl always to wipe her bottom from the front to the back. Use underpants made of cotton fiber if at all possible. Make sure the underpants fit correctly, not too tightly (i.e. they should not make a deep wedge between the legs). Treat pinworms promptly. Discourage the child from playing with the genitalia.

Consult the doctor in case the discharge becomes heavy, smelly, yellowish in color and/or bloody; or if it is associated with soreness, itchiness, and pain.

How about the inserted foreign body?

The girl tends to have a foul smelling discharge, quite often bloody and possibly profuse. The foreign body inserted by the girl into her vagina may be in the form of rolled-up wads of toilet tissue, cotton, wool, etc. It may also be glass (such as a medicine dropper), or metallic (such as a bobby pin or safety pin), or some other hard object. X-rays may be needed to help show the metallic foreign body; a rectal exam and perhaps vaginoscopy may have to be performed too.

A child who does that to herself is likely to be a repeater, and should be watched carefully to help prevent future trouble.

CHAPTER FIFTEEN

THE SKIN

the skin
dry skin
atopic dermatitis (eczema)
but it is only a rash
impetigo
boils
cellulitis and abscesses
lymphangitis (blood poisoning)
ringworm
hives
pityriasis rosea
poison ivy
paronychia (infection around the nail)
hematoma of the nail
strawberry hemangioma
athlete's foot
bee stings
bites (dogs, cats, and humans)
urticaria papulosa (the pet and the itch)
acne
warts
sunburn
scalds and burns
the bald spot
lice

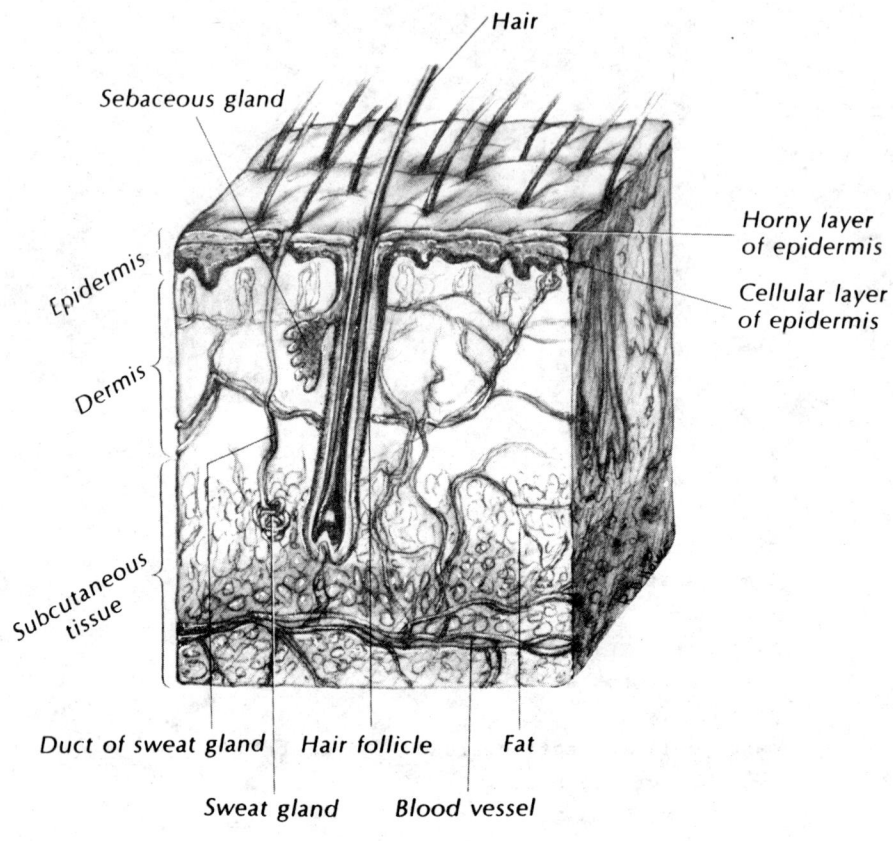

Courtesy Barbara Bates, M.D.
from a Guide to Physical Examination, p 43
Written permission from the publisher, J. B. Lippincott Co.

THE SKIN

The skin is the largest organ of the body surface-wise; it covers the whole surface area, keeps the fluids inside, evaporates moisture, and sweats when need be. It affords the pleasure of touch, the feeling of warmth and coolness, and shows the hue of health. Its integrity will have to be observed, otherwise pain, scarring, and disease may leave their imprint on it. To understand skin, we need to have an idea of what it is.

What does skin consist of?

The skin consists of many layers. On the surface there is a cornified layer covered with a very thin oily layer secreted by the sebaceous glands, which are deeply imbedded in the skin. Below that there is a thin layer which produces cells to replenish the shedding cells on the outside. These layers constitute the epidermis.

Further down there is the dermis, wherein fat is stored in loose tissue of variable thickness depending on the person's amount of fat. In this layer of fat many blood vessels branch out into tiny microscopic capillaries. Nerves abide profusely there too, thus giving us a good means to feel and react to outside environmental conditions. Along with the blood vessels and nerves, there are minute vessels (lymph vessels) that carry the lymph to the central part of the body, usually pouring into the lymph nodes first, but eventually ending in the blood circulation. In addition, the oil glands of the skin coil on themselves like a snake, and hide in this layer of the dermis. The hair follicles too originate in this layer, and shoot upwards to go through the epidermis to appear on the skin.

What insults can the skin be exposed to?

Having such a large surface area, the skin stands to receive numerous insults. Naturally physical injuries such as cuts, lacerations, bites, and abrasions are well known to all. But besides that, infections are quite common, since bacteria and fungi are always there waiting for the opportune moment to do their dirty work. Children in particular are likely to be the victims, developing things like impetigo, pyoderma, boils and carbuncles, ringworm, diaper rashes, etc.

The skin may also suffer along with other organs in certain diseases, such as chickenpox, measles, German measles (rubella), roseola, meningitis, and purpura among many others. Diseases of some of the individual components of the skin can be troublesome too. Acne is a good example, or trouble of the pigment of the skin as in leukoderma.

An individual's skin, be it inherited or otherwise, may play a part, since the skin is in contact with so many chemicals or different kinds of clothes. This may show in the form of dermatitis or eczema. Dermatitis of the feet in children is fairly common especially when their feet sweat so much while they are wearing sneakers.

DRY SKIN

Dry skin is a common phenomenon, and a good deal of it is a result of man-made products. The child's skin looks dry, even flaky. He or she may scratch and scratch, and the skin may also be rough to the touch, with tiny bumps, particularly on the surface of the outside of the arms and legs. When the condition is left uncorrected, the child may become the victim of primary irritant dermatitis.

What is that?

Primary irritant dermatitis is a special form of dermatitis where the child develops many spots on the skin. These spots are usually circular or oval in shape, flaky, and ill-defined at the edges. They may appear anywhere on the body but more commonly in the areas of the driest skin.

What causes dry skin?

The skin's several layers (see page 435) have special cells in different arrangements and with specific functions. On the surface of the skin there is a thin oily film secreted by the oil glands. This oily film will help the outer cells of the skin to keep their integrity and will prevent the skin from drying out too fast. The film is essential for the skin's good function and integrity. It is affected by several parameters, some of which are inherited, others are caused by us.

When the oily film is diminished or even removed by frequent bathing or washing, naturally dry skin will be the result. Frequent bathing (especially with hot water), staying in the tub for prolonged periods (twenty minutes or longer), along with vigorous use of soap and bubble bath, are the main adversaries of the oily film and the integrity of the skin. They form the main and most frequent causes of dry skin; yet they can easily be corrected.

Hereditary dry skin can be helped, but not cured; in these cases the oil glands are simply less active than usual. Luckily, hereditary dry skin is not very common.

Are there other causes for dry skin?

Yes, there are many others, but one of them stands out. It is important during wintertime. When the central heating system starts working, the relative humidity of the house drops greatly and may reach even the ten to twenty percent level. This will be an important contributing factor for dry skin and (furniture).

What can we do about dry skin?

Because taking frequent baths is one of the causes of dry skin, bathing twice a week or even once a week is recommended along with washing feet, bottoms, and dirty areas whenever needed. Being in the bathtub for as short a time as possible, or preferably taking a shower instead, is a good practice. Tepid water is better than hot.

Use "soapless soap" such as Neutrogena, Lowilla, Alpha Keri, instead of regular soap. Aveeno Oilated or Aveeno Colloidal, Alpha Keri, and the like are also acceptable as a soap substitute.

When the child is out of the tub, you may want to put Alpha Keri on his or her skin. You may continue to apply Alpha Keri directly to the skin, daily, until the skin looks supple enough. This may take anywhere from one to five weeks, depending on how dry the skin was to begin with.

Keri lotion, Lubriderm, Eucerin, or some powders like Caldesene or Talcum, are worth using after a bath too.

Can we prevent dry skin?

The above-mentioned bath and shower techniques will also help as preventive measures. These preventive measures are important especially when started in the fall and continued through winter and spring. Your measure of success may be much greater than you expect.

How about humidifiers?

A central humidifier is a very good thing to install. It should put the level of humidity at around forty to forty-five percent. This will help prevent dry skin significantly. It will also help reduce the chance for upper respiratory infections (see page 307). Besides all that, even your furniture, doors, wood, etc., will benefit from a normal moisture.

ATOPIC DERMATITIS
(ECZEMA)

Atopic dermatitis is not an uncommon condition. The child's skin tends to be dry, somewhat rough and red, and may be scaly or even ooze at times. In an infant, the cheeks are quite prone to show this condition, but as he or she grows older, a number of areas (especially the front of the elbows and the back of the knee joints) may also develop this condition.

In more severe instances the condition may become generalized, affecting large areas of the skin, but it may also show up in patches.

A common problem to all the above is a very itchy feeling, sometimes severe. The trouble is that the more the child scratches, the more the area will become irritated.

What causes atopic dermatitis?

Quite often the child is born with a tendency to develop atopic dermatitis. He or she is most likely to be the allergic child, who has respiratory or gastrointestinal allergy. You may even be able to discover some relationship between a kind of food and a worsening of the skin condition (food allergy). Not only that, but you often find the skin to react differently than normal skin to many things.

How does this kind of skin react to other things?

The skin of a child with atopic dermatitis tends to overreact, so to speak. Rubbing, itching, contact with wool and synthetic fiber (such as nylon and polyester), and dry, hot weather that leads to too much sweating are all likely to make the condition worse.

Worst of all, bathing especially with strong soaps can play havoc with affected skin. In fact, any contact with water, particularly when frequent, can be quite troublesome, especially if soap is used (see page 436).

Can we do anything to relieve atopic dermatitis?

Yes, a good deal can be done by you, but above all you have to be patient and understanding. Anything that is likely to irritate the skin should be avoided.

Bathing should be at minimum, once a week or less, and the bath should be very brief (a shower is preferable). The child is to be patted dry (not rubbed), and the soap used should be one of the very mild ones such as Neutrogena, Lowilla, Alpha Keri, Aveeno, Basis, etc.

If possible, the undershirts, underpants, bedsheets, pillowcases, pajamas, and other underwear should all be made of cotton. Cotton is the least irritating of the fibers. Avoid fabrics made of wool, nylon, and polyester, since they can lead to trouble. This precaution includes preventing the child from resting his or her cheeks against your coat, sweater, or any other clothing made of such fibers, and it may even include preventing him or her from crawling on a carpeted floor.

A dry, hot indoor climate during wintertime may lead to too much sweating, thus making the condition worse. A room temperature of 68 degrees F during wintertime, with a relative humidity of forty to forty-five percent (by a central humidifier) must be your goal. An air-conditioned environment during summertime will also help a lot.

Will these precautions cure the child's condition?

No, they will simply help prevent any more of the skin from becoming more itchy, irritated and inflamed, and they will help make the existing condition milder. There is no cure for this condition, and the child will often pass through many different stages in the development of this disease, throughout life.

Sooner or later you will be in need of medical help, not only for the diagnosis but also for treatment. The doctor will determine the degree and extent of the condition, give you the proper ointment or an internal medicine, and may suggest a good many points not mentioned above. He or she may also recommend that the child be seen by a dermatologist, if the atopic dermatitis is more advanced or very extensive.

By helping keep this condition under control, there will be less chance for complications, and even an upswing in the child's temperament and well-being.

Contact dermatitis is not a contagious condition, but it is genetic; it is fairly common for the parents or someone else in the family to have suffered from it in their earlier years.

BUT IT IS ONLY A RASH

A parent cannot be expected to know every kind of rash children get. There are numerous diseases associated with rash. Some are common and some are rare. The same disease may not show up with rash except on rare occasions. Some rashes show up as tiny red spots, which blanch on pressure, others will not disappear upon pressure, some are slightly hard, others are rough to the touch, some large, others blotchy, some are itchy, many are not. Some rashes appear mainly on the trunk, others mainly on the limbs, some are localized, others are generalized. Some rashes represent skin diseases, others are part of a contagious disease. Some rashes may have a special course of their own, others are fleety, i.e. show up now but in a few hours will disappear.

As you see, there are numerous diseases with numerous kinds of rash, and it is almost impossible to diagnose the condition over the phone. The child will have to be seen to be diagnosed.

<u>What kind of contagious diseases cause rash?</u>

A few contagious diseases with rash are still seen these days. Good examples are scarlatina and chickenpox. Roseola is seen commonly but it is not that contagious. Measles and rubella (German Measles) used to be common, but not anymore due to immunization. However, they are highly contagious.

Scarlatina rash is bright red, pin point, mainly on the trunk, but not on the face (see page 155). Chickenpox rash is blistery, becomes pussy, then dries up into a scab within a few days. It shows up more on the trunk than the limbs (see page 157). Roseola rash shows up in babies, and it follows a rise of temperature of 3 days duration, the rash is pink in color and generalized (see page 153).

What about the itchy hives?

Hives are more likely to be caused by allergies (especially to food) than other causes. It may be a symptom of a viral infection, strep infection, or drug reaction.

The rash of hives is fleety. It usually has a raised edge (called a wheal) and each spot is a different shape and size. Quite often it is very itchy.

Fortunately, hives are self-limited in most cases, and treatment with an antihistamine such as benadryl will keep it under control (see page 450).

Does poison ivy rash look like hives?

No, poison ivy does not look like hives. Poison ivy is intensely itchy, but the lesions are usually red, tiny pimply elevations on the skin, which sometimes ooze a clear yellowish fluid. One very important indicator of poison ivy is the development of the lesions along the scratch marks (see page 454).

There is one more thing to remember about rashes, i.e. there is a degree of mimicry.

You mean rashes can look alike!

Some diseases mimic others, and the rash of the same disease may look different in two different patients. Sometimes different stages of the same rash occur at the same time in the same patient.

IMPETIGO

Impetigo lesions of the skin can have many shapes. Most of them are small in size, yet some can be the size of a quarter or larger. They are not particularly itchy.

The floor of the lesion is red and slightly raised, the edge even more so. On top of the lesion there may be a honey-yellow crust, often crumbly because it is brittle. On other lesions, the surface may be blistery and filled with pus.

The lesions seem to spread slowly. At first, there are one or two of them, but they insidiously multiply into several lesions clustered in the same vicinity.

Will my child suffer?

There will usually be no fever, no loss of appetite, no vomiting, or other symptoms. The child will be going on in his or her usual rambunctious manner, playing and shouting.

The lesions, however, will continue to spread slowly, the more you wait. The child may even be peppered with them on the face, trunk, arms, and even the head.

It is true that impetigo can and may disappear by itself, but that is a slow, troublesome process, and may even be dangerous, especially after having affected the child for so long. Therefore it is better to have it treated early before it spreads all over.

Does it come from dirt?

Dirty children may get it more frequently, but impetigo can affect children who are immaculately clean as well. It is caused by either the staph or strep germ. A scratch of the skin at the proper place and the proper time is likely to introduce any of these germs that happen to be at the skin, thus leading to impetigo.

Is it contagious?

Yes, it can be transmitted via contact by playing with other infected children. You don't have to separate your child completely from others, but be cautious. It is also advised not to let the infected child swim with others, or use the towels of the brothers or sisters.

Can it lead to real trouble?

Impetigo caused by strep, if not treated properly, can lead to glomerulonephritis. This is somewhat rare, but it can happen. Therefore, a culture of the skin lesion is advisable to see if there is strep or staph, and if strep is present, then an antibiotic for ten days should be started.

What is the usual treatment for impetigo?

Neosporin, Bacimycin, Neopolycin, or similar ointments are usually sufficient (all nonprescription). These are used three or four times a day for a week or so. Bathing with Phisohex (prescription) will help prevent spreading of the lesions all over the affected child. Possibly the boiling of underwear, pillow cases, or even bedsheets (to kill the germs on them) can be of help. This is to be done for a few days only. A course of an antibiotic to be given internally for five to ten days is often prescribed, depending on the results of the culture.

Does impetigo look like other skin diseases?

Though it is easy to pinpoint impetigo, in some cases it can mimic other diseases. The circular kind of impetigo may look like ringworm, or the deep kind (echthyma) can look like a deep-seated boil.

Can insect bites lead to impetigo?

An insect bite can become infected, mainly because of itching, thus introducing the infection. Ticks, especially in the scalp, can give us this trouble, as can lice.

BOILS

The child develops a small red lump, tender to the touch and somewhat painful. It may come to a head, becomes pointed at the tip, and then opens and pours out some bloody, pussy fluid. There may be a yellow core inside which may stay where it is for a day or two, or it may pop out if you press the area around the boil hard enough.

Sometimes the boil won't open up and pour out pus. Instead, in extreme cases, it may become bigger and bigger, and it develops several "eyes," each of which may have its own core. This is called a carbuncle.

What causes such a problem?

Boils and carbuncles are caused by the staph germ. Quite often there will only be one boil, and when it goes away, the trouble is over. Sometimes however, new boils will show up in different places and at different times. This may go on for a number of months, if not even for years, and it can become quite a problem.

Boils can show up just about anywhere on the body. They are quite troublesome if they are near the anus, the nose, or the upper lip and the vicinity.

If a boil is near the anus, you better let the doctor check it out, since it may indicate a deeper problem than you suspect. If it is in the area in and around the nose, make sure not to squeeze it. If you do, the infection may spread by way of the veins to the sinuses of the brain, and lead to a catastrophe.

Are boils contagious?

To some extent they are. They go from one member in the family to the other by close contact, towels, clothing and other vehicles. It is not rare to see many children in the same family with some boils at various times.

These boils may look somewhat innocent but they do carry the danger of spreading infection through the blood, thus leading to serious infection of the bones (osteomyelitis).

A child who keeps developing one boil after another should be checked for sugar diabetes.

What can I do for a boil?

If it is in its early stages and if it shows up for the first or second time, you may apply heat to it for twenty minutes three times a day. This will "ripen" the boil, so to speak. When the boil drains, make sure to "sterilize" the area around with alcohol, and to cover it with gauze or a bandage, so that the pus won't contaminate the surrounding area. Also make sure to wash your hands well, otherwise you may spread the infection.

When shall I see the doctor?
If the boil: (1) keeps coming back, (2) is quite big (i.e. if the redness is bigger than one inch in diameter), (3) looks as if it is becoming a carbuncle, (4) is in, on, or around the nose, or (5) in the area of the anus, then see the doctor.

What will the doctor do?
Some boils may have to be opened and drained. Other boils have to be cared for right away in a special manner; these include boils in and around the area of the nose (upper lip, cheek, etc.)
If the boils keep coming back, then a special regime of treatment may have to be followed. In most cases this will consist of giving a course of an antibiotic (an effective one against the staph germ). Along with this, some doctors prescribe bathing the child with Phisohex soap, and doing the same for other children in the family for a month or two. Taking special care of the underwear and garments that come in contact with the area of the boil is also important. Washing such clothes is not enough to kill most of the staph germs. Therefore, garments must be put in a pot of boiling water for twenty-five to thirty minutes. This is also true of pillowcases and sheets, if these become contaminated.
You don't have to follow all these measures in all cases, and your efforts will have to be commensurate with the individual case.
A final note: avoid the messy, smelly black ointment that your mother may have used on boils; it is of little or no value.

CELLULITIS AND ABSCESSES

Cellulitis is an inflammation of the soft tissues and has a vague nondefinable margin. It may show as a swollen area, fairly diffuse, hot to the touch, tender if handled, and painful. It does not come to a point (to a head). The child may or may not have some fever, feel out of sorts or sleepy, or lose the appetite. The cellulitis can show up anywhere.

How about abscesses?

Unlike cellulitis, abscesses are a localized form of infection; the inflammation is circumscribed and you can feel the edge and differentiate it easily from the tissues around it. Also unlike cellulitis, they usually come to a point, and often they are hard, hot to the touch, tender, and painful. They are not as deep an infection as cellulitis is, but -like cellulitis- they can show up anywhere on the body, at any age.

What causes these things?

Cellulitis is mainly caused by strep, rarely by staph or other germs. Cellulitis might be related to a disease that happens to be nearby, and can be an extension of that disease itself. On the other hand, most abscesses, be they of the tissues under the skin, the lymph nodes, the breasts, or other areas, are caused by staph.

More often than not, abscesses are solitary lesions, i.e. each lesion shows up individually. When the head of an abscess is opened, a core may come out, leaving a tunnel in its place. A large abscess may have several eyes (several inner pus-containing tunnels).

When this happens, we call the abscess a carbuncle. In either case, be sure to have the urine checked.

Why should the urine be checked?

Children who get boils often, or who have abscesses and carbuncles, may later show a tendency to have sugar in the urine, i.e. diabetes. A urinalysis is a very simple procedure that ought to be done at least once a year under these circumstances. This, however, does not apply to children who have only cellulitis.

What can be done about cellulitis?

A child with cellulitis should be brought to the doctor, since the treatment of cellulitis depends on the size, location, and relationship of the cellulitis to other conditions. Sometimes an antibiotic given internally is enough, but at other times surgical intervention is needed if the pus formation has already started.

If the child has an abscess, it is worth applying heat, preferably wet heat, four times a day at first. A heating pad will suffice, and you may apply it for 20 minutes at a time.

When the abscess comes to a head, it will be time to take the child to the doctor (it is better to do this even earlier). Usually, when the abscess is ripe, the doctor will open and drain it and will attempt to get the core or cores out in spite of the child's probable apprehension. If the abscess is fairly big, its center will have completely liquified and there will be no core inside. In such cases it will have to be opened with a wide incision to evacuate the pus completely. To do this, a surgeon may be needed, depending on the size and location of the abscess.

How can we prevent the above?

If the child is seen early, i.e. before any pus has formed, the proper use of antibiotics can often kill the offending agent (the causative germ) and the inflammation will soon subside and disappear. Some doctors use PhisoHex baths, which may help prevent the spread of the staph germ from one area to another, and from one member of the family to the other. When prescribed, it ought to be used regularly in the bath for as long as the doctor suggests. In addition, whoever handles the infected area should wash his or her hands afterwards, and any clothes that have been in touch with that area should be sterilized by boiling for about thirty minutes.

Covering the infected area with gauze will help prevent the germs of an open abscess from contaminating nearby clothes or the adjacent skin.

Applying Neosporin ointment, Mycitracin or Neopolycin (nonprescription) to the infected area is of limited value only, and so is the use of other ointments. The reason is that the infection of an abscess is too deep for such ointments to do any substantial good.

LYMPHANGITIS (BLOOD POISONING)

The child has a sore area that looks red, slightly swollen and is tender to the touch. Very possibly it is a result of a puncture wound, stepping on a nail, etc. The area may be anywhere on the body.

When you take a look at the area, you will see a red line, starting from the point of injury and inflammation, and traveling up towards the trunk of the body. It may be two to three inches long or longer but not particularly tender to the touch or painful. It looks innocent, and becomes evident a day or two following the injury, which by then will be inflamed and probably pussy. There will be no fever, and the child does not act sick.

What is lymphangitis anyway?

Lymphangitis (blood poisoning) is an inflammation of the lymphatic channels that drain the injured or inflamed area. When a rusty nail or something else punctures the skin or a soiled cut of some sort takes place, the area becomes inflamed. Next the lymph vessels draining this area become inflamed, leading to this condition. Most infections are caused by strep.

Scratches, if infected, can lead to lymphangitis. The skin is loaded with lymph vessels whose duty is to drain the area, therefore any infected skin lesions can lead to lymphangitis, though statistically the commonest cause remains the puncture wound of a nail, or similar injuries to the skin.

Is it serious?

If lymphangitis is ignored, the infection will continue to creep up. It may advance a good many inches up the limb, then infect the lymph node that drains the inflamed lymph vessel. The infection then has a chance to spread to the blood (septicemia) which is a life-threatening condition.

If recognized early, the treatment of lymphangitis is simply and uniformly effective. Since it can be serious if not treated in its early stage, you should hurry to the doctor as soon as you see a red line going from the inflamed area up the limb.

What will the doctor do?

The doctor may find it necessary to open and clean the inflamed puncture location. Sometimes dirt or a foreign body must be removed, though this is the exception rather than the rule. A culture of the infected area may have to be taken too.

A course of ten days of penicillin will be prescribed, even though the redness of the line of lymphangitis will respond to treatment in two to three days. It is extremely important that all ten days of treatment is completed (see page 145).

"Blood poisoning" used to be a dreadful disease in past years before the advent of antibiotics. Now it is regarded as a simple, easily treatable disease when diagnosed early.

RINGWORM

Ringworm is not caused by worms nor by rings, but by a certain fungus infecting the skin. It is fairly common and your child might get it even if kept immaculately clean.

Ringworm usually starts as a patch on the skin, slightly scaly and so innocuous-looking that you may easily ignore it. But as the days roll on, the patch will become bigger and bigger. The center will look as if it is healing, but the edge will be dull red, even slightly blistery or scaly, forming a "ring" around the center that seems to be healing. Ringworm is not very itchy, if at all.

Where does ringworm usually show up?

Usually on the trunk and the limbs. It may start as one patch, but if left too long, many new patches will show up. It is not unusual to see five to eight patches of ringworm scattered here and there by the time you seek medical advice. There are rarer forms of ringworm that affect the scalp, the area between fingers and toes, the creases, etc.

Is ringworm contagious?

Yes, in an insidious way. The child will have picked it up from someone with this infection, and if it is not taken care of soon, it will spread slowly but surely. Often one or two other children in the same family become infected too. Certain groups of this fungus can come from infected cats or dogs.

Can I treat it at home?

Ringworm should be seen by the doctor. There are a number of other diseases that look like ringworm. These include forms of eczema, impetigo, etc. Once your doctor confirms the diagnosis, the treatment is easy. A specific ointment will be used, making the ringworm gradually disappear in less than two weeks.

If you know for sure what the ringworm looks like, you may use Tinactin or other nonprescription antifungal ointments, four times a day, for a period of two weeks.

How about ringworm of the scalp?

In scalp ringworm the hair in the affected area looks dull and halfway broken off, usually leaving some circular bald patches. The ringworm starts as a patch slowly enlarging and spreading; it will have to be taken care of by your doctor. There is a disease (alopecia areata) that can mimic ringworm of the scalp (see page 477).

Once the diagnosis of scalp ringworm is confirmed, a prolonged treatment for several weeks is needed.

Why should we use the medicine for that long?

Fungus is a germ that has a "longlife." Fortunately, we do have medicines that can kill it. However, these medicines have to slowly smother the fungus and get rid of it. If the medicine is not used for long enough, the fungus may recur.

Can I prevent ring worm?

By prompt and conscientious treatment you will help prevent ringworm from spreading in your family. If there is a child with ringworm in your neighborhood or in school, then your child should avoid playing much with him or her; in fact, the infected child should be urged to have treatment instituted. Ringworm is only fairly contagious, so don't panic if your child gets in touch with such a patient on occasions.

If there are pet animals at home, such as cats or dogs, and you suspect that they are the source of the ringworm, take them to the veterinarian to make sure. Treating an infected pet animal can remove the source of such an infection.

HIVES

The child sometimes goes wild with itching. The rash is in the form of welts (wheals), usually slightly raised, pink in color, often with a pale center. Its shape is variable; it may be smaller than a dime or bigger than a half dollar. When severe, it may cover a big area of the skin.

The rash of hives tends to come and go; a big itchy welt in one area may disappear in just a few hours, only for some other areas to be affected. The welts may also have irregular shapes and irregular edges.

What is hives caused by?

Hives is a form of an allergy. You may be lucky to find the source of this allergy, but more likely than not, you will not be able to pinpoint the cause with certainty.

Certain foods are usually the allergenic factors. You will have to think hard about what the child had eaten the previous day or two, and whether there was any new food introduced. If you can point your finger to a certain food, it is worth giving the food in question once again some time later when the child is healthy, just to see if the child will develop the hives a second time, thus proving the connection without a doubt.

Of course, there are many allergic factors other than foods that can lead to hives. The list of the causes is long and confusing, but certain conditions are worth mentioning:

A patient allergic to certain medicines may develop hives as a reaction. Allergy to bee stings is well known for producing welts and itching. A good number of viral infections can produce hives-like reaction. There are also some bacterial infections that can produce hives.

Besides these, there are a number of diseases which can produce a rash that mimics hives, thus confusing the issue.

Is hives contagious?

No, it is not; your child can mix with others. In certain cases, however, the agent causing the hives can be contagious, such as a viral infection.

Can I diagnose hives at home?

Possibly, but if you are not sure, see your doctor. There are many diseases that can produce a rash of the nature of hives. These diseases may require specific treatment, close observation, or tests and cultures, so don't be lulled into false security.

How long does it take for hives to go away?

Since hives is so foxy and variable, so is its course. Mild ones may come and go in a matter of a day or two, others may take a week or two, and chronic ones can be recurrent and even take years. The duration largely depends on the cause of the hives and whether it can be avoided or not.

Can I do anything about it?

Many people try calamine lotion or Caladryl to relieve the itching. This is O.K. if it is used temporarily until you see the doctor, or if the affected area is a small spot.

When your doctor checks the child and makes certain of the diagnosis, he or she will give you an antihistamine (usually Benadryl) or other appropriate medication. But still, searching for the offending cause of the hives and avoiding that agent is the best way to stop them and prevent them from coming back.

Is there any urgency about seeing the doctor?

In most cases, there is no urgency. However certain forms of hives require immediate attention by the doctor, e.g. the hives that accompanies some swelling of the lips and a hoarse voice after the child has been stung by a bee. Other symptoms in this category are difficulty breathing, swelling of the eyelids, and the occurrence of welts all over (see page 464).

PITYRIASIS ROSEA

Pityriasis rosea consists of a rash which is rosy in color, showing up in small spots, slightly oval in shape, and is arranged mainly on the chest and back along lines of the ribs. It may show up on the neck and shoulders, and on the hips too, but not on the distal (far) part of the upper or lower limbs. The rash may have some fine scaling on top, and it may itch to a slight extent. The child doesn't seem to be bothered in any other way, and there will be no fever, cough or other symptoms.

A pediatrician sees only a few such cases in a year's time. Pityriasis rosea usually scares the parents because they think it is measles or something else dreadful.

It usually affects a child of the school age and beyond.

Is pityriasis rosea contagious?

Generally speaking, it is safe to say that the child can go to school. If there is any degree of contagiousness, it is almost nil.

No one knows the cause of it, but it is good to know about its course.

Tell me about its course:

Before the disease shows up, the child might develop a patch that looks like a ringworm, almost as big as a quarter; it is called a "herald patch" because it heralds the coming of this disease. This patch may show up for as long as one to two weeks before the child breaks out with the rash.

It usually takes about two weeks for the rash to reach full bloom and to be distributed as mentioned above, i.e. to show up on the trunk and maybe on the neck, shoulders, and hips. This will be followed by two more weeks during which the rash stays put without any changes. This is in turn followed by about two weeks during which the rash gradually fades, the spots slowly lose their color, the scaling slowly goes away, and the number of spots gradually becomes smaller and smaller until the spots are completely gone.

This means that the rash takes an average of about six weeks from beginning to end.

What is to be done about pityriasis rosea?

There is no way you can prevent this disease, and there is no specific treatment for it. However, the condition is mild in most cases, and no treatment is needed anyway. When the doctor sees this condition, he will simply explain it to you, and your understanding of what is to be expected is all that is needed. You should avoid irritants, however, such as hot or cold baths, exposure to sunlight on the beach, etc. Such irritants might make the rash itchy to a bothersome degree. If itching becomes more pronounced than usual, an internal medicine may be prescribed, but this is rarely needed.

Are there other kinds of pityriasis too?

There is pityriasis versicolor, and pityriasis alba. The skin rash in the versicolor variety is brown in color and looks like dirty skin. In fact, parents often wash the area over and over again, befuddled at the stubbornness of the "dirt spots!"

Pityriasis versicolor is caused by a certain fungus and is easily treatable, and the dirty-looking neck or chest may look as clean as ever afterwards. This disease is hardly contagious, and you don't have to worry about school children or other members in the family catching it. It can be controlled easily with an antifungal medication or other modes of treatment such as a bath with selsun shampoo, used directly on the skin.

Pityriasis alba appears as white spots, usually on the face. They are dime-sized and somewhat scaly. They usually go away in a few months by themselves, especially if the child avoids irritating them. Irritation of these spots is caused by rubbing the cheeks against something rough such as the sleeves of a coat, or by too much wetness and soap. Occasionally a special ointment might be needed for the treatment.

Pityriasis alba is also a disease that is mild and not contagious. It tends to go away by itself without treatment but only after a period of a few weeks, perhaps extending to months. Patience is needed here, but once you understand it, you will stop worrying about it.

POISON IVY

The child will scratch and scratch, and the itchy skin will look red and may feel rough. Poison ivy can show up anywhere on the body; be it on the face, arms, legs, or the genitalia. Poison ivy may be acute, generalized (all over), and severe, but mild cases are common and often show up in patches.

If the poison ivy shows up in patches, these patches will vary in size and shape, and the appearance will depend on how recently it was acquired and how severe it is, among other things. If it affects the genitalia, there may be a good deal of swelling, especially of the penis and scrotum. If it affects the face, the eyelids may become swollen, sometimes to the degree of shutting the eye(s).

What does it mean when the poison ivy is acute?

Acute poison ivy means a rapidly progressing, fresh appearance of the poison ivy on the skin. It is usually bright red in color, rough in appearance and very itchy. If it is severe, the affected skin becomes blistery, and the blisters may open up and lead to some oozing of clear yellow fluid. This is called the "weeping poison ivy."

It is best to treat poison ivy in its earliest stages, before it becomes oozy or even blistery. The early condition responds much better and faster to local or internal treatment. When the poison ivy becomes blistery or weepy, it will need more medication for a longer time, and the response to the treatment will not be as prompt or as good.

When the poison ivy is not treated properly or is left alone without treatment, it may go to the subacute or even the chronic stage. When this happens the skin becomes infiltrated and thickened, and the treatment will take a much longer time (several weeks) before the skin is reasonably back to normal.

Can a person be immune to poison ivy?

By far the great majority of people are susceptible to poison ivy. It is a fortunate and extremely rare person who is not susceptible to it. Some people seem to get only mild cases upon exposure, but every once in a while such a person might get a whammy of a case.

Because of their frequent outdoor activity, children are more exposed to the plant, thereby "catching" the disease quite often. It is not rare to see them get it two or three times a summer. Because adults are less active than children and less likely to go in the same places, they will catch poison ivy less frequently and often less severely. However, everyone should be on guard not to get near this plant.

Why is the poison ivy plant so bad, and how can we recognize it?

The poison ivy plant is a vine, and it may come up sneakily in many areas in the backyard. However, it is especially prevalent in woods and heavily wooded areas. The vine has three leaves coming out of the same spot of the stem. The leaves are fairly shiny and they usually have one notched edge.

The reason poison ivy is such a pest is that it contains an oleoresin, not only in its leaves but also in the stems and even in the roots. Skin that comes in contact with this oleoresin will absorb it within about thirty minutes. Once the oleoresin is absorbed, it will produce the itchy, inflammatory condition.

Poison ivy spreads fast because the child scratches the affected area, and thus spreads the oleoresin. It can also be spread by rubbing of the clothes, or by dogs and cats which carry the oleoresin in their hair.

Can we prevent poison ivy?

If you can recognize the plant when you see it, do your best to spray Weed-B-Gone or some similar chemical on it. After ten to fourteen days, spray the same plant once more, and the withering vine will die.

If inadvertently you come in contact with the poison ivy plant, wash the skin area that has touched it as soon as possible. Use soap and water. You have a period of only about half an hour within which you can help prevent the disease by simply using the soap and water, after which it is too late. For preventive oral medication, many preparations are available, being over-the-counter, and of questionable value.

What do you do for treatment?

That depends on the severity, location, and distribution of the affected skin. If it is only a small area, and not so severe, you may use over-the-counter cortisone creams such as Cortaid and the like. Calamine lotion may also be used. Don't use Calydryl since this medicine can be sensitizing.

If there are many patches here and there, you should see your doctor, since he or she may have to use one of the stronger steroid ointments and "anti-itch" medicines. If the poison ivy is on the face or genitalia, the doctor may even have to use a stronger medicine. This is also true of acute generalized poison ivy, for which an internal medicine or a shot (steroid) may have to be given.

INFECTION AROUND THE NAIL (PARONYCHIA)

There is pain and soreness near a fingernail or a toenail. The flesh in that area looks red, angry, sore, tender and slightly swollen. In advanced cases some pus will ooze out, more likely at the junction of the inflamed area with the nail. Quite often the nail itself looks O.K., though occasionally the pus digs deep and seems to go under it. In that case the pus will look like a "lake" under part of the nail.

The infection looks mild in its early days, but when left unattended and untreated, the swelling may become worse, and pus may keep coming out, devitalizing the nail, and the child seems to get nowhere.

What causes paronychia?

In most cases, paronychia is caused by the staph germ which enters the area if the child plays with or pulls out a hangnail. The same will happen if the child has a habit of picking the fingers, thus providing a port of entry for the germs.

Paronychia of the big toe is a different story; usually is related to the way the nail of the big toe is cut. If the toenail is not cut in a straight line, and if it is cut in an arch that makes the sides of the nail recede into the adjacent flesh, and if tight shoes are used, the chance for paronychia will be greater. The reason is that the tight shoes will press the flesh of the big toe against the side of the nail, interfering with its blood supply and making it very receptive to infection. This condition can fool anybody, especially the unsuspecting parents.

What will the doctor do?

For early infections, an internal antibiotic along with Neosporin ointment (nonprescription) and heat application is sufficient. If pus has formed it has to be drained.

For paronychia of the big toe, the doctor will follow the same medical treatment used for paronychia of the finger nails. However, he or she will suggest using sandals to relieve the pressure of the shoes on the inflamed tissue.

If the paronychia is more advanced, the doctor will try to see if there is a dead piece of the nail, and of course will remove it. In some cases the condition is such that a surgeon or a podiatrist has to be consulted. Minor surgery may have to be done, the area opened and cleaned.

Can we prevent these problems?

Prevention is very simple. Don't let the child pick at the nail, or don't let him or her pull a hangnail. Cut the hangnail as soon as you see it. Early redness of the flesh around the nail deserves an application of Neosporin, Neopolycin or similar ointments (nonprescription).

Fitting the child with wide enough shoes is most important, as is cutting the toe nails in a straight line so that the edges of the nail don't become imbedded in the adjacent flesh. The condition is quite messy to treat, but so easy to prevent.

HEMATOMA OF THE NAIL

The child jumps with pain, having hurt one of the fingers or toes. A young child may scream for a while. The hurt toe or finger may have received a poorly aimed hit with a hammer, a slam of the car door, or a heavy fallen object. The pain is instantaneous and often severe, and when you first look at the finger or toe, there will be few if any changes.

You apply ice to the area and give comfort to the screaming child, and the pain will gradually subside. However, he or she will favor the affected hand or foot. Soon, too, you will discover that the nail of the hurt finger or toe will have become red in color, as if floating on blood.

What has happened?

With a sudden force hitting the nail, one of the fragile blood vessels under the nail breaks. Having no place to go, the blood will accumulate under the nail, building pressure and lifting it off its bed, so to speak. This causes a great deal of pain because this sensitive area is under so much pressure.

If left alone, the flesh around the nail will react by swelling and changing color, since it will be reacting to the bleeding under the nail. The end of the finger or toe may even take the shape of a club.

What can be done about it?

You can leave it and suffer the consequences, or treat it and relieve the pain right away, and preserve the nail in the process. If the hematoma is seen within a day, the doctor may use a special tiny drill. If it is no more than just a hematoma under the nail, the doctor will drill one tiny hole in the nail. You will be amazed to see how much blood and serum come out of that hole. The pain will immediately stop, and the swelling of the flesh around the nail will slowly recede. The color of the nail will be back to normal to some extent, since air and serum will have filled the space by now. For a few days there may be some drainage of serum from the hole, but the healing will be swift. Drilling the hole causes no pain.

Some doctors don't even use a drill. Instead, they will open a paper clip, heat it, put the hot end in the nail, and burn a hole. This sounds gruesome, especially when you see a scared, resisting child; however, the whole procedure is not that difficult or complicated.

What if I leave it alone?

If the hematoma is not treated, the area will continue to be sore for some time. Gradually the swelling of the flesh around the nail will subside. The color of the nail, looking at first bright red, will change to chocolate brown, and the nail, being devitalized, will separate after some more time. Over a period of many months a new nail will take its place. For a big toe this takes about nine months.

Do we lose the nail in all-nail hematomas?

This happens only if the hit was hard and the hematoma had occupied the whole area under the nail. However, if the hit is not that severe, and only part of the nail seems to sit on a lake of blood, the pain will be moderate, and there will be less tenderness. The adjacent flesh will hardly react. The rest of the nail will look normal, and the soreness will slowly subside over a period of a day or two.

Shall we see a doctor for the above cases too?

Most such cases do not need the help of a doctor. The application of ice packs for the first half-hour may help the soreness and degree of tissue reaction. You may immobilize the finger too, and give it time to heal.

Some people think Epsom salt's applications will help, but this is doubtful and it is better not to apply them.

Since only part of the nail is devitalized (the part sitting on the lake of blood), the healthy part will look normal. With time, the affected area will move outward as the nail grows. Eventually the part with the bleeding underneath will reach the nail-trimming stage, and be gone for good.

STRAWBERRY HEMANGIOMA

At first the baby looks O.K., though there may be a faint pink spot somewhere on the skin. By the time the baby is a few weeks-old, this pink spot may have become bright red and elevated, with a surface not unlike that of a strawberry. Not all strawberry hemangiomas appear in this manner. Many seem to appear from nowhere.

These skin "lesions" can vary in size too. Some of them can be gigantic; they can cover half the face, or be over the whole arm. Most of them, however, are between the sizes of a dime and a quarter. Tiny ones may also look like a spider hemangioma to the untrained eye.

Where will they appear?

Strawberry hemangiomas can show up anywhere. If they show up on the arms, legs, or trunk, they should not cause much concern. Sometimes, however, they appear in sensitive areas, such as the tip of the nose, near the eyelids, or genitalia.

What is a spider hemangioma?

This behaves differently from strawberry hemangioma. A spider hemangioma appears later in life, and usually there will be several of them at the same time. The face and trunk are the preferred sites. By looking closely, you will see a red, pinpoint-sized center, and from this center, thin, tiny blood vessels will radiate, looking like a spider. Unlike strawberry hemangiomas, spider hemangiomas take many, many years before they disappear. They ought to be left alone.

What will happen to the strawberry hemangiomas?

They often take a predictable course. Most strawberry hemangiomas reach their mature size soon, and continue to look dark red, without any pain or discomfort. In most cases they will go away by themselves (it is hard for parents to believe the doctor's word in this regard, since hemangiomas look unshapely and out of place). Nevertheless, in a matter of a few months these hemangiomas will develop whitening of their surface. Slowly but surely, the whitening will spread more and more to replace the red surface. The lesions will tend to shrink in size too. By the time the baby is one to two years old, most such lesions will have withered and disappeared.

By the time the lesion is gone, all that will be left is flat skin with a few blood vessels showing through; the color of the area will be slightly "off" but acceptably so.

Can these hemangiomas cause any problems?

In the majority of cases there will be no problems if they are left alone. Don't monkey around with them. Don't "treat" them. Rarely do they ulcerate or bleed, and rarely do they scab. Only in the case of a hemangioma that lasts for a few years, will it have to be treated.

ATHLETE'S FOOT

Athlete's foot is fairly rare in children until they become adolescents. From then on it becomes somewhat common.

It may be mild and appear as flaking between the toes, with or without mild redness and slight soreness. Or it may be more acute than that; the flaking may develop into red sore skin, mainly between the toes and the surrounding area. There may even be a slight swelling of the area, and the skin can be oozy and wet.

In some, the athlete's foot may be acute; the area may ooze some pussy material, become swollen a lot, and be quite sore and painful.

What causes athlete's foot?

It is caused by a fungus. This fungus likes dark, moist areas, where there will be little or no air. The feet, being in shoes for so long, are fairly ideal for the growth of this fungus. If we ventilate our feet out of the shoes - especially if we go barefoot - there will be less likelihood to get athlete's foot.

How can I prevent it?

If you clean the skin between the toes, dry it well, and if you allow the child to go barefoot for a while, you will have done a very good job in preventing this menace. The feet can be powdered with Enzactin (nonprescription) if there is a mild athlete's foot, and even if not. Using potassium permanganate may be good, but it is messy. If the inflammation seems to be severe, go to the doctor, since strong antifungal medications are needed.

My child is not a teenager, but has some rash on the feet?

This is very common and many people mistakenly call it athlete's foot. It is a special condition that affects the feet (even the hands) of children, mainly near and in between the toes. If you look carefully, you may see tiny blisters. It may feel and look sore; in some cases it can be very sore, oozy, mean-looking, and the skin around is all inflamed.

Some of these lesions may show up at the sides of the soles and even on top of the foot, but in the majority it affects the sole, near the toes and around.

<u>If this is not athlete's foot, what is it?</u>
Most doctors think it is a form of allergy to some chemical in the socks or shoes; some dispute the theory and have their own.

<u>Are any of the above conditions catching?</u>
No, athlete's foot is rarely as contagious as many people think, and the other condition is not contagious at all.

<u>How is this allergy of the feet treated?</u>
In most cases the child will benefit from walking barefoot as much as possible. This will work well because the feet will be aired, the skin of the sole will be stimulated and will thicken, and best of all the feet will not be in contact with a chemical from socks or shoes. For city dwellers, taking their feet out of shoes and socks, cleaning them well, and walking barefoot on the carpet, is an alternative.

When mild, this is all you have to do. In more advanced cases, you will have to have treatment with special ointment from your doctor. At times, some of the blisters have to be popped by your doctor with a lancet, especially if the blisters are deep and fairly big. Every once in a while, these lesions become infected and may need to be cultured and a local or internal antibiotic used.

<u>But I don't like to see my child walking barefoot:</u>
Being barefoot or in sandals doesn't hurt if the child is careful. Being in shoes all the time will practically "choke" the feet; they will sweat and become soggy, thereby developing this condition.

By walking barefoot, the child's feet will be dirty and there will be a chance of receiving a cut, you may say. Sandals are the answer to that.

By the way, a small child who walks barefoot will strengthen the arches of the feet and be less likely to develop flat feet.

BEE STINGS

The area looks red, swollen and itchy. It is quite painful for a while. The swelling is usually limited to a few inches in diameter, though occasionally it may become larger, given enough time. A sting on the palms or soles often leads to swelling of the back of the hands or feet. The swelling will disappear gradually in a number of days.

What other insects can do this?

Troublesome insects related to bees are yellow jackets, wasps and hornets. Some are aggressive, all are nasty when disturbed, and all give a very painful sting causing swelling of the tissues for a few days. This swelling is usually not an allergy reaction, it is more related to the chemicals injected. It is innocuous, being no more than a local reaction, and it tends to go away in a few days.

What can I do for it?

Apply ice to numb the sting area, and give the child sympathy. The child will slowly calm down. Look at the area and see if the stinger is in the center. Only honey bees leave stingers, other insects don't. If the stinger is still in, try to pull it out. You may use tweezers, but use them carefully, with light pressure. If you press hard on the tweezers, you may squeeze the poison sac which is still attached to the stinger, and this will make things worse for the child. Another method is to lift it out with the edge of your fingernail with a flicking motion.

Soaking the area with baking soda and water is of questionable value. If you want to use this kind of soaking, add one teaspoon of baking soda to one pint of water, soak a washcloth in it, then put the washcloth on the area of the bee sting. However, the ice application is better and makes more sense.

Some parents wonder about using Benadryl. As long as the swelling remains limited, there is no need to use any medicine. Benadryl is good if generalized reaction has begun. If this is the case -or if there are numerous stings- get in touch with the doctor, and if he or she is not available, go to the emergency room of a nearby hospital. Multiple stings are more likely to lead to trouble.

What is a generalized reaction?

Children who develop sensitivity to stings of the bee family, stand to have what is called a generalized or systemic reaction. This is a warning for future dangerous reactions that can even lead to death.

Look for hives; they are in the form of wheals (welts), are itchy, have a fairly well-demarcated edge, are rosy or pale-rosy in color, are of multiple size and shape, and appear anywhere on the skin. See if the child is restless, has developed a swelling of the eyelids or lips, or has a hoarse voice.

Once such reactions show up, see the doctor immediately or go to the emergency room of the nearest hospital. Such reactions can progress, sometimes quickly, and can be life-threatening.

What will the doctor do for the generalized reaction?

Once the child is checked, a shot or several shots of epinephrine may have to be given. Antihistamines, such as Benadryl, are often prescribed. Cortisone may be needed too. The child is admitted to the hospital if there seems to have been much of a reaction to the sting.

If none of these reactions show up, but the whole arm is swollen because of the sting, the excessive swelling is a forewarning that a generalized reaction will be in the wind for future stings. Benadryl may be used in such cases.

Once I saw a child who had a total of 365 stings! His scalp was loaded with stings, numerous stingers were carefully removed from his body, and he was in shock. He was treated in the hospital, and he came out smelling like a rose. Yes, bee stings can be a mess at times.

How about the bee sting kit?

This is a nice thing to have if your child is prone to having a generalized reaction. Full instructions are inside. Have the kit even when the child goes on vacation with you or goes to camp. There is no need for a kit if the child has nothing but a local reaction since a local reaction to bee stings is mainly not allergic in nature.

We have heard of desensitization:
 This is available and should be used on every person proving to have allergy to the stings of the bee family. Such allergy is shown in the form of a generalized reaction to a bee sting.
 For desensitization, an allergist will be needed. Shots are given over a certain period of time. Eventually one shot a month will be given. It is said that this is to be done for many years if not for life. Although this may sound awful, it is better to go through it than have a child in shock or risk a loss of life.
 The vaccines will give immunity not only to bee stings but also to the stings of the yellow jacket, wasp, and hornet.

BITES (DOGS, CATS AND HUMANS)

 The area of the animal bite might be no more than a nick, a puncture wound, or a simple abrasion. On the other extreme, it may be quite severe, with a jagged laceration, mutilation, and damage to the deep tissue that may require a plastic surgeon. Yet, lying between these two extremes there are numerous variations in the degree of the damage done to the tissues by a bite.

How do bites differ in severity?
 A dog's bite is usually more severe, more damaging, and more upsetting than a cat's bite. A dog's bite is also more likely to have the severity that requires the help of a surgeon or even a plastic surgeon. On the other hand, a cat's bite is often mild, but it may be associated with a deep cat scratch, and the possibility for a cat-scratch disease.
 Human bites are mostly superficial, usually mild, and nonbleeding. Many of the mild bites will be no more than a bruise or a contusion, needing very little treatment.

Are these bites dangerous?
 Usually they are not dangerous, though every once in a while we have to be on the alert. Besides the occasional need for surgery, a bite can lead to some rare but dangerous diseases that may threaten

the life of the patient. The reason is that the saliva of animals or humans is loaded with bacteria and viruses of numerous varieties and strains. The bacteria include tetanus and gas gangrene, and the viruses include rabies and the cat-scratch. This is why tetanus shots are often given to bite victims, and the bitten area is often observed for local infection or development of other diseases.

What is to be done?
　　The doctor will assess the degree of damage, and may have to send the child to a surgeon or even a plastic surgeon. A plastic surgeon is needed in special situations such as nasty bites on the face.
　　A tetanus shot will be given if the child needs one. Besides the tetanus shot, rabies shots may have to be given in some rare circumstances. Gas gangrene is quite rare, as is cat-scratch disease.

Will there be a good chance for local infection?
　　Yes; since the mouth is full of many varieties of bacteria, the chance for local infection is certainly there. This of course depends on the type of the bite and its severity, on whether dirt and clothes have contaminated the wounded area, and on the site of the bite. An antibiotic may have to be given if the bite seems to be deep and contaminated. If the bite is only superficial (has hardly broken the skin), an antibiotic might not have to be used at all. However, a deep laceration, a contaminated or dirty wound, a case of multiple bites, etc., may all have to have an antibiotic coverage for a variable period of time.

Is it possible to prevent some of these bites?
　　Of course prevention is superior to cure (where surgery, antibiotics, expense, and emotional turmoil are involved). To help in this regard, it is good to follow these rules if at all possible:

1. Avoid antagonizing the animal, especially a dog, and more so if the animal is suspicious or angry;
2. Avoid depriving the animal from something it is eating;
3. As much as you can, correct the child who likes to bite;

4. Completely avoid a sick looking dog or cat.

Shall I call the doctor for every bite?

Yes, please do. Though the doctor might be able to assess the condition on the phone, often he or she may want to see the child and evaluate the degree of the bite, the possibility of its chance for infection, the child's need for tetanus shot, etc. In some you may want to take the child directly to the emergency room of the nearest hospital, especially if you think a surgeon may have to be called.

URTICARIA PAPULOSA OR THE PETS AND THE ITCH

The name is scary, but the disease is not. It is fairly common, and is seen more often in children of preschool age and slightly beyond. In most cases there is a dog or a cat at home, and if not at home, then in the neighborhood. Preschool children (three, four, or five years old) are most susceptible to this disease. The disease can still show up in older children, but this is rare, and the older the child the less likely he or she will get the disease. It is exceptional for the adults to get this disease.

Why the dog or the cat?

This disease is actually an allergy to fleas, lice, ticks, or mites which infest dogs or cats. In experiments, children have developed this disease even when they were exposed to such pests that had been pulverized!

Any long-haired pet is likely to be infested with fleas or other pests, thus be a means for this disease. However, dogs and cats are the favorite pets of most families, and they are the animals most likely to be the target of the pests. Because of these two factors, and because of the close contact these pets have with the members of the family, it is less likely that pets other than dogs or cats are a major cause of this disease.

What is this disease?

The poor child will have lots of small red spots, each being the size of a split pea or slightly larger. The spots may have a raw area in the center to indicate a small ruptured blister, and they usually affect the legs or the arms, but not that often the trunk or the face.

One common thing about them is that they are intensely itchy. The itching may drive the child to distraction. The itching may lead to infection of the spots, thus complicating the treatment.

What can be done about urticaria papulosa?

To treat such a condition the dog or cat has to be taken care of first; i.e. "debugged" as thoroughly as possible. Unless this first step is taken, the rest of the treatment will be meaningless.

To rid the pet of its fleas, ticks and other bugs, you will have to treat it with any of the special sprays or powders designed for this purpose -they are available in drug stores, pet shops, etc.- or you can ask the veterinarian for suggestions. Follow the directions carefully.

Treating the dog or the cat is not enough by itself, however. You have to treat the areas or corners of the rooms where the dog or cat sleeps, plays, rests, or eats. Don't forget the basement if the pet happens to use it often. The reason for the cleaning is that many fleas or ticks separate from the pet, prefering dark, cool, damp areas. Even when these pests die the remains of their body can still produce this disease. Thus, the areas mentioned have to be treated with the same material used to treat the pet. This is to be followed by a thorough cleaning job afterwards. The more thorough you are about debugging the animal and the house, the better the chance will be for your child to recover from this disease.

What will the doctor do for the child?

Ointments with cortisone are usually prescribed, and any local skin infection will have to be treated too. At times, internal medicine for the itching is prescribed.

In some children, the disease can last a long time, sometimes two months or longer. The disease is more bothersome and unsightly than dangerous. Treating the child will not be successful without treating the pet or the places the pets occupy.

ACNE: TREATABLE BUT NOT CURABLE

Acne is familiar to everybody. Better than four out of five teenagers will have it, quite often badly enough to need some medical help. It comes in four degrees of severity, discernible mainly to the eyes of the doctor; the first two to three degrees can usually be managed by you and the pediatrician. The fourth degree (and some cases of the third degree) usually belong to the dermatologist.

Fortunately, the majority of acne cases are of the first and second degree of severity.

What is acne anyway?

It is a condition of troubled "oil" glands of the skin, mainly of the face, but many times the shoulder area and upper chest and back too. For some special reasons, it shows up during the teenage period and often continues until the early twenties.

Some are more likely to suffer from it than others, and occasional victims end up with many resultant scars.

Acne can be treated with various degrees of success, but it truly is a condition that cannot be completely cured -it has to run its course.

What would you do for mild acne?

For the simple cases of blackheads and the whiteheads, wash the face thoroughly twice a day; this will remove the excess oil on the skin and help open up the pores of the affected glands. Too vigorous and more frequent washing of the face, however, ought to be avoided, since this may give rise to some problems. This is true too of squeezing the pimples.

If the above doesn't help, washing with some of the medicated soaps may be of value. There are numerous varieties of such soaps, Fostex being a good example. Most of these over-the-counter acne medications can help only to a certain degree, and if it seems that the acne is too stubborn, you better call your doctor.

What will the doctor do?

The doctor may try Retin-A gel or cream, with or without benzoyl peroxide gel (prescription). Both medications are effective if used alone; if not, they can be combined. They may take a period of some time (two to three weeks) before they show a visible effect, and they may have to be used for months on end. The treated area may initially look slightly red, and it may have an uncomfortable burning feeling. Upon using such gels, the acne may seem to become worse during the first two weeks, then it begins to show signs of improvement. Your patience will count.

Another good point about these medications is that they should be used only once a day, and occasionally only once every second day.

An antibiotic such as tetracycline is often needed. It is usually started on the basis of three to four times a day, then tapered off until one dose a day is required (or even one every second day). Erythrocin or some other antibiotic can be used instead, however.

What if the acne doesn't seem to respond?

If giving the above treatment doesn't seem to help much, the patient must see the dermatologist. There are many other ways of treatment not mentioned above; the dermatologist will be able to choose one appropriate to the severity of the case.

You ought to bear in mind that dealing with acne means persistence, patience, many visits to the doctor's office, and having an open mind.

How about diet?

In spite of many claims about fats, chocolate, and other foods, acne is usually not influenced by the diet. It is rare to see a definite relationship between one particular food and acne, but if one is seen, then that food ought to be avoided.

How about makeup?

Girls who use heavy makeup may make their acne worse; it is better to take it easy with the use of makeup. If special medicated creams and gels are to be used, the makeup must be washed off thoroughly before they are applied.

WARTS

Warts are very common in children, and they disappear usually before the child reaches adolescence.

They are familiar to just about everyone. They vary in size, may become clustered as if seeding themselves, and every once in a while they seem to spread along a line.

In most children they give no trouble other than being unsightly. However, in some, they may become troublesome.

How are warts troublesome?

If the wart is at the edge of a fingernail, it may cause some pain, or the child will develop a habit of picking at it until it bleeds or even cracks. When the wart shows up at the soles of the feet (plantar wart), it can also become fairly painful, more so when it becomes big and deep.

What causes warts?

Warts are caused by a slow-spreading virus. By having the wart over a long period of time, an immunity will slowly develop. This explains why children are the most likely to get it, because they lack the immunity against it. This also explains why warts usually disappear by about the time the child becomes a teenager.

Shall we treat the wart as soon as it shows up?

No, it is better to leave it alone. By simply leaving it alone for one year, you stand a fifty percent chance that the wart will disappear by itself without treatment. If you wait for two years, the chances are seventy percent that the wart will disappear spontaneously. However, keep in mind that the wart may seed itself in the meantime.

Can I use a home remedy for the purpose?

You may buy Vergo ointment or Compound W liquid (nonprescription). Follow the directions on the package carefully.

When using such medicines, your chances for success are only thirty to forty percent, but they are worth the try. If they are not successful and the warts remain troublesome, then see the doctor.

What will the doctor do?

This depends on the doctor and the wart itself. The doctor may use liquid Nitrogen, Bichloracetic acid, an electrodesiccator, or some other method to get rid of it.

How can I treat planter warts?

Planter warts can be big, tender upon pressure, and quite painful. They show up at pressure points of the foot, and are far more bothersome than warts at most other sites.

Try at first the various over-the-counter medications, such as Dr. Scholl's patches or liquids. Read the instructions carefully, and pick up what seems to fit the situation.

If you are not successful, you may use salicylic acid plasters forty percent (nonprescription). You may stick the plasters on the wart after cutting the plasters to be the exact size of the plantar wart. You leave the plaster in place for one day, then replace it with a fresh piece daily, for a total of four days. After that you skip a day, then repeat the course for four more days. When these two courses are done, the doctor can then fray the wart and remove the dead tissue, which will be soft and pliable by then. He or she may even be able to get the core out, leaving a deep hole.

More often than not, after fraying the plantar wart and removing the dead tissue, you may find out that you have to apply the salicylic acid plaster once more for two more courses. Then you will visit the doctor once again for more trimming and searing; in most the corn has just about had it, and the trouble is almost over.

One thing to remember; when you use the salicylic acid plasters, don't let the foot get wet. The wetness may react with the chemical and produce too much irritation.

Will any scars be left after the wart?

Happily, most warts (including plantar warts) disappear without a trace, even the warts that are removed by the dermatologist. This is also true of plantar callouses, which are treated the same way as plantar warts.

SUNBURN

Sunburn is caused by the ultraviolet component of the sunlight. The skin will react to protect itself and you. If the exposure is sudden, a sunburn will be the result, especially in a fair-skinned person.

By the way, even indirect sunlight can give trouble with sunburn. If you are on the beach and it is cloudy, don't be lulled into false security. The ultraviolet rays that give sunburn will penetrate the humid, cloudy air. These rays can even reflect in the water or sand and reach you even if you are shaded under a beach umbrella!

Are there any precautions against sunburn?

Yes, there are certain rules worth observing:

1. Don't make your first exposure to the sunlight (on the beach or anywhere else) prolonged. It is best to be exposed repeatedly and for gradually longer periods over a few days.
2. Exposure to sunlight in the early morning (before 9 am) or evening (after 4 pm) will not give you a sunburn. The burning rays are usually concentrated during the 10 am to 2 pm hours.
3. Suntan lotions can be of great help. Those particularly useful are Uval, Sunscreen and PreSun lotion, be it PreSun 4, 8, or 15. Read the instructions on the bottle to pick up the strength that suits you. If used on the areas of the body most exposed, they will help prevent the expected sunburn. But even if you have already had the sunburn, these lotions or creams will help take away the sting and relieve some of the misery. They do, however, wash away to some extent as you swim, so reapply them after you have come out of the water.

Can sunburn be dangerous?

In mild cases it is no more than a nuisance. In severe ones however, it can be blistery, stinging, slightly itchy, and it may make you suffer. For these situations, use Domeboro solution, in the form of soothing packs. Put a tablet or a packet of Domeboro (nonprescription) in one pint of water. Soak a washtowel in it, then put the wet towel on the burnt area. Keep doing that as often as you think you need it.

A severe sunburn can be associated with fever and achiness, and can even cause delirium and subsequent "wacky" behavior. In such severe but rare cases, call the doctor for help, of course.

Remember to be particularly careful with babies. Their skin is quite tender and they are particularly the ones to suffer.

What kind of precautions should I take for the baby?

Babies only a few months old should not be allowed too much exposure to the sunlight, especially on the beach. Take them out late in the day or during the early morning, when there will be much less of a chance of a sunburn.

Put light clothes on them, covering much of their bodies, if you think they will be in places with high chance of a sunburn. Also shade them from the burning rays as much as possible. Of course use the creams and lotions mentioned before.

It is unfortunate when we come across three- to four-week-old babies who have been brought to the beach, only to end up looking like lobsters afterwards.

Be smart, be cautious, and have a nice vacation!

SCALDS AND BURNS

Burns affecting only the superficial layer of the skin are called first-degree burns. When the deeper layer of the skin is also involved, it is a second-degree burn. When more severe, affecting the whole thickness of the skin, it is called third-degree burn. This latter is the severest form of burns and the most difficult to treat.

Fortunately, scalds are mostly first degree burns and they are of various sizes. When they happen, they need immediate treatment to remove the pain and to help restore the integrity of the damaged area. In some however, they can lead to second degree burns, ending with a number of blistery lesions that contain clear fluid inside.

Why all this differentiation between burn degrees?

This has an important bearing on the final outcome of the scalded or burned area of the skin, and on the treatment necessary. A first-degree burn will lead to red, tender skin without blisters, it will heal fairly fast, and there will be no scarring left. A scald or burn leading to blistery or denuded skin will take longer to heal, is more likely to get infected, and needs more care, although the skin will more or less look normal in the final outcome. A third-degree burn is more difficult to treat, and it leads to scarring and disfigurement of the area. This may interfere with the function of the area affected (i.e., hands, joints, neck, etc.), and may also severely affect the psychology of the person involved.

What shall I do when a burn happens?

Temporarily you can cover the area with a sterile gauze or at least a piece of clean cloth, put loosely over the affected area.

If the scalded area is not blistery or denuded, and if it is small, you may want to soothe the pain by applying ice at first, to be followed by applying cream (any kind of cream, even butter). If the area is blistery or denuded, it is better to keep hands off, cover it with a sterile piece of gauze or clean cloth, and have the child seen by the doctor or taken to the emergency room of the nearest hospital.

What will be done there?

It is important that the doctor checks the affected area, to assess the extent of damage to the skin, the degree of burn, and the need for specific treatment.

If the burn is extensive and/or if some areas prove to be of the third-degree, the child will have to be admitted to the hospital, put on intravenous fluids, and started on a prolonged specialized treatment as deemed necessary.

What steps shall we take in prevention?

Educate the young child about the meaning of "hot"; warn about the hot pan , hot cups of coffee, the lighted cigarette, etc. He or she may even touch certain things to learn (be sure the pan is not too hot!).

Have firm rules and discipline early in life to avoid stoves, open fires, vaporizers, hot liquids, matches, lighters, etc. At the same time teach the child to use fire sensibly by letting him or her blow out matches, help build a fire in a fireplace, plug and unplug electrical equipment, etc.

Also keep matches and lighters out of reach, keep hot pans on the back of the stove, and protect the child from wall plugs, frayed cords and light sockets, or dangling electrical cords.

How bad are electrical burns?

An electrical burn is much worse than a regular burn, and it often leads to necrosis (death) of the tissues. Because it kills tissue cells, it will lead to deep scarring of the affected area. Such scarring often makes it necessary to use the services of a plastic surgeon.

THE BALD SPOT

The bald spot may catch your eye, and when you look more carefully, you will see that the hair has fallen off in one spot in the child's scalp. The bald area doesn't seem to be painful or itchy. It may look clear and shiny, the size of a quarter or even a half dollar, and the hair at the periphery seems to be normal in looks and texture. In some you may also be able to discover a second or third spot in other areas of the scalp. The whole scene will of course make you worried and concerned.

What is this condition?

It is called alopecia areata. It is not as rare as you may think. Older children are more apt to get it. The cause is unknown. The bald spot may soon progress to its biggest size and stay that way for a number of months. Then, gradually, a few fuzzy hairs will start appearing in the bald area. This is followed by more normal looking hairs, eventually making the area well covered with hairs and as normal looking as the rest of the scalp.

This may take as long as six to nine months from beginning to end.

What would you do about it?

For most of them you do nothing. The alopecia areata will take its course and disappear. In severe cases however, there are certain medications to be given.

A visit to the doctor is mandatory for two reasons; to find whether or not the child does indeed have this disease, and to make sure that the bald spot is not caused by some other disease.

What other diseases can it be caused by?

Bald spots can also be caused by ringworm of the scalp, or tinia capitis. This is a disease caused by a certain fungus.

To the untrained eye, alopecia areata looks the same as ringworm of the scalp. However, if you look carefully, you may see stubs of hairs projecting at the base of the bald spot in cases of the scalp ringworm. This is not the case with alopecia areata, wherein the scalp at the bald spot is clear, smooth and maybe even shiny.

What can be done if it is ringworm?

If the doctor suspects ringworm of the scalp, he or she may examine the scalp under a special light called Wood's lamp, and may also do a culture for the fungus that causes the ringworm.

Having done that, the child will be put on oral medication for a prolonged period (many weeks), after which new healthy hairs will have come up and filled the bald spot slowly but surely.

In the past, they used to use X-rays or give some medication to make all the hair of the head fall off, then wait until new hair came anew to cover the whole scalp. As you may suspect, this led to embarrassment of the child and the family alike. Fortunately, this is not done anymore, since the oral medication is quite effective.

What are some other diseases that affect the scalp?

Occasionally a child's bald spot will prove to be caused by him or her pulling the hair, or by a fall that caused the hair to be pulled out.

Impetigo of the scalp may also be mistaken for the above diseases. In scalp impetigo, there is usually a fairly thick crust that makes the hair sticky and messy-looking. Some degree of itching may also be present. Two, three, or more spots of impetigo may also be present at the same time (see page 441).

LICE

Lice usually infest children and the children react by scratching their heads over and over again, as if unable to satisfy the itchy feeling. The itching is worse around the ears and at the back of the head. It is not rare either to see one or two family members to start scratching their heads incessantly, after having become infested through the child.

What shall I look for when I suspect lice infestation?

The louse is smaller than a tick, is oblong in shape, and has tiny legs on both sides. It is quite active and may move fairly fast. If it is a head louse, it is dark greyish brown in color. If it is a body louse, it is greyish white in color, and tends to be bigger than the head louse.

The head louse prefers the scalp, more so the areas around the ears and the back of the head. These areas become itchy because the hungry louse lives by sucking the blood from the scalp by piercing and irritating it.

You may not be able to see the lice if the infestation is not heavy. Much easier is to look for their nits.

The nits are the eggs of the louse (which she lays by the hundreds), and they are attached to the hairs by a special glue secreted by the mother. Each looks like a tiny, dark oval spot, smaller than a pinhead, attached to the hair at an angle of about forty-five degrees. If you can crush it between two fingernails, it will pop audibly; this is a simple way to differentiate between the nit and a mere flake of dandruff.

How does a clean child get it?

Usually lice spread through contact in schools, and from there to different members in the family. The close contact of being together and playing together, is the usual manner for lice to go from one person to another. Boys and girls with long hair, especially if they don't take care of it, are often the source of the trouble. It takes only a few such boys and girls to infest many other children.

What can I do about lice infestation?

The doctor will recommend or prescribe either Kwell shampoo (prescription) or Rid shampoo (nonprescription), to kill the lice and the nits. Be sure to follow the instructions on the bottle carefully.

It is better if the whole family uses the above shampoo. Shampoo the head once or two nights in a row. Repeat shampooing the head of the infested child a week later, also once or two nights in a row, depending on the severity of the infestation. The lice and the nits will be dead by then. The nit shells will still be seen, but they cannot be popped because they are not alive any more. These "shells" still adhere to the hair and can be removed with a fine toothed comb using a warm vinegar water solution.

How about towels, hats, and bed linens?

If it is dry-cleanable, have it dry-cleaned. If it is washable, put it in boiling water for twenty-five to thirty minutes. This includes towels, pillowcases, combs, brushes, and in case of body lice, undershirts, pants, shirts, pajamas, etc. This way you are more likely to prevent reinfestation by stray lice and save yourself a good deal of "anxiety" in the weeks to follow.

Look for lice especially if the school authorities notify you, and if your child has it, please notify the school. The experience might understandably jar you, but the problem is controllable.

How about body lice?

They are less frequent than head lice, and the treatment is with a similar cream or lotion that is just as strong as the shampoo is for head lice. For body lice, however, pay more attention to the clothes, and kill the lice on them by boiling them. The body lice like to hide in the seams of shirts and undershirts, pants, and pajamas, particularly in the pubic area and near the armpits, where the areas are warm and cozy.

Lice are revolting, but they cause more annoyance than serious trouble. Because of the incessant itching, they may lead to scalp impetigo at times, with enlargement of the lymph nodes of the corresponding area. In some countries, typhus can be transferred through lice, but fortunately this disease is hardly seen in this country, thanks to good public health measures.

Do lice fly?

No, they don't. Also, they cannot jump as fleas do. If they are separated from the body for two to three days, they will die of starvation.

CHAPTER SIXTEEN

THE HEAD

the head
headache
migraine headache
fainting spells
epileptic fits
the nervous tics
the hyperkinetic child (attention deficit disorder)
concussion
Down's Syndrome
meningitis

THE HEAD

Secure inside the skull lies the most delicate and the most complex organ in our bodies, the brain. To keep it well protected, spinal fluid surrounds the brain, thus making it less likely to suffer from sudden jarring movements, thereby preserving the continuity of the brain's functions in an ideal manner. The brain is covered by three thin sheets of tissues called meninges.

The skull consists of many bones. These bones are firmly interlocked to form a rigid "box" that holds and protects the brain, its coverings, and the fluid. In a baby, however, the skull is not that rigid.

How is a baby's head different?

In a baby, the bones of the skull are much thinner than those in an adult's, and they do not interlock within each other until the baby has grown to be a few years old. The sites where these bones interlock, when fully developed, are called sutures; in a baby you can easily feel them as ridges, some in the midline of the head, others horizontal or oblique.

The head of the baby has a fairly big soft spot almost in the center of the top, and a few other soft spots in the back part of the skull. The soft spot scares many parents, making them avoid touching it for fear of hurting the baby. This fear is not warranted, because the soft spot consists of a few layers of tissues, be they the scalp, the fibrous tissue, or the meninges.

The large soft spot (called the anterior fontanelle) can give the doctor some valuable information. In some major diseases, such as in meningitis, it may bulge and become tense; in dehydration it may be sunken and depressed; in ricketts it may become very large; and it may close too soon in craniostenosis.

In normal babies you may be able to feel the soft spot become tense when the baby cries, or even slightly depressed when the baby takes a deep breath. It also varies in size from baby to baby, and as the baby grows up, the soft spot will tend to become smaller and smaller until the age of eighteen months, give or take a few months, when the spot will close completely.

How else is the head of a baby different from that of an adult?

The size of a baby's head in relation to the face and body is much larger than that of an adult's. The head of a baby enlarges a good deal during the first twelve months of life, then the rate of its growth will slow down, and it will have attained almost adult size around the age of five years. All of these changes, in size or configuration, are to accommodate the fast-growing brain.

Besides the changes in size and the presence of the soft spots, the baby's head will display ridges that later on become sutures. The bones of a baby's skull are "soft" and thin compared to those of an adult's, and this makes them more malleable and less likely to fracture upon sudden injury. Linear fractures and cracks can be detected, especially when swelling under the scalp raises your suspicion, yet the baby will look happy, smiling, and content!

Can the variation in head size and shape be of value to diagnose certain diseases?

Yes. A rapidly enlarging head is the hallmark of hydrocephalus. This usually means an excess amount of spinal fluid within the skull, caused either by obstruction to the flow of the spinal fluid or some other reasons.

A baby's head not growing as fast as expected is often a serious problem, indicating microcephaly or other major problems with the brain or the skull.

Changes in configuration of the face and head are fairly common, usually during the first two or three months of life. These can give the appearance of a lopsided head and face, flat on one side and round on the other (see page 82).

HEADACHE

Not every headache is the same; a headache is merely a symptom, and may be one of the manifestations of a disease. Children are likely to suffer from headaches far more than expected. This is especially true of migraine headache. But when the headache is one of the symptoms of a disease it makes the diagnosis easier.

What kind of diseases are headaches symptomatic of?

There are many diseases wherein the presence of a headache is fairly frequent, e.g. common diseases like tonsillitis, sore throats, respiratory infections, etc. A headache in a child with other symptoms like fever, vomiting, sore throat or cough means no more than a temporary problem which will go away when the condition subsides with treatment, or by itself. Most such headaches are described as "heavy," occur more or less in the front part of the head, become worse with movement, yet are not that severe. They present themselves in many acute diseases, and often go away in a day or two.

Headache is very important in children with a stiff neck and a high temperature (?meningitis). A child who has this disease will have difficulty or an inability to bend the head towards the chest, or to touch the chest with the chin (see page 503).

How about sinus headaches?

Most so-called sinus headaches are not caused by sinusitis (see page 278); often they are related to allergic blockage of the openings of the sinuses and/or allergic involvement of the sinuses themselves. By the way, chronic sinusitis is quite rare in children, and an X-ray of the sinuses often turns out to be normal.

How about a headache related to the eyes?

This is rare indeed, though most parents assume otherwise. On numerous occasions children have been sent to the eye doctor just to be told the eyes are O.K. and that the headache is caused by something else. It is true that farsightedness, astigmatism, and some other diseases of the eyes can cause a headache, however, this is not as common in children as many parents think.

A headache that keeps coming, often at fairly regular intervals (about once a week or two), is more likely to be a migraine headache than anything else. There are several forms of migraine headache; be it the classical, the common, the cluster, etc. These require the help of the doctor for diagnosis, investigation, and treatment. Most such headaches are only rarely associated with other symptoms, and affect children at a much higher frequency than expected by parents. They are more common in older children, especially those with highly strung perfectionist personalities, who accumulate many obligations on their shoulders.

Will a headache show up in very young children?

A young child (less than three years old) with a severe headache is more likely to have a serious disease than otherwise. A doctor's visit will be mandatory, and diagnostic work may also be necessary right away.

A severe headache that occurs almost daily, especially in the morning -in the front or back of the head- is a sign of serious disease inside the skull. This headache may be associated with bouts of vomiting, loss of coordination or trouble balancing, impaired appetite and loss of weight. The doctor should be contacted; he or she may suspect a lesion in the brain, e.g. a mass of some sort (brain tumor), or fluid collection.

Of the masses in the brain that cause such symptoms are brain tumors. Fortunately they are rare, but when they happen they are devastating, and removal depends on the kind of tumor, its place, rate of growth, etc. Many ways of easier investigation have become available, and an operation whereby the skull is opened and the mass removed can be done, but with variable degrees of success.

How do you treat headaches?

Most headaches in children are mild, and are associated with other symptoms of infectious diseases. If the disease is treated the headache will go away.

As for diseases indicating serious trouble in the brain as mentioned before, prompt treatment should be instituted once the diagnosis is determined. Headache in such conditions is an extremely important symptom; it is of a different character than others and is of great help in the diagnosis.

Headaches of migraine are of different nature, and they are not always easy to control (see below).

MIGRAINE HEADACHE

The child complains of a-headache, more often than not in the temple area or above either eye, though sometimes it can be on both sides. The headache may be severe, usually occurring regularly but infrequently at first. After several months, the headache will become more frequent, perhaps once or twice a week or more often.

Before the onset of the headache, the child may occasionally see things like a bright zigzag line, stars, etc. This is more common in adults, however.

In addition to the headache, he or she may have nausea and vomiting, though this is not the rule, especially when the migraine headache is mild. More often, however, the child goes to sleep after having the headache for a while, and wakes up without it.

How is a migraine headache different from other kinds of headache?

Migraine headaches run in the family; often they affect siblings, parents, or other close relatives of affected children.

Migraine headaches usually affect smart children who are high strung, perfectionists and who tend to compete. A sudden heavy load of obligations may act as a contributing factor.

Are there other differences?

Yes there are. Migraine headache comes much more regularly than other types of headaches. It shows up more often in one temporal area of the head, and it may end up with nausea and vomiting; that is why some people call it "sick headache." Another point to be emphasized is that a migraine headache very often goes away after the child has slept for a while.

What can we do about it?

If aspirin, Tylenol, etc. have not helped much, and a migraine headache is suspected, call the doctor. When the doctor is convinced that the headache is migrinous, he or she will emphasize prevention. There is no cure for migraine so far. The treatment of an acute attack of a migraine headache leaves much to be desired, and quite often the result is only half successful.

What do you do to prevent migraine headache?

Fortunately we can expect good results with prevention, especially with children.

The doctor may elect to prescribe a small dose of medicines like phenobarbital to be given once a day after breakfast over a period of one to two weeks. If the migraine headache stops, then the treatment should continue for a full course (six months). If the recurrent headache doesn't seem to have gone away, the medicine may be increased to twice a day. Inderal (prescription) is preferred by other doctors, and given in a different dosage.

What happens after the full course for prevention?
At the end of this course you stop the medication to see if the child continues to be free from those miserable headaches. If the headache comes back, you better start him or her on another course.

FAINTING SPELLS

It is often a frightening experience when you are confronted with a fainting spell. All of a sudden you see your teenage child fall to the ground, looking pale, slightly sweaty, and limp. He or she will look washed out, the mind will be foggy, and in a minute or two he or she will seem to come out of it; the color will slowly return, the limbs will have more tonicity (muscle tone), and the child may look embarrassed or scared. In some, he or she will feel nauseated and may vomit.

In no more than five to ten minutes, the child is up and around as if nothing has happened.

What causes such a trouble?
Fainting spells (syncope) are more likely to show up in teenagers and young adults, though we see them occasionally in younger children. The spells are likely to show up in special situations, such as upon being given a shot, seeing blood, being in a warm stuffy room, dancing in a hot environment, being in school or church where the thermostat is kept too high, etc. It is more likely to show up in families, and certain people are more sensitive to the condition.

What happens in such cases is that the vagus nerve dilates the blood vessels it supplies, and by action of gravity the blood is pooled down, causing the body to slump. Slumping is an attempt to gain the circulation back to the brain.

Are a good many cases psychological?

Have you ever seen a 200-pound hunk of humanity sitting on a couch to receive a teeny-weeny shot, and as soon as the procedure is done and over with, he slumps over the doctor who is half his size, like a rag? I have, to my own decided discomfort! Indeed, even the thought of the needle or the thought of seeing blood will work on the vagus nerve in some people, and precipitate syncope.

What should we do about it?

If you know that it is syncope and no more, you simply lay the patient flat on his or her back and bend the legs at the knee, and let the person remain in this position for about ten minutes. If the patient wants to get up earlier than that, do not allow it, otherwise he or she may faint again. Keep in mind that some people may need longer than ten minutes.

By so doing, the blood that was pooled by gravity will have returned in its usual manner to the brain. This will lead to the return of tonicity to the muscles, and the patient will feel fine.

Can we recognize the onset of the spell in advance?

In the special situations mentioned above, the patient may develop a queasy feeling, slight nausea, and restlessness, as if he or she is suspecting the oncoming slump. You will notice paleness in the face, along with the restlessness.

At this stage, syncope can be prevented. All that is necessary is to lay the patient on his or her back and let the legs bend at the knee. If the patient is sitting down already, bending them over with their head between the knees will also promote blood supply to the head. Not only will the attack be aborted, but the recovery will be faster.

Shall we treat all syncopes ourselves?

No. Usually the first attack will prompt your concern enough to take the child to the doctor. If the physical exam is negative, the doctor will assure and inform you about what to do in case the same thing happens again.

In some patients, the blood pressure may be found to be on the low side, and patients with low blood pressure will always have a tendency to develop syncope in the future.

Are there medicines to be used?
Yes, there are, but they are to be used immediately to revive the patient. In most cases however, the fainting spell takens place somewhere away from the doctor, and the patient gets over it in a matter of a few minutes. So, for practical reasons, medicines are not likely to be used.

By the way, there are no medicines thus far to prevent such spells, but trying to avoid the precipitating causes of such spells will help prevent them.

EPILEPTIC FITS

Fortunately epileptic fits are not that common, but when a child suffers from them, they become quite a problem. Usually there is a family history of the same or similar forms of seizures. They are not the same as febrile seizures (see page 134), though they may look the same. Only a very small percentage of febrile convulsions become persistent and eventually prove to be epileptic.

How many kinds of epileptic fits are there?
Epileptic fits come in different forms. Unfortunately, it is not unusual for a child to start with one type of epilepsy for some time, just to end up with another type in addition.

The most prevalent form is called grand mal epilepsy. In the latter, the convulsions are similar to those of febrile convulsions. The seizure may last for as little as one or two minutes, or for longer than twenty. Both sides of the body jerk, the face twitches and becomes blue, the breathing becomes almost imperceptible, and finally the patient will take a deep breath with a sigh, just as the fit comes to an end. The victim may sleep for a while afterwards, and may involuntarily urinate. Convulsions of one side of the body, or one limb only, can happen too.

Naturally, this is scary, but what is worse is that it can happen at unexpected moments, and may lead to dangerous consequences.

Certain things can precipitate these attacks and the doctor will certainly discuss them with the child and parents.

Besides the above, there are petit mal or absence fits.

What are these?

Petit mal or absence fits, are more likely to affect older children and pre-adolescents. The child will become still, look at a corner, seem to lose contact with the surrounding, may smack his or her lips, and then come out of it all in a few seconds. It is rare for the victim to sag to the ground or fall; usually he or she stays still. It can happen at night during sleep too, just as grand mal epilepsy can. The two may show up together in the same patient.

Are there other kinds of epilepsy?

Yes there are, though not as common as the above ones. Some affect babies; these are called salaam fits, or myoclonic seizures. They are more dangerous than other kinds of epilepsy. Also there are myoclonic jerks, sudden jerky movement all over, making the body stiff for a short while. Abdominal epilepsy is rare.

Besides the above, there is a form difficult to diagnose called psychomotor seizures. The child will have unusual behavior for a short time -unusual movements of one of the arms, making half a turn, etc.-then fall to the ground. He or she may look pale. After a few minutes of unconsciousness, the child may be up and around.

How are febrile convulsions related to epilepsy?

Febrile convulsions are related to a sudden high temperature; most cases occur in young children. Febrile convulsions are by far the commonest form of fits, but they should not be regarded as a form of epilepsy. The two look alike, but they have different outcomes. Only a small percent of children with febrile convulsions develop epilepsy (see page 134).

To see a convulsion for the first time, be it febrile or epileptic, is a very scary experience for anyone. A child who has fallen to the floor, with repetitious jerky movements all over, seemingly unable to breathe, will unnerve every parent. But it is important that the following be done to the convulsing child right away:

1. Turn the head of the convulsing child to one side,
2. Put something between his or her teeth so that the tongue is not bitten,
3. Let someone call the doctor.

Fortunately most such convulsions, be they febrile or grand mal epilepsy, will take a short time and stop spontaneously.

What can be done about it?

The doctor or neurologist will have to do the investigation. Brain-wave test (EEG), CAT scan, blood tests, etc., may all be indicated. Once the diagnosis is determined, treatment will be initiated.

Just as important, is the need to understand epilepsy, not only by parents but also by the child, if he or she is old enough. Some points of extreme importance are taking the medicine regularly, taking special precautions when swimming or bicycle riding, and finding out whether or not the child will be able to drive.

How about treatment?

Once the form of epilepsy is diagnosed, certain medicines or even a combination of medicines have to be used. They will help prevent further fits, or make them less frequent. Medications should preferably be prescribed by a neurologist or someone experienced in this field. Often they are used for a good many years, and the patient has to be seen by the doctor regularly for special blood tests. Such measures are necessary to prevent these fits and let the patient lead as normal a life as possible. If the child fails to take the medicines regularly, this may precipitate convulsions and epileptic fits, some of which may be so prolonged as to go into status epilepticus, which in itself is a true emergency.

NERVOUS TICS

Your child seems to have a nasty habit of twitching and moving the shoulder, on and off. It is more evident when he or she is watched, or under tension. You may break your silence and say "stop that," and with a twitch of the shoulder the child will say, "stop what?"

What causes nervous ticks?

No one really knows. Many a child will go through such a stage and come out of it without any recurrence. A high-strung and competitive child stands a greater chance of developing nervous tics, and so does a sensitive or self-conscious one.

Nervous tics go through phases; they may start at one location, subside weeks or months later, and then reappear in a different form or location.

How can the nervous tic change?

It may go to the eye or eyes: the child may blink incessantly, or lift the eyebrow. This may drive you batty, and the more you look at the poor soul, the more you feel like holding the affected area still. It may also take a few weeks to a few months before it subsides. Just as you start to count your blessings, the habit may then go to the nose and throat: twitching the nose or twirling it, clearing the throat, moving the neck as if there is something agonizing inside, and even making seal-like noises.

These are but a few examples of nervous tics. A combination of different forms of tics can also show up, leading to some truly bizarre movements. Mild ones usually disappear after a few months. More severe ones may go from one form to another, but they eventually disappear after a year or two. It is not rare for these tics to continue to come and go for years, but in most they disappear after adolescence. Only exceptionally do they persist in adulthood.

Won't this look funny in front of people?

Naturally, people will see the tic, but they are less likely to make fun of the child than the parents themselves are. For some reason, other children may imitate him out of sympathy, but rarely do they make fun of him.

What can I do about the tic, then?

Don't badger the poor child; control yourself. Shift the child's attention (thus breaking the cycle of tics) by asking him or her to do certain things for you, thus keeping his or her mind off it.

Don't overschedule the child. Don't overcommit him or her in school or otherwise. Allow competition but don't push too much; allow participation in athletics. Love but don't smother the child.

Remember, there is no medicine that is truly helpful. It is a stage in life many children go through, and although it is bothersome, it will pass.

How about a tranquilizer?

Although the tics are called "nervous", medicines such as tranquilizers are usually useless. Calming the nerves, making the child dopy and less alert, will not reduce the degree of frequency of the nervous tics.

Unfortunately there is no specific medicine up to this date that can help a child with nervous tics. Social and cultural pressure, especially in a sensitive and self-conscious child, combine to produce this problem. Those bizarre movements are in essence a release of tension by the central nervous system. We must learn to live with it, and make it easier for the child.

Is it catching?

No it is not, unless your child is quite suggestible, and inclined to nervous tics anyway. Upon seeing another child with the tics, your child may start his or her own, mimicking the other twitchy child.

THE HYPERKINETIC CHILD
ATTENTION DEFICIT DISORDER

They act differently from others, are quite overactive and tend to be restless, have a short span of attention and are easily distracted. They tend to be impulsive and inconsistent, or emotionally high-strung, and can easily panic. Some parents call them "hyperactive".

They may have difficulty in learning, especially in arithmetic, reading, and spelling. They may also have difficulty in other aspects such as visual and auditory perception; this may manifest itself in poor handwriting, printing, and drawing. They are difficult to manage, in school or at home.

Not only that, but at times their general coordination seems to be affected. They appear to be clumsy and awkward, and this may show in the way they walk, ride their bicycles, button their shirts, etc. This is a problem of attention, what is called "attention deficit defect, or ADD". The child will have difficulty sitting still and listening.

Does this mean they have some trouble with the brain?

No one is sure of the cause of this condition, and there are many theories. It is good to know that this condition is quite common; about one out of ten children is affected. The degree of severity varies a great deal from child to child, but mostly tends to be mild. It is more common in boys than in girls. The most reasonable theory about its cause is that it is a delay in the maturation process of certain functions of the brain.

How does this affect school performance?

They may have low, normal or superior intelligence. Therefore, they may do quite well in school. However, slow learning can result if the child cannot keep still to pay attention.

These children are often quite frustrated; they may become depressed and have low self-esteem because of their repeated failures. They want to sit still and listen, and they want to learn as much or more than anyone else in the class, but they cannot. There seems to be something inside them that keeps their motor running and highly charged. They will need a specialized approach, good understanding of the problems by others, and sympathetic and very patient ears.

How will the teacher react?

Most teachers are familiar with this condition since it is so common. The experienced teacher will accept the child and try to help as best as he or she can. However, if the child is too distractible or tends to disrupt the class too often, the teacher will certainly notify the authorities and the parents.

What is to be done?

The child ought to see the doctor first to make sure there is nothing wrong physically. If the condition is very mild, your doctor might explain the condition to you and offer some suggestions. If the condition is fairly severe, the doctor might send the child to a specialist who will analyze the home and school situation, and offer many good recommendations.

Using medicines may help sometimes but we should not resort to them until the situation is analyzed by the pediatrician or specialist. If medicines are to be used, you will have to use them over a prolonged period.

Recently, coffee has been discovered to be of help in some; it is certainly worth a try. It doesn't hurt to give the child a cup of coffee at breakfast and after school, and see if he or she improves in general. Decaffeinated coffee won't do, and coffee with cream is O.K.

How long will the child have this condition?

Most, if not all, hyperkinetic children are born with this condition. They are the more difficult ones to discipline and raise. They are difficult in the school for the first few years, and by the pre-teenage period they will have matured some. However, a bit of this condition will be with them the rest of their lives.

Tell me more about the medicines:

As said before, it is far better to have the child and the home/school environment analyzed first. By so doing, you will gain a deeper insight into the problem, and you will be better able to cope with it.

If the doctor (not you or the teacher) feels that medicines are indicated, they can be used for prolonged periods. Most are used once or twice a day. They can prolong the span of attention; the child will be relatively still, and likely to learn somewhat closer to his or her potential.

Medicines don't treat the basic cause of the problem however, and they are likely to produce some side effects. They are expected to help in fifty to seventy-five percent of the cases.

If the child is tested in the school and found to have learning disability and/or psychological repercussions, proper handling in the school will become mandatory. Placement under teachers with special expertise will help a lot.

You may have heard of the Feingold diet, and it is worth a try. It is difficult to follow, but if the results are good, it is worth sticking to it.

CONCUSSION

A concussion may follow a fall or a hit on the head. Generally the more severe the fall or hit is, the more severe the concussion. Sometimes, however, the fall or the hit may be insignificant in severity, yet it may result in a concussion. And, of course, many severe falls cause no concussion whatsoever.

Concussion is a reaction of the brain when the skull is jarred.

<u>What does a concussion mean?</u>

When a concussion shows up, it means nothing beyond a sudden temporary reaction of the brain to the situation, and the child will be perfectly all right afterwards.

However, a concussion and its aftermath may be warnings of some important changes in the skull or the brain itself. Although this is not so common, we should always be on the look out for such possibilities.

<u>What symptoms shall we expect?</u>

After the fall or the hit on the head, the child may lose consciousness for a few seconds, become limp, pale, and unresponsive to anything around.

The child may continue to be pale for some time after regaining consciousness and may want to go to sleep. He or she may sleep for variable periods of time (from fifteen minutes or more). The child's color may gradually come back to normal too.

When the child wakes up, he or she may complain of a headache, even though the headache will not seem to be that severe. This may also be accompanied or followed by one or two bouts of vomiting.

This sequence of events may not be as orderly as mentioned above and some of its components may not even show up. As a matter of fact, a concussion may be much milder than the above.

<u>What symptoms indicate a mild concussion?</u>

There may not be any vomiting, but nausea instead, or not even that. The headache may be very mild, or the period of sleep that follows may be almost absent. In some, loss of conciousness may not even have occurred.

The milder the concussion the less severe the symptoms.

<u>When shall I worry?</u>

Call the doctor, of course, if the child has all the manifestations of concussion; he or she may want to see the child and perhaps take an X-ray of the skull.

Call the doctor also if any of the following occurs:

1. a loss of conciousness,
2. and/or headache,
3. and/or prolonged sleep,
4. and/or vomiting.

<u>What can we do?</u>

The local swelling of the hit area may take a few days to go away. Applying ice packs for the first half-hour will help. This should be followed by applying heat for twenty to thirty minutes, three to four times a day. The cold application will help prevent the swelling from enlarging, but applying the heat afterwards will help make it go away faster.

The doctor will probably tell you to:

1. Give your child liquids or a light meal;
2. Wake your child through the night every one to two hours depending on how severe the concussion is. This is done to make sure that the child can respond to being awakened and that he or she is not in a coma. You wake the child up to the extent that a question can be answered;

3. Try to avoid aspirin unless the headache is really severe enough.

Will any trouble follow concussions?

Most children with a concussion will snap out of it without any aftereffects. However, a few children will develop some trouble.

The amount of trouble usually depends on the severity of the fall or the hit. In some it may not be more than a local swelling of the area hit. Yet a crack of the skull, or even some damage to some of the tissues inside the skull, can result if the fall or the hit is quite severe. This is the reason for all the fuss about checking, taking skull X-rays, waking up the child, etc. But remember, if the fall or hit is prevented, the concussion will never show up to begin with, and you will have saved yourself all the worries.

Remember please, a child with a prolonged headache, dizziness, or any unusual symptoms that immediately follow a fall -or develop some time after the fall- should see the doctor.

DOWN'S SYNDROME (MONGOLISM)

The child is born with certain features, and as he or she grows up, the looks will be very much like others who have the same condition. Down's syndrome is probably the largest cause of mental retardation; as much as ten percent of the children in an institution for the mentally retarded are children with this affliction. It usually, but not always affects children born to older mothers.

How is that?

Pregnancies beyond the age of thirty-five years and especially after the age of forty, are more likely to result in a baby with this problem. The older the expecting mother is, the more likely she is to have such a baby. On the other hand, some young mothers (in their teens) can have a baby with such a problem too. Also some families seem to have the tendencies for it.

The cause is troubled chromosomes, and since such chromosomes can be detected in the amniotic fluid during pregnancy, it is easy now to take preventive measures.

The amniotic fluid, as you know, is the fluid in which the baby "bathes" while inside the uterus. This fluid contains many cells which the baby sheds. A sample of such fluid can be obtained by the obstetrician and sent to the lab for chromosome analysis. If the analysis shows the abnormal chromosomes of Down's syndrome, the parents may agree to have a therapeutic abortion, terminating the pregnancy.

How will the child look?

A child who has Down's syndrome is usually easy-going, agreeable, and does not cause problems. The face shows slanting eyes and a low bridge of the nose; often the tongue protrudes slightly, the ears look slightly defective and the head seems small and a bit flat.

The hands are chubby, with somewhat short fingers, and the fifth finger is slightly curved. When the child walks, the abdomen protrudes, and frequently he or she has an umbilical hernia. The doctor will listen carefully to the heart, since these babies carry a high chance of congenital heart disease.

What about their development?

Because they are always mentally retarded, their development is delayed; e.g. they begin to sit up late and they walk late, much later than the usual age of twelve to thirteen months. The same applies to other physical development. Talking will also be delayed, depending on the severity of the condition, as will the degree of emotional maturity and power of reasoning.

It is important to know that not all cases of Down's syndrome are of the same severity. The children with mild ones are quite educable, and they can be trained to do certain jobs. Of course the severe cases are quite a load on the family, and it may be so severe that the family will prefer to put the child in an institution. But at home, such a child often easily earns the love and care of parents, brothers, and sisters, and each will cater to the child's needs.

Is there not any treatment?

No, unfortunately there is not, because the trouble is in the structure of the cells themselves. However, prevention can be done by now, thanks to our ability to check the amniotic fluid.

Will their health suffer?

Most children with Down's syndrome are likely to have frequent, repeated infections, especially upper respiratory infection. Pneumonia is not that uncommon. Many will have frequent ear infections, sore throats, etc. Many of these infections are preventable, especially when the parental care is of good quality. Prevention of exposure to such diseases, well-cared-for skin, a humidified environment during winter, will go a long way in minimizing such infections.

How will they be when they grow up?

A child with Down's syndrome will have the condition throughout life. The features will continue to be the same, as will the degree of mental retardation. The care given by the family, especially an understanding family, with the help of some specialized schools and perhaps even some institutions, will help in giving the best opportunity to develop the limited potential of such unfortunate but lovable persons. Adults with mild cases may even be able to hold minor jobs, but with some degree of supervision.

MENINGITIS

Meningitis is a dreaded disease, and once it is there, immediate treatment has to be initiated, otherwise a good deal of serious trouble can result. Meningitis means inflammation of the meninges, or the covering of the brain. The inflammation is caused by a variety of germs that prefer different ages.

How are the different ages affected?

Tiny babies in the neonatal (newborn) stage often have a completely different meningitis than older children. A meningitis caused by pneumococcus or H. influenzae is far more common in infants and older children than newborn.

Also a germ by the name of meningococcus can be the cause. Meningitis by this germ is quite contagious, and when this is the case, special precautions have to be taken by those in contact.

What precautions should be taken?

A child with meningitis caused by the germ meningococcus is more contagious than one with other forms of meningitis. Therefore those in contact with the sick child have to be put on certain medications to prevent them from getting meningitis. Your doctor will be the one to take such a step.

The "contacts" mean those who have been in close contact with the child for the previous few days. Therefore mother, father, other children, and other people living in the same house must receive the medications. If one of these members had only a momentary contact with the patient, it is unnecessary to put him or her on any prophylactic medication.

How will we know the child has meningitis?

In most cases the child is very sick, though in the early stages of the disease he or she may not be that sick-looking. A high temperature with or without convulsions is the usual first symptom, with headache, sleepiness, or an unusual inability to be aroused. The latter is a very important point. The neck usually becomes stiff in an older child (but not necessarily in an infant). The stiffness is usually such that the child cannot bend the head toward the chest, or touch the chest with the chin. If this seems to be the case, get in touch with your doctor.

Other symptoms such as vomiting, refusing to eat, staring, convulsions, etc., may all be present.

What will the doctor do?

Once the doctor suspects meningitis, he or she will send the child to the hospital immediately. A spinal tap will be done, as will cultures and other tests, and if positive for meningitis, intravenous treatment will be initiated. The culture of the spinal fluid is very important since it determines what kind of antibiotic has to be used, and for how long.

In most, a ten-day or longer course of antibiotics, mostly intravenously, has to be given. Usually within a day or two of the treatment, the child will look and feel better, and the temperature comes down. In a baby, the soft spot on the head will not feel tense anymore. In case of complications, the progress will not be as good, and a second or even third spinal tap may have to be done.

Will the child be O.K. afterwards?

If treated promptly and early enough, meningitis will go away without aftereffects in most children. If treated late, or if complications arise, there will be a danger for later problems.

If meningitis is not discovered until two or three days have passed (or even longer), if it is of a certain severity or form, or it occurs in certain age group, there will be a chance for possible later consequences: the child should be examined by a neurologist, the hearing should be tested, and even the psychological status may have to be assessed at a future time.

How common is meningitis?

Meningitis is not that common; every few years a pediatrician may see one. The treatment has to be in the hospital, and should be prompt, to avoid the aforementioned consequences.

It is fortunate that present day treatment, if given early, can result in a prompt improvement and a normal child within about two weeks.

Unfortunately there is no way to prevent meningitis as of yet; that is, except for those who are in close contact with an already established case.

CHAPTER SEVENTEEN

ORTHOPEDICS

bones and growth of the child
growing pains, fact or fiction
sprains of the joints
fractures
the swollen joint
flat feet and knock-knee
pigeon toe
Osgood Schlatter disease
toxic synovitis of the hip joint
radial subluxation
scoliosis or the curved back
kyphosis and lordosis (the round-back and the sway-back)
congenital dislocation of the hip joint

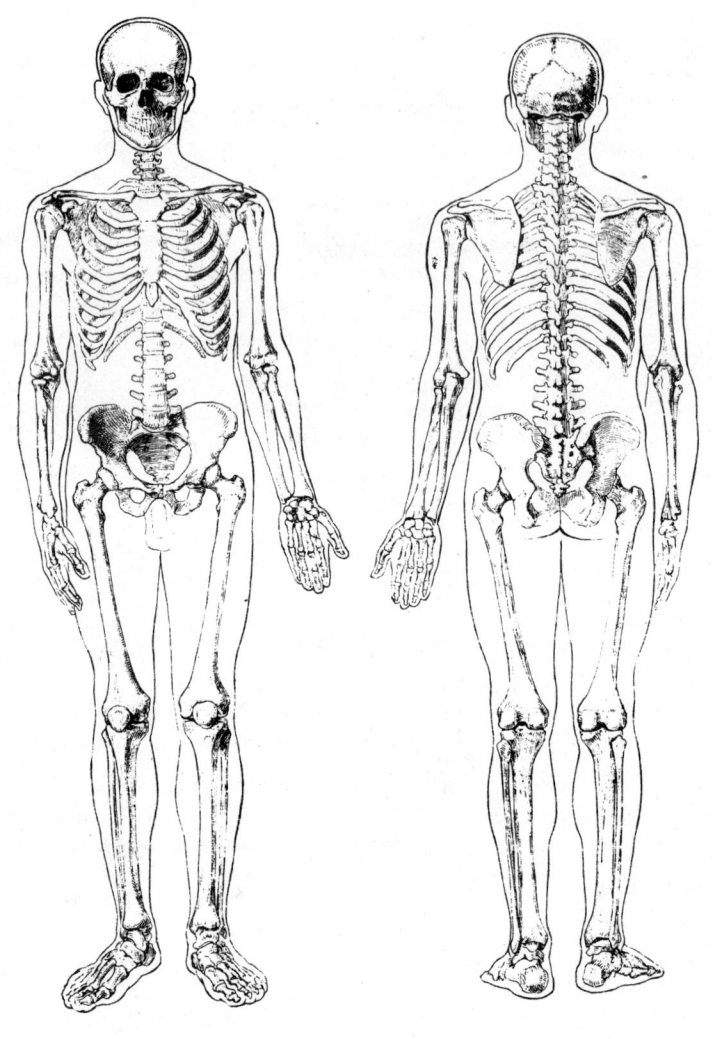

Gray's anatomy, p 135, fig 144, 26th Ed 1954
Courtesy Eycleshymer & Jones
Written permission from the publisher, Lea & Febiger, Philadelphia

BONES AND GROWTH OF THE CHILD

Some bones serve for walking, others for using the arms, some for the dexterity of the fingers and toes, others to hold us erect, some to shape our faces, and others to protect our most important organ, the brain. Some bones are long, others are flat, some are cuboid or oddly shaped. Some bones meet at the joints to make it possible for movements, and others are so closely enmeshed with their next bone that they are immobile.

A baby has pliable bones, with abundant cartilage; the bones have growth centers situated in certain areas. Not only that, but as the baby grows so will the degree of ossification, or solidification, of the bone. The process continues at various rates until the child reaches maturity.

The bones also contain the marrow, which is the site of most blood formation in a baby, and all of it in a child or adult. That is the reason why in certain blood diseases a doctor may have to do a bone marrow tap.

The bone marrow is fully active producing blood in a baby, but as the baby grows up there will be less need for that much blood formation. When this stage is reached, the blood forming bone marrow will be exclusively in the flat bones and the ends of the long bones.

A growing child has soft bones which can change shape depending on the stresses put on those bones.

How do the bones change shape?

Because the bones are malleable in a growing child, and because of variable degrees of growth, the bone may shape itself according to the degree of stress put on it, if given long enough time. A good example is that of the baby who sleeps on his or her back with the head turned to one side. After two or three months, the face and the skull will become flattened on one side, and the face may even look lopsided (see page 82).

A baby who sleeps on his or her stomach and keeps his or her feet turned in, will cause the shinbone to curve to accommodate the stress of the weight of the legs, leading to some degree of pigeon toe (see page 521). In an older child, the habit of sitting on the floor with the feet by the side of the buttocks can lead to rotation of the head of the femur (thigh bone). This will also lead to inward turning of the legs, a more difficult form of pigeon toe to treat and correct (see page 521).

Even teenagers are not exempt from such problems. Because of their fast growth, the bones can do some accommodating too. The teenager who habitually reclines on his or her side while watching TV, or sits in a classroom chair leaning towards one side, will cause the spine to curve towards that side after a few months. This may lead to what is called postural scoliosis (see page 528).

Not only that, but a teenager who hunches his or her back and droops all the time, can develop some degree of postural kyphosis. This is especially true of teenage girls who are embarrassed and shy because of the budding of their breasts (see page 530).

What can we do about all these things?

All the above conditions can be prevented if the position of the child is corrected early. Usually the doctor has to notify you since it is very easy for the parents to miss the implications. If the bone changes are left for too long, they often become permanent. Early and persistent attempts at correcting the position of the child, from infancy through teenage, can prevent a good deal of worry, treatment and expense.

Are vitamins good for the growth of the bones?

Growth of the bones is governed by the growth hormone, thyroid hormone, gonadal hormone (during the teenage growth spurt), and many other things. Vitamins are essential for the body, and they should be given when there is suspicion that they may be deficient. But for the bones, even during the period of fast growth, the administration of vitamins is not as important as a well-rounded diet. In such a diet, an ample supply of calcium, protein, and vitamins is quite available.

The availability of calcium, protein, and vitamin D is essential, since they are needed by the growing bone. Many diseases can show up if any of the above factors is deficient. A pint of milk a day usually gives an ample supply of not only calcium but also protein and vitamin D. In an older child, the well-rounded diet will easily supply all the essential constituants the bones need; therefore, even the pint of milk a day may not be needed that badly.

If vitamin D is not present adequately, be it in milk or food, a disease called rickets may show up. This used to be common in days gone by, but with better nutrition and with the addition of vitamin D to milk, this disease has almost disappeared from the scene. Rickets is probably still prevalent in countries where nourishment and sunshine are deficient. (Vitamin D can be synthesized in the skin upon exposure to sunlight.)

"GROWING PAINS": FACT OR FICTION

By the time children are a few years old, they are active and vigorous. They jump a lot, are constantly on the run, and show many bruises on their legs as a testimony to all of that. Their parents repeatedly mention that they cannot keep up with them. The children are on the go from the time they wake up until they go to bed.

But often these children wake up at night complaining of pains in the legs. The pains may be severe enough at times to make them cry. The pains don't come regularly. When you ask where it hurts, the children will point to the legs, but not to any specific point. Somehow the location of the pain is vague and variable, but it is in the legs. There is no fever or any other symptoms. You look for swelling or other signs of trouble in the legs, but you find none. Because of the recurrence of this experience, you take the child to the doctor, and ask if the child has "growing pains."

The doctor will check the child, paying special attention to the joints, feeling the muscles, trying to see if there are any points of tenderness, check the legs for alignment, and will check the arches of the feet.

Though everything is O.K., the doctor will still say that there is no such thing as "growing pains."

If "growing pains" are a myth, what are these pains then?

Growing pains are a myth, and the term used to be used often in the days gone by, by doctors and parents alike, for lack of a better description. Such pains are felt by very active children who are constantly on the go, jumping and running much of their waking hours.

Naturally this "strains" the muscles, mainly the muscles of the legs. The "strained," weary muscles then have to repair themselves and be in shape for next day's activities. When the child goes to bed, the muscles will have that welcome period of rest and repair. As they do so, the pains in the legs will be felt and this may wake up the child.

The irony of the term "growing pains" is that these pains show up at a period when the rate of growth is quite slow (if not the slowest) during childhood.

Why check the child?

It is wise to make sure that there are no other causes for these pains. That is why the doctor will look for flat feet, knock knees, bow legs, pigeon toes or other orthopedic problems. The doctor will also try to rule out the presence of other diseases. If all the findings are negative, the pain will be blamed on the activity of the eager beaver. Such pains are fairly common; their severity varies from child to child, and in the same child from day to day. They may show up for a while, just to go away by themselves for a few weeks, then reappear again. In most they are not severe enough to make the child cry, although this can happen, and mainly at night.

What can I do for the pains?

When confronted with the child's complaints, it is wise to give the child some assurances and comforting words. Administer aspirin, and massage the area that hurts. You may elect to rub in Ben Gay or Myoflex Cream (nonprescription). Also application of heat (or a hot bath) may be necessary. These measures often ease the pain and give comfort to the aching muscles.

Can we prevent such pains?

Because these pains are related to the amount and level of activity, and to the frequent constant stress put on the muscles, if the child cuts down on the activity, the pains will probably not show up. This of course is easier said than done, since the world is very exciting in the eyes of young children, and it is more fun to jump or run than to think of preventive measures.

However, if the parent devises ways to curb the child's activity to some extent, and to let him or her rest during daytime, the frequency of these pains may diminish. If the child sits down, watches TV, is read to, or plays sedentary games, the muscles will be spared some, and there will be respite for his or her body and parents alike.

At what ages do the pains show up?

They often show up when the child goes wild with activity at ages three, four, and five years. Before and after that the pains will hardly be there.

The mild cases are often cared for by the parents, and the doctor is rarely consulted. Severe ones are a different story; they require medical advice. When the condition is diagnosed and treatment is given, it will be reassuring to the whole family that no dreadful disease is in the winds, and that a simple approach is all that is needed.

SPRAINS OF THE JOINTS

The child comes to you with pain in the joint; if it happens to be in the knee or ankle, he or she will come with a limp. The pain may or may not be severe, and he or she may scream at your attempts to move the painful joint.

The swelling at the joint may progress rapidly, over a period of several hours, to become easily noticeable. Often there is some degree of discoloration.

The child may have twisted the foot rapidly and sprained the ankle, or hurt the knee suddenly while playing a sport. Sprain of the wrist or finger joints may occur while trying to catch a fast-moving ball, or some similar manner.

What shall I do right away?

Apply an ice pack to the area. This is more important for the first half-hour of the injury. It will help prevent the swelling from becoming very large, and it may also help ease the pain. In the meantime, call the doctor to see whether or not the child should be seen right away.

Will the child need to be seen for that?

In most cases yes. The main reason is that a small percentage will prove to have a fracture in one of the bones of the sprained joint. The doctor will also be able to evaluate the severity and the degree of the injury, and will try to see if there are associated injuries to the other structures. The treatment will of course depend on the severity of the injury and on whether or not there is any associated fracture. Therefore, quite often an X-ray will have to be taken.

Why does the joint swell so much?

The bones composing a joint are connected to each other by a capsule of various thickness and strength. Some bones are also connected to each other by ligaments of various strength and thickness. When there is a sudden injury of a severe enough degree, there will be a break of some of the fibers of the soft tissues of and around the joint. On rare occasions the ligaments may also suffer.

When this happens, the tissues around will react to heal the injury, and in the process they will swell. The injury and the swelling will cause the pain, and the pain may force the immobilization of the joint.

What will the doctor do?

That depends on the degree of the sprain, on the joint involved, on whether there are associated injuries, and especially on whether there is a fracture nearby.

Application of ice packs for the first half-hour (to reduce the swelling) to be followed by application of heat to the area involved will help promote the healing.

The principle of treatment, however, will remain the same. Resting the joint for an appropriate amount of time is the most important point. To rest the joint, you will have to immobilize it to a certain extent. Application of an ace bandage or some similar support can be used for certain joints. This will add support to the area, keep the heat, and insure a fair degree of immobilization. To restrict the movement of the injured joint, or even to prevent it from moving for a while will go a long way to speed up the recovery. For a sprained ankle or knee, a crutch may be necessary; this will help a lot in resting the joint.

For a finger or wrist, immobilization can be done with various devices too, and for the sprained elbow joint, the arm has to have a sling.

How long will this have to be done?

This depends on many factors too. Most sprains need about seven to fourteen days of treatment, though more severe ones will need longer. The tissues of a sprained joint need a longer time to heal than many other tissues because of the very nature of the joint tissues themselves.

Fortunately, most sprains will go away without residual trouble, complications, or defects.

FRACTURES

A broken bone of some sort, is an experience that many families go through. Mostly it is a product of an accident, be it a fall, a hit, or otherwise. It can show up in any age. When it happens or is suspected, immediate attention is to be sought. Fractures in babies or young children may behave differently than those in older children or adults.

How do fractures behave differently for different age groups?

The bones of a baby and a young child are like the green branches of a tree; they are softer and not as brittle as the bones of an adult. When a fracture in a baby or a small child takes place, it may be incomplete (green-stick fracture), just as a green stick of a tree, will only break in part, while the adjacent part will remain intact. This is the usual in fractures of the collarbone (clavicle), which are seen mostly in newborns and young children.

Chips, cracks, and linear fractures of the small bones, long bones, or the skull, occur more often in the very young than in older children or adults, and healing takes place at a faster rate. This goes hand in hand with the fast growth of the very young, and the adaptability of their agile bodies.

Even after treatment, and even if the ends of the bones do not seem to be in perfect alignment, the bones will straighten themselves out within a few months afterwards, thanks to the diligent work of mother nature.

What can we do when we suspect a fracture?

If it is obvious that the child has a fracture, or even if you suspect that there is a fracture, see the orthopedic surgeon right away. If he or she is not available, take the child to the emergency room of the nearest hospital.

Be careful not to disturb the injured part. Movement of the injured part may make it more difficult for the doctor to fix the fracture, or may lead to some complications.

An X-ray will be taken to ascertain the type and degree of fracture.

What will the doctor do?

That depends on the type of bone fractured, and on the extent of the fracture. A fracture of the skull may not need anything done, if the skull has been cracked but has remained in perfect alignment. If the skull fracture is depressed or has developed some complications, the proper treatment will have to be done.

A "green-stick" fracture of the collarbone may need only a figure-eight strapping, or a similar brace. After a number of weeks, the bone will have healed nicely, and the strapping will not be needed anymore. Actually, this type of fracture in a newborn will need to be left alone, and it will heal nicely by itself within about three week's time.

Minor cracks or chips of the finger and toe bones, and of some bones of the hands and feet, may need immobilization for only two to three weeks.

Fractures of the arms and legs need casts, as you well know. The cast will immobilize the injured part, and this will be required for a few weeks to a few months, until the bone is fully healed. The length of time depends on how bad the fracture is, where it is, what type it is, and at what age it takes place. Some fractures may need hospitalization. This is especially true in case of fractures of the back, the thigh bone (femur), the hip, etc. Various bizarre-looking modes of management may have to be used, from pins through the bones, to traction or slings, to special body casts, etc.

Should we take any precautions during the period of treatment?

Generally speaking, the fracture area should be handled as little as possible, especially when the fractured part is not in a cast (such as fractures of the collarbone and the ribs) or is splinted (such as fractures of the finger bones and hands).

While fractures of the arms and legs are safely secured in a cast, exercise of the toes and fingers are very important. The reason is that without such exercises, the muscles inside the cast will atrophy.

Do fractures always come from accidents?

In the majority, fractures come from accidents of sufficient severity. Sometimes, however, they come from bone diseases, or generalized diseases such as osteogenesis imperfecta. In some such diseases fractures may seem to come from nowhere. Fortunately, these diseases are quite rare.

THE SWOLLEN JOINT

The child complains of a dull and continuous pain in a joint that may become sharp when a movement of that joint is attempted. You take a look and you will find out that the joint has become swollen, and it may have some discoloration.

As you know, there are big joints and small joints. Examples of the big joints are the knees, ankles, hips, shoulders, elbows and wrists; examples of the small joints are the joints of the fingers, toes, and some others.

Accidents can lead to a sprain of any of the joints above. Of course the small joints as well as the large joints can become sprained if that particular joint has endured the accidental injury. Therefore, a sprain can affect almost any joint, large or small, and the degree of swelling or pain will depend on the type and severity of the injury (see page 513).

Besides sprains, other diseases can also lead to swelling of the joints; some affect mainly the large joints and others affect mainly the small ones.

What diseases usually lead to a large-joint swelling?

Large joints can become swollen, painful, and tender due to diseases such as rheumatic fever (see page 166), which can affect a large joint at one time only to affect another joint in a few days. Another disease that likes large joints is anaphylactoid purpura (see page 403). This disease affects the ankle joints, making them swollen, hard, tender to the touch, and painful. Most likely there will be rash in that area, and quite often the trouble takes longer than a week or two before going away.

There are other diseases besides the above that affect big joints but these diseases are rare. It is good to know however, that the arthritis common in older people does not show in children except on very rare occasions, and only when related to some specific circumstances.

What makes a small joint swell?

Of course, a sprain of such joints is the commonest cause of their swelling, but there are some other diseases that can do the same. A noteworthy example is rheumatoid arthritis. This is not a common disease, but when it affects a child it tends to affect the joints of the fingers and/or toes in particular (less commonly it can affect big joints too). In this disease, the joints tend to become stiff and moderately painful; the swelling feels rubbery to the touch, and a finger may look like a spindle, being swollen in the middle. The swelling tends to come insidiously, advancing gradually and lingering for weeks before subsiding.

What shall I do when my child has a swollen joint?

Whenever a child has a swollen joint of any type and shape, he or she should see the doctor. If it is a sprained joint, the area has to be immobilized, and if the swelling is caused by some other disease, it is very important that a diagnosis be established and treatment initiated as soon as possible. Make sure not to use aspirin before seeing the doctor, since aspirin may mask the symptoms of the troubled joint.

Naturally there are many rare diseases other than the above that lead to swelling of a joint or a number of joints, and a good many tests and X-rays may have to be done before reaching a diagnosis. Occasionally such diseases may prove to be serious.

FLAT FEET AND KNOCK-KNEE

Flat feet are fairly common, especially the mild variety. However, they cannot be detected with certainty until the child is around the age of one-and-a-half years.

Why is that?

Most babies' feet have the appearance of flat feet, but as the babies reach the age of around twelve months, a doctor can have a fairly good idea about whether or not the baby will actually develop flat feet. The little one has to be kept under observation for a few months, and if he or she has flat feet, they will show clearly around the age of eighteen months. If you discover it as early as this, it is fairly easy to correct.

What would you do for flat feet?

In all the early cases, you should encourage the child to walk barefoot -if possible, on rough uneven surfaces. This will not only let the toes "dig in," but will also force the muscles that control the legs, ankles, and feet to work extra hard. This will tend to pull up the arch of the feet. The more the child does this, the better; it should also be done for a long period, i.e. several years.

Another good exercise is to encourage them to walk on tiptoe. This will make the calf muscles contract hard, pulling at the arch of the foot.

What would you do for the shoes?

In mild and moderate degrees of flat feet, a doctor usually prescribes "wedges" to be put on the inside margin of the soles and heels. The shoes with the wedges will have to be used for several years, and the feet have to be checked every six to twelve months. In most cases an arch "cookie" and/or Thomas Heel shoes are not desirable.

Another point to be remembered is that the flat-footed child should not use sneakers on regular basis, even if someone sells you on the idea of putting the arch "cookie" in the tennis shoe. Tennis shoes with arch cookies will give a negative support to the foot and a false sense of security to you. When the child is older and wants to play tennis, he or she may use the tennis shoes for that occasion, but not as a matter of routine.

How long will it take to correct the flat feet?

It usually takes a few years to correct flat feet. In most cases the foot corrects itself spontaneously. The special "corrective" shoes do one useful function: they put the flat-footed legs in the proper alignment. This will help prevent any painful muscle spasm resulting from being flat-footed.

What will flat feet do?

If left uncorrected, it will lead probably to pain and tension of the leg muscles. It may also lead to some degree of knock-knee. Various degrees of flat feet and knock-knees can be seen together in one child. Knock-knee is easy to discover. To do so, just sit the child and hold his or her legs together until the inside of both knees touch each other. Look at the distance between the two bones above the inside of the ankles. If the distance permits four finger-breadths or more, then the child has knock-knee.

What would you do for knock-knee?

Knock-knees can be helped with the same procedure used for flat feet. Likewise, when given time, most cases of knock-knee correct themselves spontaneously. Occasionally a knock-kneed child may even become bow-legged no more than a few years later! And that may also correct itself spontaneously!

Are flat feet inherited?

Only to some extent. Some babies are born with eversion of the feet and this will lead to a tendency for flat feet. This happens in particular if the baby is left to sleep on his or her stomach all the time. In such cases, you may be able to effect some prevention if you encourage the child to sleep on his or her back.

Are flat feet the business of the orthopedic surgeon?

Most flat feet should be evaluated by the child's doctor. If the flat feet and/or knock-knee is mild to moderate, the doctor will manage it accordingly. If it is severe and if there is a chance of other kinds of trouble in addition, he or she will refer you to an orthopedic surgeon.

PIGEON TOE

Pigeon toe is a fairly common condition. The feet (and sometimes especially the big toes) seem to point inward. It can be detected soon after birth, and it can persist long after that in some cases. When mild it can disappear without any treatment.

What causes pigeon toe?

Pigeon toe can originate at three important sites:

1. The front part of the foot, when the foot points towards the middle line.
2. The tibia (shin bone) when it is rotated inward. You can detect this easily if you sit up the child, have the leg extended, hold the kneecap in a horizontal manner, and see if the tibia (shin bone) curves sharply toward the middle line. You may want to mark the edge of the tibia with a felt pen and see how it curves. The result may surprise you.
3. The head of the femur (thigh bone) when it is the culprit, especially in girls. This leads to turning of the whole leg inward.

What do you do if the pigeon toe originates at the feet?

Mild ones may be left alone. Other cases may require special shoes, such as the kind known as straight-last or reverse-last. This may have to be used early and for a long time. In severe degrees of this kind of pigeon toe an orthopedic surgeon may have to apply a cast to begin with. Fortunately this doesn't happen very often.

What would you do if the pigeon toe happens to be at the tibia?

This is what we call internal tibial torsion. Fortunately, most cases gradually correct themselves over a period of four to five years, without any special treatment. Luckily too, the majority of pigeon toe are of this kind.

Only severe cases of internal tibial torsion need specialized treatment with the orthopedic surgeon, early if possible, and usually through the use of casts.

Can I help in correcting the above problems?

In most mild pigeon toes originating in the feet, the tibias, or both (but not the femur), you can follow a simple procedure to help the legs correct themselves.

Most parents tend to let their babies sleep on the stomach. This position tends to keep the legs and the feet turned in. On top of that, the weight of the legs will tend to put pressure on the legs and feet, thus enhancing the pigeon toe! This will prolong the period of spontaneous correction of the pigeon toe.

Therefore, common sense dictates that such babies should be encouraged to sleep on their sides and backs. By so doing the legs and feet will be freer to straighten themselves, and will attain faster spontaneous correction.

Won't that position make my baby choke upon spitting up?

This is an unfounded fear. If the baby spits up, the material will roll out the side of the mouth, and the baby may swallow whatever remains in the mouth.

It usually takes three or four days of trying before the baby adjusts to sleeping on the back or sides. The best age to start such an attempt is between one to three months. The baby will resent the change of position, and may cry and fuss, but persistence will pay off.

What if the trouble of the pigeon toe is at the head of the femur?

Your doctor will be able to detect this trouble. In severe cases, you will have to pay several visits to the orthopedic surgeon. Mild cases may require nothing except adjusting the manner of sitting down.

In general, as a female child grows up closer to "budding" age, the hips will change shape and size and the thigh bones will correct themselves spontaneously.

What do you mean by "sitting down"?

Many a child (especially girls) takes to the habit of sitting on the floor in such a manner that her legs will be folded by the side of her buttocks, like a frog. This tends to worsen the femur-caused pigeon toe, or at least it may stand in the way of spontaneous improvement.

So to help in this matter, the child should be educated to sit crosslegged, and if possible to avoid sitting like a frog. This is easier said than done, and it may take six months to two years until this new habit sinks in.

OSGOOD SCHLATTER DISEASE

Within the age group of nine to fifteen years, sometimes the child complains of pain in his or her knee. The pain is not that severe, not throbbing or shooting; it is dull, and sometimes it may make him or her limp a little.

When you ask the child to pinpoint the pain, he or she will point to below the knee joint, to an area which appears swollen.

When you press at this area, there will be some tenderness, yet it is not that severe as to make the child jump with pain.

What causes such a disease?

No one knows for sure, but it is thought by many that Osgood Schlatter disease is the result of the excessive pull of the muscles that straighten the leg at the knee.

There is a bulge of the shinbone located just below the knee joint. To this bulge is attached a ligament connecting it to the kneecap. It is this bulge (the tibial tubercle) that becomes affected in Osgood Schlatter disease.

Is Osgood Schlatter a serious disease?

No, it is not serious, but it is bothersome, because it takes such a long time before it goes away. Because of this, you will have to curb the physical activity of the child. It is not a cancerous growth; it is simply a self-limited disease.

Is it contagious?

No, Osgood Schlatter disease is not contagious. If two children of the same family are affected, it is a coincidence.

Since it is not contagious, the child may go to school as usual.

Does it affect one leg or both?

It can affect one leg or both at the same time. We have seen a number of children recover from the disease in one leg; only to have it occur in the other leg. Of course this meant a repeat treatment all over again.

What kind of treatment?

Most doctors don't use casts, though there are some who do.

Physical activity should be limited. This means no football, soccer, basketball, horseback riding, bicycling, running, or any other activity that puts much stress on the knee.

It is very hard to oblige, and if the child "cheats," the area will simply take longer to heal.

As said before, the disease can take a good many months before subsiding. It may even take a year or so before it is over, though six to nine months is the average.

Should anything be done for the affected area?

An Ace bandage may be used to cover the lower half of the thigh, the knee, and the upper half of the calf muscles. The child is told to take off the Ace bandage twice a day and reapply it, tightening it slightly. The Ace bandage will act as a reminder to our active child to avoid stressful activity. Applying heat, doing massage, etc., is not helpful.

Some doctors ask for revisits every eight to ten weeks to check on the progress of the disease and the degree of the child's activity.

TOXIC SYNOVITIS OF THE HIP JOINT

The child is seen limping, or favoring one leg. He or she doesn't complain much about it, but may nevertheless refuse to walk. It shows up in an insidious way, and there is no letup even after a day or two or longer. There are no bruises or other evidence of a fall. The joints do not look swollen either. You become worried and bring the child to the doctor.

What will the doctor do?

The doctor will pay special attention to the child's manner of walking. The joints will be checked carefully, especially the knee and the hip. Then the doctor will explain all about toxic synovitis and what to do about it.

What age group is likely to get this disease?

Toxic synovitis is seen more often in younger children, around the ages of two, three, or four years old. In other words, this disease is seen more often in the active, jumpy, "wild" age group, in which the joint is likely to be under a good deal of stress.

What causes toxic synovitis?

There are many theories advanced, but none of them can be accepted as explanation for all cases of toxic synovitis.

Extreme activity, with a lot of jumping, may account for a good percentage of them. When the child is that active, the lining of the hip joint may suffer through some sudden jarring movements. When this happens, the lining becomes slightly "inflamed" and will hurt if the child moves the leg. Another theory postulates that since an upper respiratory infection often precedes such cases, the two conditions may be related.

Does the doctor do any tests?

In mild ones, tests are not needed. In more severe cases, or in prolonged ones, X-rays and some blood tests may have to be done. It all depends on the severity of the condition, the age of the child, the doctor, and whether there is suspicion of a different disease.

How do you treat it?

When the hip joint is painful to move, it means it needs rest, so that the troubled elements inside can go back to normal. This means taking the child off his or her feet. This is easier said than done. The little one wants to dart here and there, run, and climb. Alas, all these movements will delay the healing of the joint, sometimes as long as several weeks!

The parents are usually asked to forgo house chores, and instead concentrate on carrying the child if at all practical to keep him or her off the feet as long as possible. At the least, the child should be forbidden from too much activity; parents should read to the child, play jigsaw puzzles with the child, let the child watch TV, etc.

Applying heat, specifically putting the child in a tub of hot water for twenty minutes two or three times a day, may be of some help too.

Even with such a degree of care, this disease may take as long as one to two weeks before going away. Antibiotics, sedatives, aspirins, etc., are of little help if any.

Are there any diseases that look like the above?

Yes, there are. A mean disease called Legg-Perthes disease can act and look like toxic synovitis. However, it affects older children. It takes a long time (many months) before it goes away, and it needs special treatment and a number of X-rays to follow the course.

Diseases like rheumatic fever, rheumatoid arthritis, regular arthritis, etc., should all be considered and ruled out. They may all look like toxic synovitis, at times.

RADIAL SUBLUXATION

Radial subluxation affects children in the age group between eighteen months and five years. Their problem is that suddenly they have stopped using their forearm. They don't want to use the fingers of that arm, and don't want to make a fist or pick up something that interests them.

They prefer to protect their forearm too, from the elbow down. It seems as if they have some pain in the area, but the pain is not severe enough to make them scream. When you look at their elbow or hand, you will see no swelling, no bruising, nor any evidence of injury, and you will see that they are able to move their affected arm freely at the shoulder joint.

What causes radial subluxation?

There are two bones in the forearm, the radius and the ulna. The end of the radius at the elbow joint is shaped like a small cup on top of a constriction, making it look like a mushroom. This is held to the other bone (ulna) by a collar of tissue which looks almost like a ring.

When the young child walks holding your hand, and trips or falls while still holding on, the head of the radius bone will slip out of the collar of tissue holding it. This happens mainly if he or she suddenly buckles under while the parent reflexly jerks the arm up, attempting to prevent the fall.

Another way in which radial subluxation occurs is when you suddenly jerk the child up by one of the wrists.

As you can see, anything that suddenly pulls the head of the radius out of the ring of tissue around it, is likely to produce this problem.

Is this very common?

Yes, common enough and it will need to be fixed. It is seen most often in the aforementioned age group, and girls can get it as often as boys.

How can radial subluxation be fixed?

A child with this problem should be seen by the doctor. You cannot fix it yourself, and if you attempt to, trouble might arise. Another point to be brought to your attention is that rarely an X-ray has to be taken, since the clinical diagnosis is sufficient in most.

What the doctor does may look and sound simple enough for you to do, but don't be fooled by that. The doctor will hold the hand and the elbow of the affected area in a certain manner. While twisting the hand inward, he will gradually move it with the forearm towards the body, as if flexing the muscle. He will feel a click (you may even hear it) which will mean that the subluxation has been reduced. No anesthesia is needed.

You will be startled to see that once this procedure is done, the child will start using the hand and forearm immediately, as if nothing has happened.

Can we prevent such a problem?

Yes you can, and you may be prompted to if you know that radial subluxation can show up a second and a third time if not more often. A repeated subluxation may become a source of trouble, and that is why we should try our best to prevent it from happening.

One popular way to lift a small child is to lift up by pulling at the wrist. If you do that suddenly and jerkingly, it may lead to this problem of subluxation. So don't do it; make a habit of lifting the child by the arms themselves or by his or her sides. Avoid any sudden jerky movements applied to the wrist of the child.

This condition is quite rare after the age of five to six years, and the precautions can be relaxed then.

Can this condition show up simultaneously on both sides?

There is little likelihood, if any at all, for radial subluxation to show up on both sides. The odds are that when you suddenly lift the child up by both wrists, arm muscles will be contracting at the same time, and this will prevent the head of the radius bone from slipping out of the collar of tissue around it. For subluxation to occur, the arm has to be relaxed, and the jerk applied to the wrist must be sudden and strong.

SCOLIOSIS, OR THE CURVED BACK

Scoliosis is not a rare condition; it is estimated that five to ten percent of all children have a certain degree of it, and one to two percent need active treatment.

Usually it shows up in the pre-adolescent age group and beyond-in other words, in those who are ten years old and older. This is a period of rapid growth which is susceptible to this kind of problem.

What is scoliosis anyway?

Simply stated, it is a curvature of the spine. It can be of various degrees and severity, and it can be to the right or to the left. Better than eighty percent of scoliosis are postural (functional); in other words, related to faulty posture. Whereas structural scoliosis is caused by a defect in the spine.

When detected early and offered correctional exercises, or simply observed over a period of time, such cases of scoliosis will improve and the back will look straight later on.

How do we look for it?

Let the child take off his or her shirt and undershirt. Let him or her stand up with the back toward you, bend over as if to touch the toes with the fingers, i.e. to make a ninety degree angle (with a flat back), and make sure that the arms hang down pointing towards the floor.

Look at the back while the child is in that position. You will see the tips of the spines of the vertebrae. They come out from the small of the back up to the base of the neck. They are supposed to be in one straight line. There should be no curvature whatsoever, and both sides of the back symmetrical. Also, see if the level of the shoulder blades is the same.

If the above points are not met, it will mean scoliosis.

What would you do for the postural scoliosis?

If you or your doctor discovers this problem, the doctor may tell the child about posture and to do certain kinds of exercises. Some cases may not even require those; the doctor will merely want to observe it again in a few months. An X-ray is taken for an accurate comparison's sake except for the very mild ones.

In most postural scoliosis, the deformity may disappear over a period of several years.

What causes "structural" scoliosis?

If the scoliosis is structural, it will mean problems in the bones (the vertebrae), or perhaps in the muscles of the spine or some of the structures nearby.

This usually means that many changes, potentially serious, will have taken place in the integrity of the structure of the back. The important point here is that structural scoliosis can become progressively worse unless you do something to halt the changes. The earlier you can discover it, the easier the treatment will be.

What can be done for structural scoliosis?

It depends on the kind and degree of severity of the scoliosis. In many early ones certain braces may have to be put on for a good many years. These braces do a great deal in halting the scoliosis, thus preventing further deterioration. It is safe to say that such braces cannot correct the condition to look normal.

In severe degrees of scoliosis, an operation might have to be done. When done, the back will become stiff, but the scoliosis will not progress as to endanger the life of the patient as sometimes it may.

Is structural scoliosis hereditary?

Certain types are. It is not rare to see a mother and two daughters to have a varying degree of that problem, and often the condition becomes known only after the scoliosis in one of the children has been discovered.

As you can see, to discover scoliosis you do an easy test, and if found, it is easy to treat; but the key to the whole problem is to discover it early. It is also good to know that four out of every five cases of scoliosis prove to be postural, and this is easy to correct with posture correction.

KYPHOSIS & LORDOSIS:
THE ROUND-BACK AND THE SWAY-BACK

Kyphosis and lordosis are two conditions that are not as rare as you think, and they are more likely to be discovered in pre-adolescent children. Along with the curved backs (scoliosis), it is said that five to ten percent of school children have either kyphosis or lordosis, and one to two percent will need corrective treatment.

The child is not aware of it because there is usually no pain, and the condition comes on so insidiously. The condition may be missed if the child doesn't come for checkups, or if the parents don't look for it.

How can we discover them?

It is simple. If you suspect kyphosis (round back) by noticing that the upper back seems too round, you ask the child to lie down on his or her stomach. Let the arms be by the sides of the body. Ask the child to arch the body by raising the head and straightening the legs. If he or she does that and the rounded back seems to disappear, then there is no kyphosis; otherwise there is a good possibility that it exists.

If you suspect lordosis (sway-back) by seeing an excessively curved small of the back, there is a simple test to do. Let the child lie down on his or her back and bring the knees as close to the chest as possible. When the child is in that position, see if you can slip your hand under the small of the back. If you can do so, then it is positive for lordosis.

What causes such problems?

The majority are postural or functional. In other words, a round back is more of a habit than anything else; many a pre-adolescent tends to hold himself or herself in that posture. The same can be said with sway backs. As time passes by, the condition is likely to become worse and worse unless steps are taken to correct these conditions.

Of course, there are many diseases that can cause such problems too; one in particular is Scheuermann's disease of the back. To discover any of these, an X-ray of the spine will have to be taken.

What can be done about these conditions?

Kyphosis and lordosis can be divided into two groups, the postural (functional) and the structural. In the latter, there is some trouble in the structure of the spine, such as Scheuermann's disease, congenital trouble in the vertebrae, etc. The treatment here depends on the particular disease and its degree of severity. Fortunately, structural kyphosis and lordosis are not as common as postural (functional) kyphosis and lordosis.

Postural (functional) kyphosis and lordosis are related to bad habits of holding the back hunched, or holding the small of the back protruding forward.

For such cases not only are certain forms of exercise important, but the adolescent should be made quite conscious of the nasty habit. If the child keeps holding the posture correctly and exercises the muscles of the back well, he or she stands a good chance of recovery over a period of time. In the case of postural kyphosis, the child must also lie down on the stomach holding the chin up with the palms of the hands, mainly during studying or watching TV.

For lordosis, situp exercises, once or twice a day, as many as twenty-five times at each setting, may prove to be of help. This is to be done over a period of several months, inspite of any objections or lack of cooperation from the child. Chinups, pushups, and swimming should be encouraged.

Early discovery of such problems will necessitate very little treatment compared to late discovery.

Are these conditions inherited?

Cases of postural kyphosis and lordosis are usually not inherited, although some structural ones prove to be congenital. An example is a child who is born with a defect in a vertebra.

It is good to remember that trouble with the spine comes not only from trouble in the bones of the spine, but also from some troublesome diseases of the muscles and other structures that support the spine. That is why some require extensive investigation.

Fortunately, such diseases are not that common. Your being aware of such possibilities, however, will make you an active partner with the doctor to look for and detect such problems early.

CONGENITAL DISLOCATION OF THE HIP JOINT

Congenital dislocation of the hip joint is fairly common, but if present, early diagnosis is important; thus preventing many troublesome consequences.

Most cases can be discovered at birth or within the first few months of life. This is usually diagnosed by your doctor during the newborn exam or the baby checkups afterwards.

What does congenital dislocation of the hip do?

As the name indicates, congenital dislocation of the hip joint(s) is a condition in which the head of the thigh bone (femur) is not stable in its socket (the hip bone). It may even be partly or completely out of the socket. It usually affects one joint, but both joints can be affected too, though not that often.

If not discovered and left untreated, the hip joint will develop in an improper way during the baby's fast period of growth. If this happens, the head of the femur will slip out of its socket when the child stands or walks. The child will have a waddling gait (almost like a duck), if both hips are affected; or a limp to one side in case one hip is affected.

Not only that, but a chain of events may follow, such as the inability to run or to use the legs properly, difficulty going upstairs or downstairs, pain or trouble in the back, etc.

How can we detect congenital dislocation of the hip?

The test is simple and you may easily learn how to do it during the baby's first few months of life.

To examine the hip joint, place the baby on the back, with the legs bent at the knees and the thighs held vertically. You hold the inner surface of the thigh with your thumb while the palm of your hand and the rest of your fingers are on the thigh's outer surface. You hold each thigh firmly with your corresponding hand and try to move and separate the thighs apart so that they go from the vertical position to a horizontal level.

If you can do so, the hip joints are O.K. If the thigh does not move easily from a vertical to a horizontal plane, or if you feel or hear a click or a snap upon doing this, it means the joints are not OK. Verify this with your doctor.

The above signs are easily detectable in the majority of infants born with this defect. However, a small percentage may be difficult to detect early; the condition may not show up clearly until the infants are nearing the standing or even the walking age. In this situation, the condition is more difficult to treat and it takes longer to correct.

How about the folds of the thighs?

Some people claim that if the folds (fat rolls) of the thighs are not equal in number on both sides, the baby may be having a congenital dislocation of the hip. This is not a reliable sign; quite often a perfectly normal baby will show it.

What can be done about this problem?

When discovered during early infancy or in a newborn, the treatment is simple and often very successful.

Your doctor will explain the line of treatment. This simply consists of positioning the legs in a certain manner and keeping them that way for several months. Repeated checkups are required to monitor the progress of the condition.

Casts, splints, and other methods of treatment are not needed if this condition is discovered at an early age.

What if it is discovered late?

If the congenital dislocation of the hip is discovered late, say at the age of one year or later, the treatment will be more complicated, difficult, and costly. Casts and often surgery may be needed; two, three, or even more operations may have to be done. The treatment may seem endless and the child may have to go through quite an ordeal.

GLOSSARY

ABO incompatibility: a condition leading to jaundice in a newborn, caused by incompatibility between the mother's and the baby's blood type.
acetone: material occurring in blood and urine in minute amount, but greatly increased in diabetes.
acute: sharp, severe, having a rapid onset and a short course and pronounced symptoms.
adenoids: a mass of lymphoid tissue present in the nasopharynx.
adenoid facies: characteristic open-mouthed and pinched-nose appearance associated with enlarged adenoids.
adolescent goiter: diffuse enlargement of thyroid gland, most frequently seen during adolescence.
alopecia areata: loss of hair in circumscribed patches usually of scalp.
amblyopia: dimness of vision, may be congenital or acquired.
amino acids: components of protein, some can be synthesized by the body, others cannot and have to be available in the diet.
amniocentesis: procedure for getting a sample of aminiotic fluid in a pregnant woman.
anemia: below normal reduction in red blood cells, hemoglobin, or hematocrit.
anterior fontanelle (the soft spot): the membranous area at the top of the head of a baby, usually closing during the second year.
antihistamine: A substance capable of preventing, counteracting or diminishing the effects of histamin. Allergic persons may secrete excess histamin which leads to some allergy symptoms.
antipyretic: a substance that reduces or tends to reduce fever.
appendectomy: operation removing the appendix.
astigmatism: an irregularity in the curvature of the cornea and surfaces of the lens, leading to defective vision.
atrophy: an acquired reduction in the size of a tissue, organ, or region of the body.
auditory canal: the external ear canal.
auricle: the projecting part of the external (outer) ear.
axillary: of or pertaining to the armpit.

baby food: cereal, fruits, vegetables and meat specially processed to be used by babies.
base study: tests or other studies done to establish values for similar future comparison's sake.
balanitis: inflammation of the glans penis.
bone age: age as judged by X-ray of bone development.
bronchial tubes: branches of the trachea to the lung.
bronchiolitis: disease caused by inflammation of bronchioles, most often in babies.
bronchoscopy: a procedure to visualize the interior of the bronchi.

caliber of the voice: natural or essential character of the voice.
callus: a callosity, especially of palm or sole.
callosity: a circumscribed area of thickened skin caused by friction or pressure.
canker sore: a small ulceration of the mucous membrane of the mouth.
carbuncle: a painful, localized, pus producing lesion of the skin, discharging pus through multiple external openings.
carotene: a substance occurring in carrots, beets and some other plants, converted to vitamin A by the liver.
carotenemia: the presence of carotene in the circulating blood.
CAT scan: X-ray scan by computer-assisted tomography.
cauterize: 1. to apply a caustic to 2. to apply a cauterizing agent to tissue.
cell indices: blood studies of the size of and relative concentration of hemoglobin in the red blood cells.
chalazion: a chronic localized inflammation of the eyelid occurring as the result of blockage of a tarsal gland.
cholesterol: A constituent of all animal fats and oils, of bile, nervous tissue, egg yolk and blood. It is important in metabolism.
chromosome: microscopic bodies that carry hereditary factors, present in the nucleus, numbering 46 in man.
chronic: long-continued, of long duration.
cilia: threadlike cytoplasmic processes of cells, which beat rhythmically.
coarctation of the aorta: narrowing or stricture of the aorta.
cochlea: spiral structure of the inner ear containing nerve ends essential for hearing.
colony count (urine): a special method of counting the number of colonies of bacteria in one ml. of urine.
coming to a head: an abscess, pointing and ready to rupture.
contrast material: a substance that permits radiographic demonstration of an organ or space.
corn: a cone shaped, horny thickening of the skin, usually on or near a toe, resulting from friction or pressure.
cornea: the transparent anterior portion of the eyeball.
cornified layer (skin): a thickened skin with horny squames on its surface.

corona of penis: crown or ridge of the glans penis.
cryptic: having a surface with small pits and recesses.
cystoscopy: the procedure of looking into the bladder by an instrument called cystoscope.

decongestant: an agent that reduces hyperemia (congestion).
definitive urine culture: complete or fully developed culture.
demulcent: soothing, allaying irritation of surfaces especially mucous membrane.
depressed fracture: A skull fracture whereby one side of the broken skull is at a lower level than the rest.
dermis: The layer of the skin below the epidermis, bearing the appendages (hair apparatus, oil glands, etc.)
diastolic blood pressure: minimum arterial blood pressure during ventricular diastole (when heart muscle is not actively contracting).
distal: farther from the point of origin or median plane; nearest the end.
dormant: quiescent, inactive.
double pneumonia: pneumonia involving both lungs.

ecthyma: ulcerated crusted persistent inflammation of the skin, usually appear on the knee area.
EEG (brain wave): electroencephalogram.
electrolytes: a substance that dissociates into ions in solution or when fused, thereby becoming electrically conducting.
encephalitis: inflammation of the brain.
enzymes: a substance formed by living cells and having a specific action in promoting a chemical change.
epidermis: the superficial portion of the skin, consisting of several layers.
essential hypertension: a familial and possibly a genetic form of elevation of blood pressure of unknown origin.
ethmoidal sinus: either of the paranasal sinuses in the ethmoidal bone.
eustachian tube: a tube connecting the middle ear to the nasopharynx.
eversion: turning outward.
exacerbation: increase in manifestation or severity of disease or symptom
exchange transfusion: the replacement of much of the recipient's blood in small amounts at a time from a donnor.

fasting blood sugar: a test for blood sugar level after an overnight's period of fasting.
fauces of the tonsils: the space occupied mainly by the tonsils.
femur: thighbone
fissure in ano: anal fissure.
fleety: moving swiftly; showing temporarily.
fovea: a small pit or depression.
frenulum: any small fold of mucous membrane or tissue that restrains a structure or part.
frontal sinus: the paranasal sinus situated in the frontal bone.
fulminant: sudden, severe, intense, and rapid in course.
fundi: the part farthest removed from the opening (exit) of the organ.
funnel chest: a defromity of sternum and nearby structures producing a depression of the lower portion of the chest.

gamma globulin: immunoglobulin processed from blood, containing protective antibodies, used clinically in viral hepatitis, measles and a few other diseases.
glans: the conical body that forms the distal end of the penis or clitoris.
glossitis: inflammation of the tongue.
glucose tolerance test: a series of blood tests at specific times to determine the level of glucose in the blood, after intake of glucose by the patient.
gonococcus: the germ causing gonorrhea.
grand mal epilepsy: a form of epilepsy characterized by severe seizures involving spasms and loss of consciousness.
granulation tissue: newly formed fragile tissue representing a stage in repair of damage associated with inflammation.
green stick fracture: An incomplete fracture of a long bone affecting part of bone's shaft.

hematoma: a circumscribed collection of blood, usually clotted, which forms a mass.
hemoglobin: the oxygen bearing, iron containing protein in the blood (usually in the red blood cells.)
hemoglobin SS, SC and SA: various forms of hemoglobin found in sickle cell disease.
heel stick: the process of taking blood by sticking the heel of a baby with a blood lancet.
hormones: a specific chemical product of an organ or of certain cells of an organ, transported by the blood or other body fluids, and having a specific regulatory effect upon cells remote from its origin.

hydrocephalus: distension of the brain ventricles with spinal fluid due to obstruction to the flow of the spinal fluid.
hypoglycemia: the clinical status associated with decreased level of blood sugar (below normal).

incarcerated hernia: the abnormal imprisonment of the hernia.
induration: the hardening of a tissue or part, resulting from inflammation or infiltration.
infiltration: a process by which cells, fluid or other substances pass into tissue spaces or into cells.
internal tibial torsion: the internal rotation of the shaft of the tibia seen mainly in babies.
intussusception: the receiving of one part within another; the invagination, slipping or passage of one part of the intestine into another.
invagination: the infolding of a part, to become ensheathed.
iris: the pigmented, round, contractile membrane of the eye, and perforated by the pupil.
IVP: abreviation of intravenous pyelogram.

labile: unstable, readily changed by other factors.
lactose: a form of sugar present in milk.
larval: pertaining to or in condition of an immature and independent developmental stage in the life cycle of worms, insects or animals.
larynx: the organ of voice, voice-box.
Legg-Perthes disease: a disease of the head of the femur of a long duration (osteochondritis deformans).
leukoderma: loss of skin pigment (melanin) secondary to a cause.
lipids: Anyone of a group of fats and fatlike substances having in common the insolubility in water and solubility in fat solvents. Examples are fats, fatty acids, fatty oils and waxes.
lumbar area: pertaining to the loin.
lumbar puncture: puncture of the spinal canal in the lumbar area for the removal of cerebrospinal fluid, or for introducing medication.
lymph: a clear watery sometimes faintly yellowish liquid.
lymph node: Any of innumerous oval or round bodies which supply lymphocytes to the circulatory system, and remove bacteria and foreign particles from the lymph.
lymph vessel: tiny tube, hair like in size, transporting lymph to the lymphnodes.

macerate: to soften a tissue, or remove therefrom certain constituants, by steeping in a fluid.
macerated skin: soggy skin.
malleable bone: capable of being shaped or formed.
malocclusion: any deviation from a normal alignment of the teeth; faulty closure of the teeth.
mastoiditis: inflammation of the mastoid bone.
maxillary sinus: the paranasal sinus in the maxilla bone.
meatatomy: incision into and enlargement of a meatus.
meatus: an opening or a passage.
mediastinum: the space left in the middle of the chest between the two pleurae.
meninges: the membranes enclosing the brain and spinal cord.
middle line: An immaginary line that divides the body into left and right sides.
microcephaly: a condition characterized by an abnormally small head often associated with mental retardation.
morbidity: 1. condition inducing disease, 2. the state of being diseased
mortality: 1. conditons leading to death, 2. death rate.
mucoid: resembling mucus.
mucous membrane: the membrane lining those cavities and canals communicating with the air, and kept moist by secretions of various types of glands.
mycoplasma: minute organisms that lack rigid cell wall, some of which cause disease.

nasal septum: The septum that separates the left from the right nasal cavities.
nasopharynx: The space behind the nasal cavities, above the level of the palate.
neonate: an infant from birth through its twenty-eighth day
nits: the eggs of a louse, usually attached to a hair.

osteogenisis imperfecta: an inherited disease with imperfect bones resulting in bone fractures with minimal trauma.
osteomyelitis: inflammation of the marrow and hard tissue of the bones, usually caused by bacteria.
otoscope: an apparatus to examine the ear and to render the ear drum visible.

pancreas: a gland, lying transversely across the back wall of the abdomen.
paraphimosis: retraction and constriction, especially of the prepuce behind the glans penis.
perianal area: area around the anus.

paroxysm: a sudden attack; a sudden outburst.
perichondrium: the fibrous tissue covering cartilage (except articular surface).
petechii: a minute rounded spot of hemorrhage on a surface such as skin, mucous membrane, serous membrane, or on an organ.
petit mal epilepsy: a form of epilepsy characterized by recurrent absence attacks.
pharynx: throat; the section of digestive tract that extends from the nasal cavity to the larynx, there becoming continuous with the esophagus.
phimosis: elongation of the prepuce and constriction of its orifice, so that the foreskin cannot be retracted to uncover the glans penis.
pituitary gland: a small round endocrine gland attached to the base of the brain.
plasma: the fluid portion of the blood (without the cells).
platelets: one of the components of blood cells about a third of the size of the red blood cell, essential for homeostasis (blood clotting and other things).
pleura: the serous membrane enveloping the lung and lining the internal surface of the chest cavity.
polyp: a smooth spherical or oval mass projecting from a membranous surface.
prepuce: foreskin of the penis.
proctoscopy: looking at the anal canal and rectum with a special device called proctoscope.
projectile vomiting: a form of vomiting in which the stomach contents are suddenly and forcefully shot forth out of the mouth to some distance, usually without nausea.
psychogenic: production or causation of illness by psychic rather than organic factors.
pubis: the portion of the hipbone forming the front of the pelvis.
pyoderma: any pus-producing skin lesion or lesions, such as pustules.
pyloric stenosis: obstruction of the pyloric orifice of the stomach.

radius: the outer of the two bones of the forearm.
rattly: with vibrating and short sharp sound.
rebound phenomenon: the stuffiness of the nose resulting from using certain nose drops for longer than three days, thus giving the opposite effect the nose drops are intended to do.
reduce a hernia: to restore a part (that of a hernia) to its previous normal relations.
resolving (pneumonia): to return to normal state after some disease process.
Rh baby: usually a jaundiced newborn whereby the jaundice is caused by adverse reaction between the baby's blood Rh factor and that of the mother.
reverse-last shoes: shoes with the forepart reversed in direction.

satellite lesions: small circular lesions appearing near the periphery of the original skin disease, as in fungus diaper rash.
sclera: the firm fibrous white layer that covers the eye except for the cornea.
screening urine culture: a culture usually done on urine of females during checkups to rule out the presence of bacteria.
scrotum: the pouch containing the testicles.
sentinel pile: the thickened wall of the anal pocket at the lower end of an anal fissure.
sebaceous glands: the glands that secrete special fatty-substance (sebum).
seborrheic blepharitis: seborrheic disease of the edge of the eyelids.
self-limited: term used to designate a disease which runs a definite course in a specific time.
semicircular canal: three loop-shaped tubes in the inner ear.
sensitivity test: tests to check the degree of sensitivity of germs to certain medicines.
septum: a partition between two spaces or cavities.
sigmoidoscopy: looking at the sigmoid colon with the aid of a special instrument (sigmoidoscope).
shiners: dark circles under the eyes usually show up in the allergic.
slough: a mass of necrotic (dead) tissue in, or separating from, living tissue.
smegma: smelly cheesy material secreted by sebaceous glands in the penis and clitoris.
spermatic cord: the cord extending from the testicle to the wall of the abdomen, containing the tube through which sperms travel.
spinal tap: see lumbar puncture.
spores: a usually single-celled reproductive structure or resting stage, as of a fungus or bacterium.
staphylococcus (staph): any of the spherical bacteria occurring in grapelike cluster and causing abscesses, boils and other infections.
status epilepticus: a condition in which generalized convulsions occur at a frequency which does not allow consciousness to be regained in the interval between seizures.
sternomastoid mass: mass or lump in sternomastoid muscle.
straight-last shoes: shoes with the forepart being straight.
strangulated hernia: a hernia in which circulation of the blood and the fecal return are blocked.
startle reflex: the reaction observed in a normal baby from birth to a few months old, consisting of abduction and extension of all extremities, followed by flexion and adduction of the extremities as in an embrace, usually in response to a sudden stimulus.
streptococcus (strep): any of various rounded bacteria occurring in pairs or chains and often causing disease.
sternum (breastbone): the flat, narrow bone in the median line in front of the chest.
subacute: 1. somewhat less acute in severity, 2. of a disease, intermediate in character,

between acute and chronic.
superadded infection: an infection affecting an already diseased area.
surgical abdomen: abdominal disease that needs immediate surgery.
sutures (of skull): a line of junction or closure between bones, as a cranial suture.
symptomatic treatment: treatment pertaining to and of the symptoms of a disease.
syncope: a faint.
systolic blood pressure: The maximum arterial blood pressure during contraction of the ventricles of the heart.

tender: painful to the touch.
thyroglossal cyst: cystic distension of the remnant of the thyroglossal cyst.
tibial tubercle: a bony bulge at the upper part of the front (arterior) surface of the tibial bone.
tinia capitis: fungus infection of the scalp and hair.
tonicity: the condition of normal tone or tension of an organ.
trachea: windpipe.
trauma: an injury caused by a mechanical or physical agent.
turbinates: three folds of mucous membrane on each side of the nasal cavity.

ulna: the bone on the inner side of the forearm.
umbilical hernia: a hernia occurring through the umbilical ring.
umbilical granuloma: proliferation of granulation tissue of the umbilicus.
upper cervical lymph nodes: a group of lymph nodes in the upper part of the neck and beneath each angle of the jaw.
ureter: long elongated tube conveying the urine from the kidney to the bladder.
urethra: the canal through which the urine is discharged.
uvula: the conical piece of tissue hanging from the free edge of the soft palate.

vagus nerve: the tenth intracranial nerve.
voiding cystourethrogram: a special procedure for taking X-ray of the urinary tract mainly to detect back pressure (reflux).
viscid: sticky, adhesive, glutinous.

walking pneumonia: a pneumonia resolving in one lobe just to appear in another lobe of the same or the other lung.
wart seeding itself: a wart that spreads in the adjacent area.
wheeze: a prolonged whistling or sighing sound produced in the act of breathing, usually upon exhalation.
Wood's lamp: a special lamp that transmits only ultraviolet light, usually used in the diagnosis of fungi such as fungus infection of the scalp.

INDEX

A and D ointment, 8
Abscess, 445
ABO incompatibility, 104
Accidents
 prevention in the young, 114
 ABC's of child safety, 117
 accidental poisoning, 118
 to the mouth, 241
Acne, 470
Actifed, 280
Actifed C, 304
Acute tonsillitis, 252
Adam's apple, 261
Adenoid facies, 231
Adenoids, 245
Adolescent goiter, 261
Air filter
 electronic, 292
Alconephrine, 274
Allergic conjunctivitis, 191
Allergic rhinitis, 278
Allergies of
 respiratory tract, 294
Allergy
 food, 349
 milk, 75
 shots, 297
Alopecia areata, 477
Alpha keri, 437
Ambenyl-D, 304
Amblyopia, 182
Anaphylactoid purpura, 403
Ancylostoma worm, 374
Anemia, iron-dificiency, 398
Anterior fontanelle, 485
Antibiotics, 151
Antipyretics, 131
Aphtha, 237
Appendicitis, 372
Appetite, 332
Arch cookie, 519
Ascaris worm, 374
Asthmatic bronchitis, 317
Astigmatism, 183
Atarax, 158
Atherosclerosis, 347
Athlete's foot, 462
Atopic dermatitis, 438
Attention deficit disorder, 496
Auditory canal, 205
Auricle, 205
Aveeno oilated, 437

Baby's
 belly button, 7
 bleeding vagina, 9
 blemishes and spots, 10
 bottoms, 8
 bowel movement, 5
 breasts, 10
 colicky pains, 4
 constipation, 6, 100
 coughs, 79
 chest trouble, 79
 earache, 78
 night feedings, 21
 nuk pacifier, 88
 orange juice, 22
 pacifier, 86
 penis, tip of, 83
 pyloric stenosis, 80

Baby's
 sentinel pile, 82
 skin care, 6
 startle reflex, 10
 stuffy, runny nose, 77
 Thum, 87
 vomiting, projectile, 80
Back
 curved-back, 528
 round-back, 530
 sway-back, 530
Balanced diet, 339
Balanitis, 107
Bald spot, 477
Balneol lotion, 110
Bed wetting, 420
Bee stings, 464
Benadryl, 452
Bentyl, 5
Benylin, 304
Benzoyl peroxide, 471
Bilirubin, 104
Bites,
 dogs, cats, and humans, 466
Black eye, 192
Blemishes, 10
Blood, 396
 in stool, 368
 in urine, 415
Blood poisoning, 447
Blood pressure
 diastolic, 394
 systolic, 394
Boils, 443
Bones, 509
Bone marrow tap, 509
Boric acid solution, 184
Bottle-feeding, 18
Brain tumor, 488
Breasts, 387
Breast-feeding, 15
Bronchial tubes, 261
Bronchiolitis, 79
Bruises, 112
Burping, 21

CBC, 397
Caldesene powder, 7
Canker sore, 237
Carbuncle, 443
Care of teeth, 93
Carotenemia, 27
Cat scratch fever, 266
Cawliflower ear, 219
Cellulitis, 445
Cereal, 24
Chalazions, 188
Checkups, 69
Cheracol, 303
Chest, 385
 cold, 307
 pains, 389
Chickenpox, 157
Chloraseptic gel, 92
Cholesterol, 347
Choroid, 181
Chromosome, 501
Chubby, child, 342
Circumcision, 107
Clean-up job, 106
Chlortrimiton, 305

Coarctation of the aorta, 396
Cochlia, 206
Colds, 273
Colony count, 414
Compound W, 472
Concussion, 499
Congenital heart disease, 393
Congenital laryngeal stridor, 311
Conjunctiva, 180
Conjunctivites, 190
Constipation
 acute, in children, 356
 baby, 6, 100
 chronic, 357
Contusions 121
Convulsions
 febrile, 134
Corn starch powder, 7
Cornia, 179
Cortaid cream, 90
Cough, 299
Cough medicines, 303
Cracked "anus", 81
Cradle cap, 88
Craniostenosis, 485
Croup, 313
Culture, 143
Cuts and lacerations, 122
Cystoscopy, 414

Debrox ear drops, 228
Dehydration, 366
Demazin, 305
Dermatitis
 atopic, 438
 primary irritant, 436
Dermis, 435
Desitin ointment, 8
Diabetes, 380
Diabetic coma, 380
Diaper
 ammoniacal rash, 83, 101
 fungus rash, 102
Diarrhea, 364
Diastolic blood pressure, 394
Digestive tract, 331
Dimetane, 305
Dimetapp, 305
Domeboro, 474
Donnatal, 5
Double pneumonia, 324
Downs' syndrome, 501
Dry skin, 436

Ear
 discharge, 217
 external, 205
 foreign body, 224
 inner, 206
 middle, 206
Earache, 209
Ear canal
 inflammation, 220
Eardrops, 222
Ears, 205
Earwax, 227
Echthyma, 443
Eczema, 438
Eggs, 29
Electronic air filter, 292
Endocrine glands, 389

541

Enzactin powder, 462
Epidermis, 435
Epilepsy
  abdominal, 493
  grand mal, 492
  myoclonic seizures, 493
  petit mal, 493
  psychomotor, 493
  salaam fits, 493
Epileptic fits, 492
Epinephrine, 465
Esophagus, 331
Essential hypertension, 395
Eucerin, 437
Eustachian tube, 205
Exchange transfusion, 105
Expectation
  age of one month, 35
  age of two months, 38
  age of three months, 40
  age of four months, 42
  age of five months, 44
  age of six months, 46
  age of eight months, 48
  age of ten months, 50
  age of one year, 52
  age of fifteen months, 54
  age of eighteen months, 56
  age of twenty one months, 58
  age of two years, 60
External ear, 205
Eye
  accidents, 198
  checkups, 181
  drops and ointments, 183
  watering, 95
Eyelid
  swollen, 194
Eyes, 179
  baby (neonate), 9
  crossed, 186
  false crossing, 182

Fainting spells, 490
Fasting blood sugar, 380
Febrile convulsions, 134
Fedahist, 280
Feingold diet, 499
Female development, 65
Femur, 521
Fer-in-sol, 400
Fever and infections, 127
Fiber Med, 355
Fifth disease, 170
Fissure in ano, 81
Flat feet, 519
Fleet enema, 356
Flu, 141
Fluorides, 94
Food allergy, 349
Foreign body
  in ear, 224
  in lung, 320
Fovea, 179
Fractures, 515
Frenulum, 242
Fruits, 26
Fungus, 136
Funnel chest, 385

Gagging, 30
Gamma Globulin, 162, 379
Gastroenteritis, 362

Gator ear plugs, 221
Geographic tongue, 233
German measles, 162
Glossitis, 243
Glucose tolerance test, 380
Gluey ear, 213
Grand mal epilepsy, 492
Green-stick fracture, 515
Growing pains, 511
Growth center, 509
Gum boil, 240

Hand, foot, and mouth disease, 256
Hashimoto's disease, 261
Head, 485
Hearing, 207
Heart murmur, 392
Hemangioma
  spider, 461
  strawberry, 460
Hematocrit, 397
Hematoma of the nail, 458
Hemic murmur, 393
Hemoglobin, 397
Hemophilia, 397
Herald patch, 453
Hernia
  direct, 371
  incarcerated, 371
  inguinal, 370
  strangulated, 371
  umbilical, 111
Herpangina, 250
Herpes Zoster, 159
High blood pressure, 394
Hip joint
  congenital dislocation, 532
  toxic synovitis, 525
Hives, 450
Hornet, 464
Horse-shoe kidney, 409
Humidifiers
  cool-mist, 290
Hydrocele, 425
Hydrocephalus, 486
Hyperactive child, 496
Hyperkinetic child, 496
Hypoglycemia, 382
Hypospadias, 425

Impetigo, 441
Incarcerated hernia, 371
Infectious hepatitis, 378
Infectious mono, 168
Inflamed middle ear, 211
Inguinal canal, 426
Inguinal hernia, 370
Inner ear, 206
Innocent murmur, 393
Internal tibial torsion, 522
Intussusception, 369
Iris, 179
IVP, 414

Jaundice, 103
Joint, swollen, 517
Junior food, 31

Kaopectate, 363
Kidney stones, 410
Knock-knee, 519
Kwell shampoo, 480

Kyphosis, 530

Labial adhesions, 84
Larva, 374
Laryngitis, 309
Larynx, 261
Legg-Perthes disease, 526
Leukoderma, 436
Lice, 479
Lipid, 338
Lobar pneumonia, 324
Lordosis, 530
Low blood, 398
Lowilla soap, 437
Lozenges, and mouth sprays, 246
Lubriderm cream, 437
Lump under the jaw, 265
Lymph vessel, 448
Lymphangitis, 447

Male development, 63
Malocclusion, 232
Maltsupex, 100
Measles, 160
Meatal stenosis, 423
Meatotomy, 424
Meats, 28
Meckel's diverticulum, 369
Mediastinum, 385
Meninges, 503
Meningitis, 503
Meningococcus, 503
Menstruation, 67
Metamucil, 355
Microcephaly, 486
Middle ear, 206
Middle ear inflammation, 211
Migraine headache, 488
Milk allergy, 75
Milkinol, 359
Modane, 359
Mol-iron, 400
Mongolian spot, 10
Mongolism, 501
Mouth-breathing, 231
Myoclonic seizures, 493
Myringotomy, 214
Mumps, 164
Murine ear drops, 228
Murmur
  heart 393
  hemic, 393
  innocent, 393
  organic, 393
  physiologic, 393
Mycostatin, 99
Myoflex cream, 512

Naldecon, 305
Nasal allergy, 278
Nasal septum, 283
Neck, 261
NeoSynephrine, 274
Nephrosis, 410
Nervous tics, 494
Neutrogena soap, 437
Nits, 479
Nose, 271
Nose
  deviated septum, 284
  fractures of, 284
Nosebleeds, 282

Novafed, 280
Novahistine, 280
Nuk pacifier, 88
Num-zit, 92
Nupercaine ointment, 82

Orajel, 92
Organic murmur, 393
Osgood schlatter disease, 523
Osteogenisis imperfecta, 517
Osteomyelitis, 138
Otitis externa, 220
Otitis media, 211
Outer ear disease, 218

Paraformaldehyde, 296
Paraphimosis, 108
Paronychia, 457
Paroxysmal tachycardia, 391
Pedameth, 102
Periactin, 158
Peri-colace, 359
Permanent teeth, 239
Petechii, 401
Petit mal, 493
Phenergan expectorant, 304
Phenobarbital, 136
Phimosis, 108
Phobia, 71
Phototherapy, 104
Physical development of
  adolescent female, 65
  adolescent male, 63
Physiologic murmur, 393
Pigeon toe, 521
Pin-hole meatus, 84
Pink eye, 190
Pinworms 376
Pityriasis
  alba, 454
  rosea, 452
  versicolor, 454
Plantar wart, 472
Platelet, 401
Playtex bottle, 19
Pleura, 290
Pleurisy, 326
  dry, 326
  wet, 327
Pneumatic otoscopy, 215
Pneumococcus, 149
Pneumohydrothorax, 327
Pneumonia, 324
  double, 324
  lobar, 324
  walking, 324
Pneumopyothorax, 327
Poison ivy, 454
Polyp, 356
Postnasal drip, 281
Povan, 378
Prepuce, 424
Presun, 474
Primary irritant dermatitis, 436
Proctoscopy, 369
Projectile vomiting, 80
Psychomotor seizures, 493
Pubis, 427
Purpura, 401
Purpura, anaphylactoid, 403

Radial subluxation, 526
Radius, 527

Rash, 440
Relatives, 11
Respiratory tract, 289
Retin-A gel, 471
Retina, 181
Reverse-last shoes, 521
Rh baby, 104
Rheumatic fever, 166
Rheumatoid arthritis, 518
Rickets, 511
Rickettsia, 173
Rid shampoo, 480
Ringworm, 449
Robitussin AC, 304
Rocky Mt spotted fever, 172
Roseola, 153
Round-back, 530
Roundworms, 374
Rubella, 162
Ryna, 305
Rynatan, 305

Salaam fits, 493
Salicylic acid plasters, 473
Salmonella, 362
Scalds and burns, 475
Scarlatina, 155
Sclera, 180
Scheuermann's disease, 531
School phobia, 71
Scoliosis, 528
Scrotum, 425
Sebaceous glands, 435
Seborrheic blepharitis, 196
Seborrheic dermatitis, 88
Semicircular canals, 206
Sensitivity tests, 414
Sentinel pile, 82
Septicemia, 448
Shigella, 362
Shoes
  arch cookies, 519
  reverse-last, 521
  straight-last, 521
Sickle cell
  anemia, 406
  crisis, 406
  disease, 405
  trait, 405
Sigmoidoscopy, 369
Sinuses
  ethmoidal, 272
  frontal, 272
  maxillary, 272
Skin, 435
Smegma, 106
Solid foods, 24
Sore bottom, 109
Sore throat, 248
Spermatic cord, 427
Spinal fluid, 485
Spinal tap, 504
Spitting-up, 4, 85
Sprains, 513
Staph, 148
Status epilepticus, 494
Sternomastoid mass, 82
Sternum, 261
Stomachache, 352
Stomatitis, 234
Stool
  bloody, 368
  normal, 354

Straight-last shoes, 521
Strangulated hernia, 371
Strawberry hemangioma, 460
Strep, 145
Strongloides worm, 374
Stuffed-up nose, 276
Styes, 188
Subconjunctival hemorrhage, 196
Sunburn, 474
Sunscreen, 474
Sutures, skull, 485
Sway-back, 530
Swimmer's ear, 220
Swollen
  eyelid, 194
  joint, 517
Syncope, 490
Syrup of Ipecac, 120
Systolic blood pressure, 394
T & A, 254
TB, 322
Table food, 28
Teeth, care of, 93
Teething, 91
Temperature
  to reduce high, 132
Testicle
  hiding, 426
  undescended, 426
Tetracyclin, 471
Throat, 244
Thrush, 98
Thum, 87
Thumb-sucking, 86
Thyroglossal cyst, 261
Thyroid gland, 261
Tics, 494
Tinactin ointment, 450
Tinia capitis, 478
Tofranil, 421
Tongue-tie, 97
Tonsillar pillar, 244
Tooth
  abscess, 240
  eruption, 91
Torticollis, 263
Toxic synovitis, 525
Trachea, 261
Tracheobronchitis, 315
Trench mouth, 237
Triaminic, 280
Trichiuris, 374
Trind, 304
Turbinates, 271

Ulna, 527
Umbilical granuloma, 7
Umbilical hernia, 111
Undescended testicle, 426
Upper respiratory infection, 307
Ureter, 409
Urethra, 409
Urinary tract, 409
  infection, 416
Urine, 411
  bloody, 415
  culture, 414
  screening culture, 414
Urinalysis, 413
Urticaria papulosa, 468
Uval, 474
Uvula, 244

Vagus nerve, 490
Vaporizers, 290
Vegetables, 27
Vergo, 472
Vermox, 378
Vicks, 291
Viral infections, 138
Viruses, bacteria, and fungi, 136
Visine, 184
Vitamins, 23, 337

Voiding cystourethrogram, 414
Vomiting, 360
VoSol drops, 221
Vulvovaginitis, 429
Walking pneumonia, 324
Warts, 472
Wasp, 464
Watery eye, 95
Weed-B-Gone, 456
Weeping poison ivy, 455

Wet pleurisy, 327
Wheals, 450
Wheeze, 318
Wilm's tumor, 410
Wood's lamp, 478
Wry neck, 82, 263

Yellow jacket, 464